The Ultimate Guide t
Our Toxic Exposures

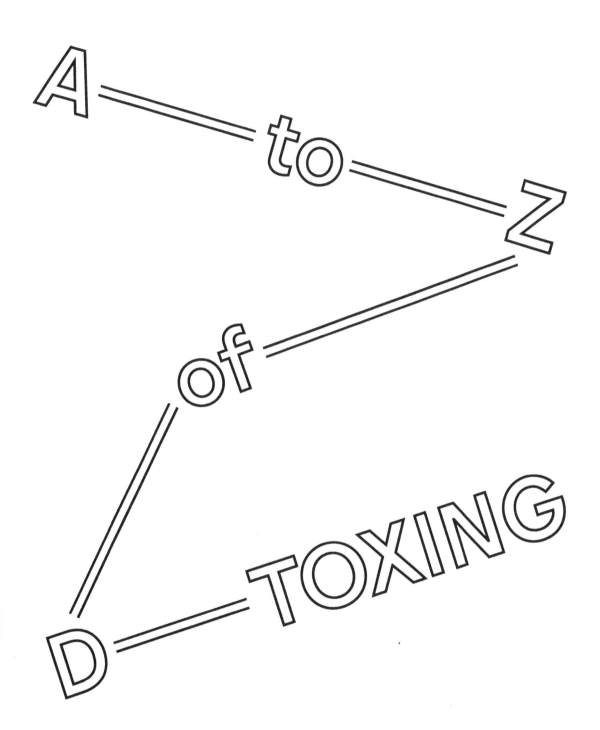

A to Z of D TOXING

Sophia Ruan Gushée

A TO Z OF D-TOXING:
THE ULTIMATE GUIDE TO REDUCING OUR TOXIC EXPOSURES

The S File Publishing, LLC
411 Lafayette Street
New York, NY 10003

Library of Congress Cataloging-in-Publication Data
ISBN-13: 978-0-9911401-0-7

First Edition:
October 2015

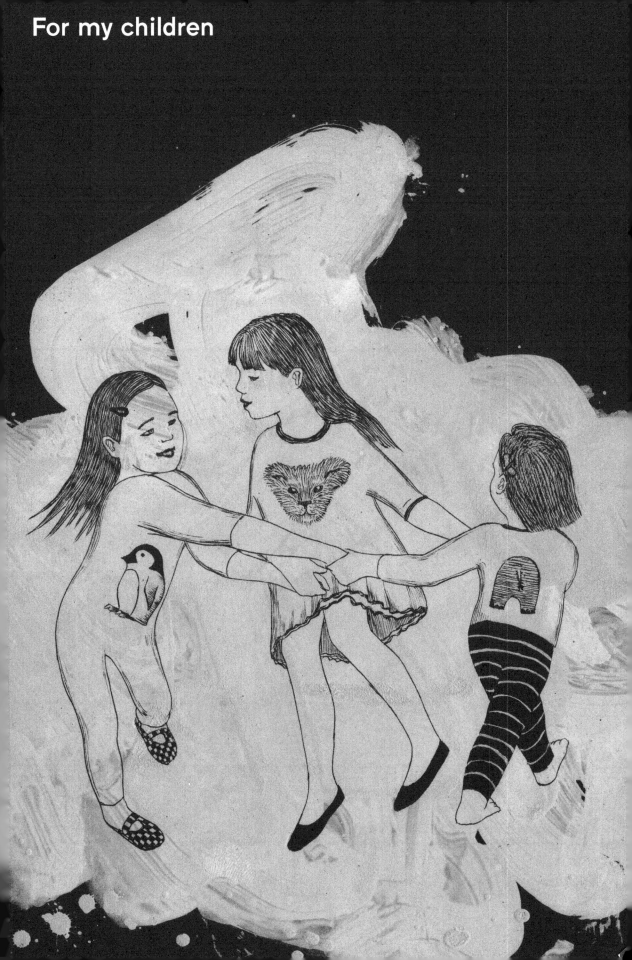

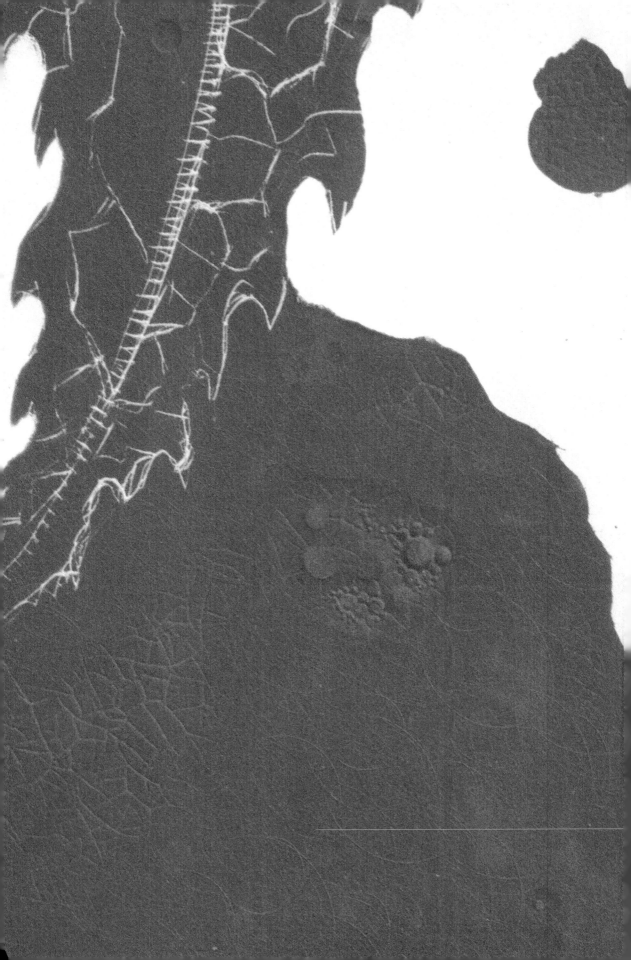

Contents

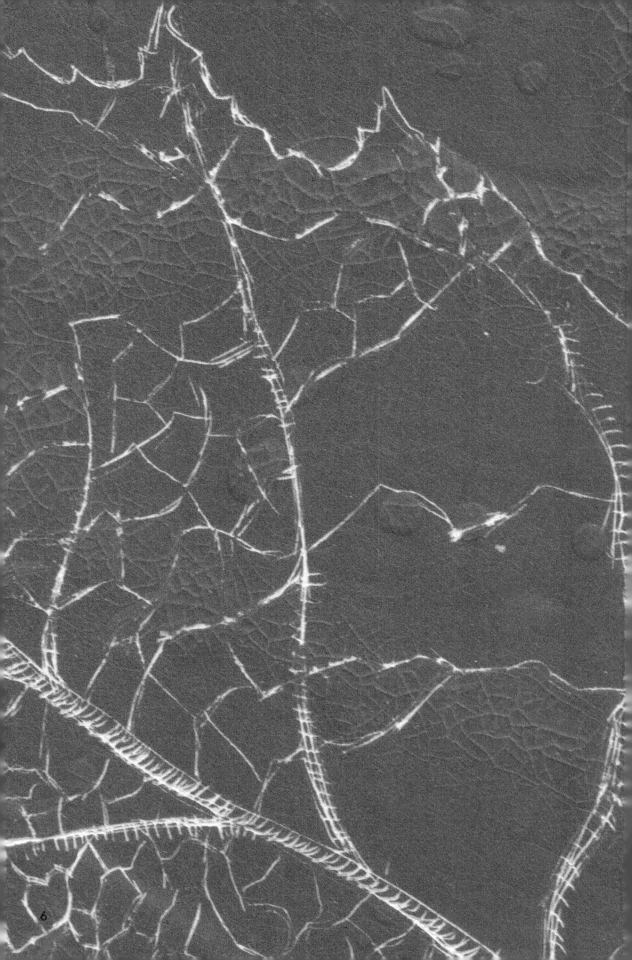

6

Introduction

Did you know that over 84,000 chemicals have been introduced into commercial use since World War II? And that the Environmental Protection Agency has been able to require safety testing for just over 200, and regulate only *five* of them? Furthermore, those numbers—on our chemical explosion, limited understanding of safety, and lack of effective regulation—refer to just the US. Every country has its own experience.

If you'd like to learn how this impacts you and your loved ones, then this book has answers. If you'd like to reduce unnecessary toxic exposures, then this book is full of detailed tips that you can incorporate and revisit as you're ready for change. If you get overwhelmed by too much information or by how to get started, just go to part IV to follow the top ten goals that I focus on.

In this section, I explain why I created this book and my key takeaways from completing it, which I hope will also be yours. If you would like to dive into why you should reduce your toxic exposures, then please start with chapter I.1.

MY FIRST EXPERIENCE

It began with bisphenol A (BPA), which may seem irrelevant in 2015 with the prevalence of BPA-free products, but it's not. Substitute chemicals are not necessarily safer, as part I explains.

It was around 12:20 a.m. I was in our New York City apartment, late in the year 2007. I was 34 years old, and our first-born was three months old. She, my husband, and our two dogs were sound asleep.

I had only recently returned to work after a maternity leave. After a long, demanding day at work—and anticipating an equally busy day to follow—I had stayed up until midnight to pump breast milk. As I finished pumping, cleaned up, and added to my small stash of frozen milk, I knew that I only had a few precious hours to sleep before I had to wake up for work the next morning—if our daughter didn't wake up even earlier.

Around 12:30 a.m., I climbed into bed. While physically tired, my mind was still racing from the day and preparing for the next. To help me wind down to sleep, I skimmed through the short pile of reading materials that I hoped would further enlighten me on how to care for my daughter.

By 12:50 a.m., on page 73 in the book *Feeding Baby Green: The Earth-Friendly Program for Healthy, Safe Nutrition* by Alan Greene MD, I came across a section that mentioned a hormone disruptor in conventional baby bottles and a carcinogen in conventional baby bottle nipples. Surprised, I found it hard to believe. That just could not be true, I thought. If that were true, then someone—my OB/GYN, pediatrician, or someone else in the maternity ward—would have warned me, I told myself.

Alarmed, because my daughter would be exposed to these conventional baby items the next day, I went to the computer to see if I could verify these claims by credible sources. By 2 a.m., I learned from information on websites of the Environmental Protection Agency and Food and Drug Administration that the claims were valid: BPA is an endocrine disruptor found in some plastics, including baby bottles; and nitrosamines are carcinogens that have been detected in some rubber nipples.

By 2:45 a.m., I couldn't determine whether my daughter's potential exposures would be harmful and I didn't think I'd be able to figure it out that night. Opinions of credible experts varied: The President's Cancer Panel, which reports to the President of the United States, expressed concerns about children's exposures; the Food and Drug Administration stated they were safe. Millions of children have been exposed to the plastic and rubber materials of baby bottles. Could they truly pose harm? Regardless, I preferred to avoid exposing my newborn to any unnecessary amounts of threatening chemicals. So I set out to find safer alternatives.

By 4 a.m., I had purchased glass baby bottles and medical-grade silicone bottle nipples. By 4:10 a.m., with the crisis addressed, I finally noticed that I was exhausted.

I was also confused. How could common baby products contain harmful chemicals? Where else did harmful chemicals hide? What other relevant information did I not know? Why hadn't I been warned of these risks sooner? I also worried about what consequences, if any, would result from my daughter's exposure thus far.

By 6 a.m., my daughter was awake and ready to start her day.

With fewer than a couple of hours of sleep, I don't know how I functioned at my job. I pretended to be mentally alert in my fast-paced work environment while exhausted. Throughout the day, I was processing my experience from the night before: Learning that I was unintentionally offering my infant a hormone disruptor and carcinogen was upsetting.

Unfortunately, the prior night's episode was just the beginning. Many future versions of that first experience lay ahead of me.

JUST THE FACTS, PLEASE

I am a fact-oriented gal. I *love* facts. Facts are unbiased, after all.

During my first pregnancy, I was running a department at an international bank that specialized in maximizing value from distressed investments—that is, investment opportunities mired in chaos and defined (or not defined) by limited reliable data. As part of my analyses, I would gather all the facts I could about a relevant opportunity while identifying gaps where information was either unavailable or questionable. An important skill was recognizing what I didn't know as well as what experts didn't know. That way, I could pursue answers to the most relevant questions, exercise better judgment about whom to trust, and decide how much weight to give various sources of information. I considered formal analyses and informed intuition, identified trends and opportunities, and applied due diligence to develop a recommendation and value creation plan. As a result of my professional experiences, I became accustomed to learning quickly, and making decisions based on the best available, albeit imperfect, information.

I *loved* my work.

However, "my first experience" started a shift. As I continued to research other potential sources of BPA, I encountered one unsettling fact after another. I became increasingly unsure about how I was committing my time: While I truly enjoyed my professional work, I was devoting myself toward *institutional* investments. What about my most important responsibility: my *infant* daughter?

Eventually, I decided to redirect my professional experience toward a new focus.

THE INSPIRATION FOR THIS BOOK

I never wanted to research this topic—the toxic burdens in our bodies, in our homes, and on our planet—as much as I have. At the same time, I couldn't ignore the alarming claims that I was encountering.

After too many experiences that were versions of "my first experience," I grew tired of this *reactive* learning curve and decided to be *proactive*. I chose to tackle this topic head-on and research to meet these objectives: Identify my family's key sources of exposures; prioritize my efforts and budget; and create a manual of what I'd need to know and what actions to take as the head of a household.

My first step was to find credible sources. Getting educated was cumbersome since the information was spread through various sources and was not always easy to find, even when I knew what to look for. Furthermore, finding agreement among authorities on various related issues was sometimes impossible. You can appreciate this more as you read, in part I, about my continued investigations of whether chronic exposures to small doses of BPA and other hormone-disrupting chemicals are safe. Considering responses by both state and foreign governments was helpful since they differed from those of some federal agencies.

The media, books, and my own investigations spotlighted concerns that fueled my research for years. I noticed that this subject shared characteristics with situations inherent in distressed investment opportunities: Information is imperfect, gaps in explanations pervade, inconsistent "facts" are common, expert opinions vary, and sound judgment is required. I found myself applying my business skills in this new area:

how to reduce unnecessary exposures to toxicants.

Gradually, I discovered a wealth of scientific studies that were relevant to me and my family, such as those in the Works Cited section. As I read, I encountered a lot of troubling information that I wished I had known sooner because I realized that *my* choices were influencing my family's exposure to many industrial chemicals, mainly through my purchases and everyday practices in caring for my family and home. As I continued to read, I also learned about other risks in our consumer products: developmental toxicants, immunotoxicants, neurotoxicants, and reproductive toxicants. Even more disturbing: They've been detected in our bodies, breast milk, and cord blood.

At the same time, I tracked health trends among the pediatric and general populations. The incidences of a wide variety of health issues have been increasing rapidly, as chapter I.1 introduces. I wondered what role toxicants might play in this.

I learned that some toxicants are so similar to the natural substances produced and used by our bodies that they can disrupt biological processes, and that consequences can be particularly serious if exposure occurs during critical stages of development. I also learned that we experience chronic exposure to toxicants from our diets and indoor environments—workplaces, homes, daycare facilities, and schools. This means that we can reduce our exposures.

Once I became convinced to change habits or possessions, figuring out the alternatives was challenging too. For example, when I tried to identify safer mattresses and crib mattresses to buy, the best information that I could find was from biased sources. When I have included those biased sources in this book, it's because the messages are consistent with my overall lessons learned from the credible, unbiased sources.

I collected facts throughout my years of research. Ultimately, I was able to connect my "fact dots" from an informed perspective, which is shared in part I. The weight of the evidence encourages me to follow a precautionary (and *balanced*) approach, which takes the position that it's better to be safe than sorry.

As General Gordon Sullivan, US Army (Ret.), explained in the May 2014 report "National Security and the Accelerating Risks of Climate Change" by the CNA Military Advisory Board, it's important to be decisive with even imperfect information:

> Speaking as a soldier, we never have 100 percent certainty. If you wait until you have 100 percent certainty, something bad is going to happen on the battlefield.

My personal challenge in becoming knowledgeable, balancing conflicting opinions, figuring out practical approaches, and sharing important information with those who help me care for my family have been the inspirations for this book. No one should have to discover these things the way I did: at unexpected times, while sacrificing needed sleep, after you've spent money on things you may want to replace, and when you feel that it's too late. As chapter I.15 discusses, it's never too late!

Considering that the claims sometimes suggest devastating outcomes—birth defects, SIDS, neurologic or reproductive damage, cancer, and more—you too may decide that a precautionary approach is worthwhile. Regardless of what you do with the information, you should have easier access to it.

OUR HOMES

When I began this book project, my main concern was human health. At the time, there were many books on how and why to be planet-friendly. But I had an infant daughter and hopes for more children, so concerns for the planet seemed less urgent to me. My top priorities were to detox our apartment, our diet, and our personal care and cleaning products.

Today I am also very concerned about our planet. I now understand that pollution is not contained within borders: No country, no region, no human body, and no life form are untouched. Moreover, while climate change wasn't on my radar at the start of my research, I now recognize that it's among the most hazardous of risks. And one of the underlying causes is our consumption/waste of resources, including electricity, gas, and consumer goods (including those in our diet).

In 2014, the CNA Military Advisory Board— an elite group of retired generals and admirals from the Army, Navy, Air Force, and Marine Corps—updated a report, "National Security and the Accelerating Risks of Climate Change." It described climate change as a serious threat to national security, explaining:

> During our decades of experience in the [US] military, we have addressed many national security challenges, from containment and deterrence of the Soviet nuclear threat during the Cold War to political extremism and transnational terrorism in recent years. The national security risks of projected climate change are as serious as any challenges we have faced.

I now see that "Home" is more than just our built environment: It also includes our bodies (the first home of our children) and our planet (our collective home). The health of these Homes—our built environments, our bodies, and our planet—are interconnected, as are the well-beings of all life forms, which part I explains.

Leaders fighting to curb climate change are urging each of us to assess how we can help because our choices matter. The disruptors of both our bodies and our planet share an important common denominator—fossil fuels, which you'll see in parts II and III. The strategies and tips throughout parts III and IV balance and serve the best interests of all our Homes.

TAKE ADVANTAGE OF MY LEARNING CURVE

A dear friend recently asked, "How did this book change you?" She proceeded to inquire with real vigor, "You quit your job because of this!" (I resigned for more than one reason.) "You didn't just work on this part-time; you pursued this study passionately as a full-time job. You spent the past five years working on this—all while bearing and nursing three children and juggling other major challenges. Why?! What kind of person does that, takes on this complex and overwhelming topic? How did this book change you?"

Inevitably, this journey has changed me profoundly. Most obvious, it has empowered me. And I hope that it empowers you.

In this book, I share the lay of the land that I wish I had sooner—a road map of a

family's potentially toxic exposures, especially those that are avoidable—so that you can formulate a *game plan* that suits your family's unique environment, lifestyle, and budget. From this educational foundation, you can adapt strategies as circumstances change, controversies arise, and new information emerges. Becoming familiar with the key issues will provide helpful perspective as you encounter alarming claims that will continue to populate the news.

This book has broadened my perspective, changed my focus, and ignited new passions. Spreading awareness, provoking productive dialogue, empowering others, fostering more compassion for our planet, and raising money for worthwhile efforts now feels like a calling. You can contribute to solutions also. Starting with yourself is huge—just one change at a time.

Please join me on my path of evolving from being an unconscious to a *conscious* consumer, who naturally considers the contamination imprint—on not just our planet but in our bodies—that our purchases create. In fact, this book is intended for the conscious consumer.

I have always believed that being proactive from a place of awareness is invaluable in creating good luck. With the practical guidance in this book, you may increase your, and our collective, odds for resilient health and a more comfortable life. We're really all in this together. D-Tox, baby!

NOTE TO READER

You are about to encounter many acronyms, capitalized terms, and in-text citations. Please remember that you can refer to the How to Use this Book section in the Appendix for further explanations.

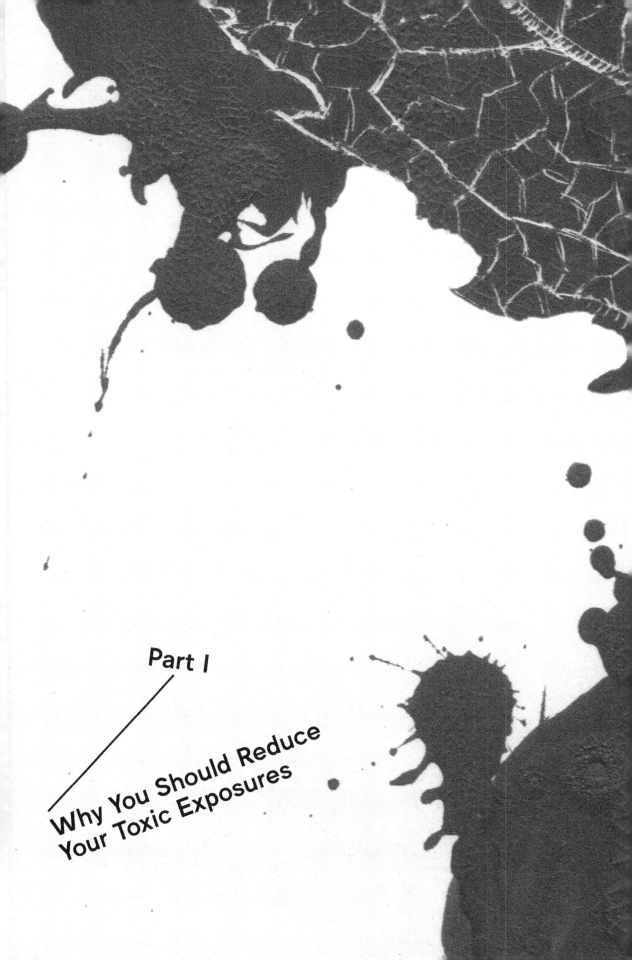

Part I

Why You Should Reduce
Your Toxic Exposures

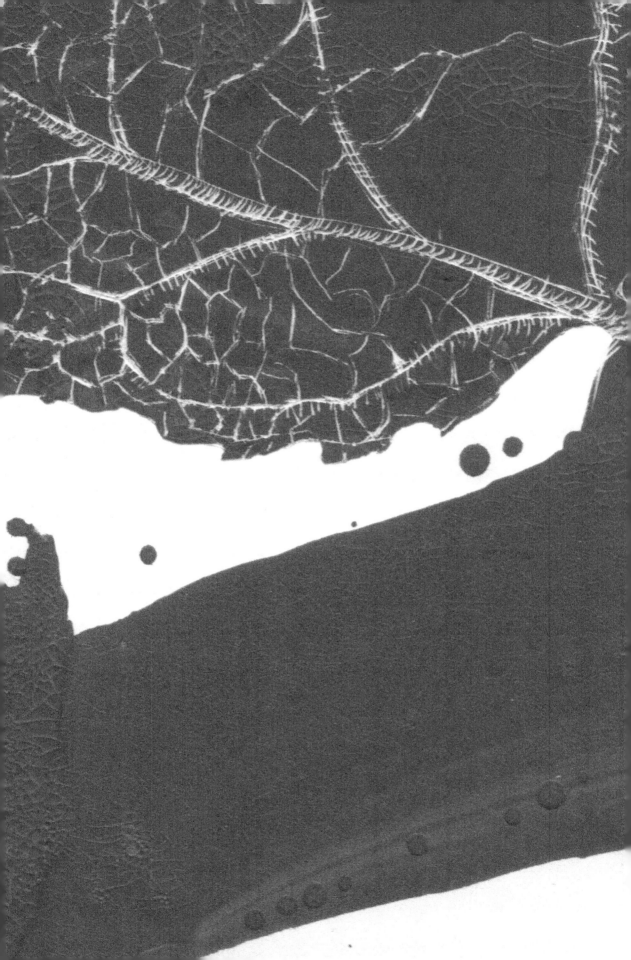

Chapter I.1
What's Going on with Us?

I grew up during the 1970s and 1980s in upstate New York—in Binghamton, a city of about 200,000 residents at the time. I attended various schools that were diverse: a Jewish nursery school with approximately 15 to 20 children per class; a public elementary school for kindergarten through second grade with class sizes of approximately 33; a Catholic school with about 33 students per class; and then a public high school with approximately 400 students per grade. I don't recall a student who had an allergy or a chronic condition worth mentioning. In fact, based on my childhood experiences, I believed that children didn't get sick, except for things like a cold, the flu, and chicken pox.

Today, a shift has occurred among all of us, but especially among our kids. As a new mother, I wanted to make sense of the endless media headlines about the alarming health trends among children. As I sought to understand the big picture while collecting statistics, the emerging portrait concerned me.

HEALTH TRENDS AMONG OUR CHILDREN
Parents of all generations have worked to protect their children from specific threats. In prior generations, threats included infectious diseases, such as polio, smallpox, whooping cough, and measles. Modern medicine has largely controlled these and other illnesses that once harmed or killed millions of children. Our current generation of children, however, faces a different set of health threats.

Pediatric health trends have attracted concern. Figure #01 provides a variety of statistics based on reports by leading organizations such as the World Health Organization (WHO) and United Nations Environment Programme (UNEP), the President's Cancer Panel (PCP), the Endocrine Disruption Exchange, the US Centers for Disease Control and Prevention (CDC), and the Children's Environmental Health Center at Mount Sinai Hospital (CEHC).

As you can surmise from the statistics in figure #01, the portion of children suffering from chronic health conditions has "increased dramatically" (Perrin, Bloom, and Gortmaker 2007). Data for 1988 to 2006 indicate that the incidence of chronic health conditions among children more than doubled during that period, from 12.8 percent to 26.6 percent, according to an article published in the *Journal of the American Medical Association*. The authors note that over the past 30 years, the most marked increases have been seen for asthma, obesity, and behavior and learning problems such as attention deficit/hyperactivity disorder (Van Cleave, Gortmaker, and Perrin 2010).

In another study, which examined data from the 2007 National Survey of Children's Health, approximately 43 percent, or 32 million, US children were estimated to have at least one of 20 chronic conditions. This estimate increased to 54.1 percent when overweight, obesity, and being at risk for developmental delays were considered (Bethell et al. 2011).

More recently, the number of children diagnosed with one or more chronic health conditions was estimated to have "quadrupled" over the past four decades (Stephens 2014).

Surely these statistics provide only part of the story, since details on the design and execution of studies and surveys, among other factors, are important in interpreting the data. However, the reality is clear: There is something unusual happening with our kids, and no one fully understands the causes.

HEALTH TRENDS AMONG ADULTS
A growing portion of adults is also suffering from a variety of health issues, as figure #02 shows. Chronic conditions afflict almost half of us, or 117 million Americans (CDC 2014c). Increasing reports of illnesses

Pediatric Health Trends

While research is still underway, experts recommend a precautionary approach towards synthetic chemicals, among other healthy habits.

Premature Births
Increased more than 30 percent since 1981 in the US, UK, and Scandinavia. These babies are more likely to develop adverse health effects later in life, such as respiratory and neurological conditions, cardiovascular disease, obesity, lung disease, and type II diabetes (WHO and UNEP 2013).

Food Allergies
Increased 50 percent from the 1997-1999 period to the 2009-2011 period, totaling 5.1 percent of children ages 0-17 years old (CDC 2013b).

Birth Defects
"Birth defects are the leading cause of infant death" and certain ones—such as undescended testicles and penile malformations—are rising in many countries or leveled off at "unfavorably high rates" (WHO and UNEP 2013; Caione 2009).

Leukemia
Increased by nearly 60 percent between 1975 and 2004 among children 14 years and younger (CEHC 2014b).

Pediatric Melanoma
"Increased by an average of 2 percent per year from 1973 to 2009" (Skin Cancer Foundation 2014; Wong et al. 2013).

Type II Diabetes
Became epidemic worldwide over the past 40 years (WHO and UNEP 2013).

Obesity
More than doubled in children over the past 10 years (CEHC 2014b) and quadrupled in adolescents over the past 30 years (CDC 2014b).

Brain Cancer
Among children 14 years and younger, primary brain cancer increased by nearly 40 percent between 1975 and 2004 (CEHC 2014b).

Precocious Puberty

Girls are starting puberty at younger ages. This has been detected in all countries studied (WHO and UNEP 2013).

Precocious puberty prolongs exposure to estrogen, increasing breast cancer risk by 30 percent (Galvez 2011), and increasing risk of advanced bone age as well as psychological and emotional challenges (Weil 2012).

Skin Allergies

Increased 69 percent from the 1997-1999 period to the 2009-2011 period, totaling 12.5 percent of children ages 0-17 years old (CDC 2013b).

Developmental Disabilities (DD): US Children Aged 3-17 Years

Children 3-17 years old were evaluated by researchers led by the CDC. The study examined data from 1997 to 2008. During this time, the incidence of DD increased 17.1 percent, which equated to 1.8 million more children than the decade prior. The numbers below highlight the percent change in certain DD from the 1997-1999 to the 2006-2008 periods.

Asthma

Increased 100+ percent in frequency since 1980 and is the leading cause of pediatric hospitalization and school absenteeism (Trasande 2008).

Percent Change Between 1997-1999 and 2006-2008

ADHD 33.0 percent
Autism 289.5 percent
Blindness 18.2 percent
Other DD 24.7 percent
Seizures 9.1 percent
(CDC 2012a; Boyle et al. 2011)

Testicular Cancer

Increased up to 400 percent among some populations of young men, especially in industrialized countries, and is occurring at younger ages. Testicular cancer is more common among those born with hypospadias (penile malformations) or cryptorchidism (undescended testicles), both of which have increased in incidence to level off "at unfavorably high rates" (WHO and UNEP 2013; Landrigan and Etzel 2014; Huyghe, Matsuda, and Thonneau 2003).

Note: Please refer to the Terms to Know and Index sections for more information on the disorders and illnesses in this figure.

FIGURE #01

15

and disorders span a wide spectrum of diagnoses: obesity, diabetes, allergies, autoimmune diseases, heart disease, cancer, inflammatory illnesses, reproductive challenges, and others. In 2010, chronic diseases accounted for seven of the top 10 causes of death in this country (CDC 2014c).

Americans aren't alone in these trends either. Chronic diseases are the main causes of sickness and death worldwide (WHO 2011b; WHO and UNEP 2013).

THE STATISTICS AND TRENDS ARE TOO HARD TO BELIEVE

When confronted by reports of increased incidence of diseases and disorders, people can't believe the data. They assume, "Oh, it must be genetics." When hearing about skyrocketing rates of autism, a common reaction is "It must be from sharper or earlier diagnoses or from broader definitions." It's just too hard to believe that the increases could be so significant.

Studies have explored these questions. In the following pages, I share what I have learned about investigations of these questions as they pertain to pediatric cancers and neurotoxicity, since these were discussed in credible sources. In short, investigators have determined that even after accounting for factors like genetics and improved diagnostic capability, the incidences of certain disorders have increased enough to raise eyebrows.

WHY HAVE THE INCIDENCES OF PEDIATRIC CANCER STEADILY INCREASED?

Although cancer in children is rare (NCI 2014), incidences have been increasing. In 2010, the PCP, which reports to the president of the US, released a report titled *Reducing Environmental Cancer Risk: What We Can Do Now*. It states that the increased incidences of pediatric cancers "have been too rapid to be of genetic origin." Improved diagnostic techniques—like computed tomography (CT) and magnetic resonance imaging (MRI)—might explain a one-time spike in rates around the time of certain events, such as the introduction of newer imaging equipment. However, something unidentified is also contributing (Reuben 2010).

Experts urge further research into the role of environmental factors. Philip J. Landrigan MD MSc, dean for Global Health at Mount Sinai Hospital, explained in a 2008 PCP meeting:

> While mortality from childhood cancer has gone sharply down, incidence rates are increasing. There has been a 55 percent increase from 1975 to 2005 in the incidence of leukemia in 0- to 14-year-olds and an 81 percent increase for acute lymphocytic leukemia—the most common type of leukemia. Incidence of cancer of the brain and nervous system has increased 39 percent. Testicular cancer, which primarily occurs in 15- to 30-year-olds, has increased by 51 percent in white males and by 45 percent in black males. The explanation for this increase may be due in part to better diagnostics, but this alone does not account for the continued inexorable rise. Serious consideration must be given to the possibility that environmental factors are involved. (Leffall 2008)

IS NEUROTOXICITY MORE PREVALENT?

Autism has increased 289.5 percent over the past 12 years, an increase that is too large to be explained by genetics (CDC 2012a; Boyle et al. 2011). In California, it increased even more: The number of people diagnosed with autistic spectrum disorder grew 1,148 percent from 1987 to 2007, while the general population in California grew just 27 percent during this time (Cavagnaro 2007). Scientists have been trying to identify the drivers behind this trend.

Researchers in the Department of Public Health Science at the University of California, Davis examined autism cases reported in California from 1990 through 2006. In 1990, 205 cases were reported. The number increased 1,363 percent to more than 3,000 cases in 2006 (Cone 2009a; Hertz-Picciotto and Delwiche 2009).

Some of the increase in reports of autism was explained by the inclusion of milder cases (56 percent increase), diagnosis at younger ages (24 percent), and changes in state reporting requirements for autism (120 percent). Collectively, however, these factors explain less than half of the reported increases during the study's time

More of Us are Sick

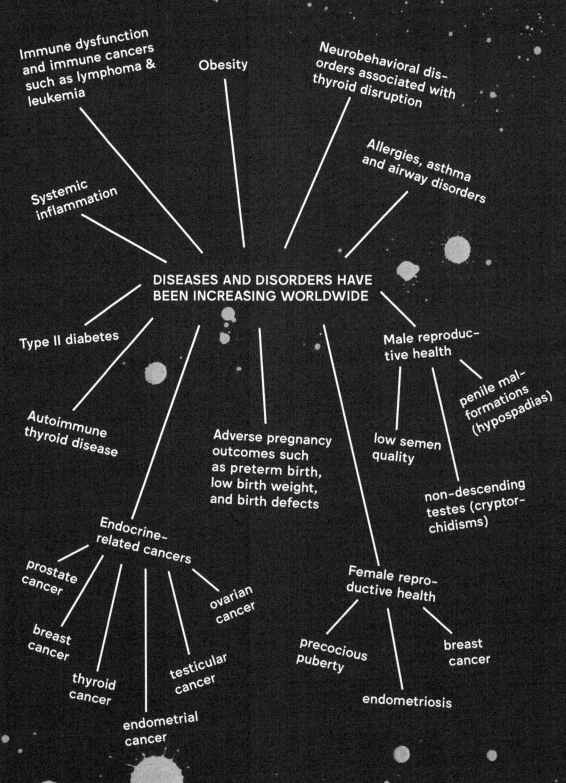

Immune dysfunction and immune cancers such as lymphoma & leukemia

Obesity

Neurobehavioral disorders associated with thyroid disruption

Allergies, asthma and airway disorders

Systemic inflammation

DISEASES AND DISORDERS HAVE BEEN INCREASING WORLDWIDE

Type II diabetes

Male reproductive health

penile malformations (hypospadias)

Autoimmune thyroid disease

Adverse pregnancy outcomes such as preterm birth, low birth weight, and birth defects

low semen quality

non-descending testes (cryptorchidisms)

Endocrine-related cancers

prostate cancer

ovarian cancer

Female reproductive health

breast cancer

breast cancer

precocious puberty

breast cancer

thyroid cancer

testicular cancer

endometriosis

endometrial cancer

(Source: WHO and UNEP 2013)

FIGURE #02

17

period (Cone 2009a; Hertz-Picciotto and Delwiche 2009).

According to information from Autism Speaks, a leading autism advocacy organization, after considering sharper diagnosis, broader diagnosis, and more awareness of the disorder, roughly half of the increase in diagnoses can't be explained (Falco 2012). The organization recognizes that a genetic predisposition, in combination with various environmental—which broadly encompass the nongenetic— factors, increases the risk of a child developing autism (Halladay 2014).

An expanding body of evidence indicates that early-life exposure to developmental neurotoxicants is probably one of several influential factors (Grandjean and Landrigan 2014; WHO 2011a; Cone 2009a; Braun et al. 2014). In fact, autism is part of a broader trend.

In March 2014, Dr. Landrigan and Philippe Grandjean MD PhD, adjunct professor at the Harvard School of Public Health, authored a seminal review, "Neurobehavioural Effects of Developmental Toxicity," in *The Lancet Neurology*, a prestigious medical journal. Focusing on the neurotoxicity of certain industrial chemicals that can undermine the normal development of the brain prenatally and during childhood, the authors describe a "global pandemic of neurodevelopmental disorders" that affects millions of children worldwide (Grandjean and Landrigan 2014).

The authors estimate that genetic factors may explain no more than 30 to 40 percent of the diagnosed cases of neurodevelopmental disorders and that nongenetic, environmental exposures may be important contributors.

UNIDENTIFIED FACTORS ARE MAKING MORE OF US SICK

The health statistics and trends, as well as the significance of the underlying studies, can be debated. And trends will change—certain illnesses will increase, others will flatten or decrease. However, the global perspective is clear: More children and adults are suffering from chronic illnesses and other health challenges. While researchers actively explore the contributing factors, the role of environmental variables seems increasingly certain.

KEY POINTS

01. We, and our children, are getting sicker and feeling more uncomfortable.
02. While the exact causes are unknown, improved diagnoses and genetics cannot fully explain our rapidly deteriorating wellness.
03. A growing body of science suggests that environmental factors exert a significant influence on our health.

Chapter I.2
The Power of Environmental Factors

In 2009, my husband experienced a carotid artery dissection, a tear in the major artery in his neck. Though the event was unusual for a 37-year-old, he was released from the hospital with no recommended changes in diet or lifestyle (aside from blood pressure and cholesterol-lowering medication).

Disappointed by the doctors' failure to push for a healthier lifestyle, I asked, in disbelief, "Really? You don't think there's anything that he should change? He has a high-stress job. Doesn't exercise. Doesn't eat until 9 p.m. Normally eats a not-so-healthy restaurant delivery or sometimes just wine and cheese for dinner. You don't think those things might have played a role in his ending up in this ER?"

The doctors replied, "No, it was just bad luck."

Since that made no sense to me, I began exploring the role of nutrition in health because I strongly suspected that improved nutrition could vastly improve my husband's vascular health. After reading *The China Study*, a book by T. Colin Campbell PhD and Thomas M. Campbell II MD (2006) that provides a comprehensive review of the scientific studies examining the role of nutrition in a variety of diseases, I persuaded my husband to try a nutrient-dense vegan diet.

Within a few months, his weight dropped from 225 to 187 pounds, his cholesterol dropped to such a low level that his physicians agreed to let him go off all medication since dietary changes had been so effective, and the damaged artery healed *completely*. His doctors were amazed by the likely role that dietary changes played.

THE ROLE OF ENVIRONMENTAL FACTORS

My husband's physicians were among the best in their respective specialties, so I was intrigued by their amazement at how powerful diet is. How could they not have considered the influence of nutrition (and other lifestyle choices) on my husband's cardiovascular health? Later, I learned that nutrition is not a substantial part of the education of a Western-trained physician.

In 1985, the National Academy of Sciences released a landmark report on the inadequate training that medical students receive in nutrition. It recommended that medical schools incorporate a minimum of 25 hours of nutrition instruction in the curriculum (Committee on Nutrition in Medical Education 1985). In 2010, researchers at the University of North Carolina at Chapel Hill published survey results that found that although all schools surveyed required instruction in nutrition, only 27 percent of 105 medical schools surveyed offered the recommended minimum of 25 hours. This is a decrease from 38 percent of 104 schools surveyed in 2004 (Chen 2010; Bein 2010; Adams, Kohlmeier, and Zeisel 2010).

Western-trained physicians receive even less instruction on how environmental factors may influence health. A 2009 report in *Environmental Health Perspectives,* a peer-reviewed journal published by the National Institute of Environmental Health Sciences, examined the efficacy of an initiative that aimed to build environmental health capacity among pediatric health professionals (Rogers et al. 2009). The article noted that in a 1996 survey of 126 US medical schools, 24 percent of respondents reported that there was no environmental medicine requirement in their curriculum. Among the schools offering it, environmental medicine instruction averaged just seven hours over the four-year medical program (Schenk et al. 1996). Moreover, less than half of US pediatric residency programs regularly cover environmental health issues, except for lead poisoning and factors that may exacerbate asthma (Rogers et al. 2009).

Yet, science is increasingly underscoring the influence of environmental factors on health. As a result, authorities—such as the Institute of Medicine, American Academy of Pediatrics, American Public Health Association, and others—are urging health care providers to learn more about environmental health issues (Rogers et al. 2009).

— *National Institute of Environmental Health Sciences (NIEHS 2011)*: 85 percent of all diseases are influenced by environmental factors.

— *The American Cancer Society (2010)*: 75 - 80 percent of cancer risk is due to environmental factors, including tobacco smoke, nutrition, physical activity, and exposure to carcinogens in the environment.

— *US National Academy of Sciences (Collaborative on Health and the Environment - Washington 2014)*: "28 percent of neurobehavioral disorders could be attributed directly or indirectly to environmental contaminants, not including alcohol, tobacco or drugs of abuse."

— *American Autoimmune Related Diseases Association (AARDA 2014) and National Institute of Allergy and Infectious Diseases (NIAID 2005)*: Genetics is estimated to contribute about 30 percent to the development of autoimmune diseases.

THE STRESSORS FROM MODERN LIVING

I live in Manhattan, an extraordinary city. Those who work here are among the most diligent, persistent, determined, talented, and resilient people in the world. However, I often think that some environmental factors seem uniquely extreme for Manhattan professionals and residents. While it's a privilege to live or work here, we arguably have less balanced lives, more stress, fewer natural retreats, urban air, and more electromagnetic fields (from cellular and wireless technologies) due to our population density.

Manhattan residents aren't alone, however. Modern living and our modern environment pose unique stresses on the biology of everyone and every life-form around the world. The "load" of environmental stresses on our bodies' natural resilience to fight, repair, and restore is unprecedented, as figure #03 depicts and the rest of part I explains.

THE ROLE OF TOXICANTS

While the causation of diseases and disorders is highly complex, multifactorial, and not entirely understood, their onset can result from a perfect storm of many variables that interact with our genes. In this book, I focus on the environmental factors that can be reduced through our purchases, behaviors, and habits: the toxicants in our consumer products. (Please note: Toxins refer to naturally occurring poisons, while toxicants generally refer to man-made poisons. When I use the term toxicant, I include both man-made poisons and naturally occurring toxins that exist in our environment at significantly higher-than-normal levels due to human activities.)

An abundance of scientific studies exist on the threat of toxicants from consumer products, and they have attracted major reviews in recent years. In addition to the 2010 report from the PCP, reviews of the current science have been published by leading organizations such as the European Environment Agency (EEA), the WHO, and the UNEP. Collectively, they report that science is proving that synthetic chemicals found in our average consumer products not only persist throughout our air, water, and soil, but also pervade our bodies. These toxicants have been linked to cancer, neurotoxicity, reproductive challenges, and a wide range of conditions that may be associated with endocrine disruption. And these risks arise from everyday exposures, as the following points make clear:

— Hundreds of substances have been definitively linked to cancer in people (Physicians for Social Responsibility 2014; Scorecard 2014), and thousands more have not been studied enough for us to understand their effects. The PCP reported that scientific evidence increasingly shows that exposure to low levels of chemicals in our everyday environment is contributing to the country's cancer burden (Reuben 2010). This higher cancer risk can come from repeated exposures to low levels of toxicants or from exposure during a vulnerable biological stage. For example, a child can be exposed to low, chronic levels of formaldehyde (a known human carcinogen) from various sources in the bedroom, including wooden furniture, drapes, mattresses, and carpets.

— Industrial chemicals commonly found in our environment can injure the developing brain. The March 2014 article by Grandjean and Landrigan, mentioned in chapter I.1, reported that "strong evidence" exists that certain commonly found industrial chemicals are "important contributors" to the increasing prevalence of neurodevelopmental

Our Bodies are Overwhelmed with Modern-Day Stressors

The interplay between these stressors and genetics adversely affects our health.

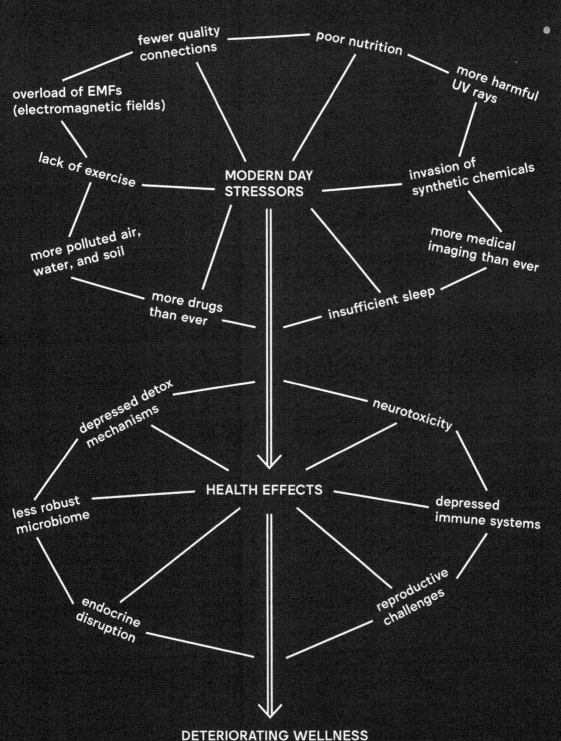

FIGURE #03

21

toxicity. For example, children are exposed to arsenic, a developmental neurotoxicant that is created both naturally and artificially, through multiple dietary sources.

— Scientists have found infertility (and, therefore, population declines), malformed reproductive organs, and other reproductive challenges among certain human and wildlife populations. According to the 2013 WHO and UNEP 2013 report titled *State of the Science of Endocrine Disrupting Chemicals—2012,* Scandinavian studies have found a correlation between genital abnormalities in male babies and decreased sperm quality in adulthood. In fact, 20 to 40 percent of young men in the general population of Denmark, Finland, Germany, Norway, and Sweden are estimated to have sperm counts in the subfertile range. "There is more evidence from laboratory studies now than in 2002 that chemical exposures can interfere with endocrine signaling of pubertal timing, fecundity [the ability to reproduce], and fertility and with menopause" (WHO and UNEP 2013). Endocrine disrupting chemicals are found in a wide range of consumer products and food packaging.

My perspective on health has significantly broadened. Today, I think about my family's exposure to toxicants as frequently as I think about how to provide them with a nourishing diet and restorative sleep.

STEER YOUR HEALTH TOWARDS BETTER LUCK

I learned a great deal from the experience of my husband's carotid artery dissection. It gave me additional context for my understanding of health and wellness, partially because I realized the limited perspective of experts with even the most impressive credentials.

I learned that the health of my family is, ultimately, my responsibility. No one will decide on groceries and other household items as frequently as I do. And no one will better know our family medical history, lifestyle, diet, and other environmental factors.

Not wanting my husband to return to the hospital, I placed new importance on learning how to proactively position my family for more resilient health. Motherhood further broadened this interest.

Since then, I have continued to learn more about all factors—both proven and suspected—that may prevent disease and help improve our health. I have learned that just because beliefs are common doesn't mean they're true, just because products are popular doesn't mean they're harmless, and just because habits are widespread doesn't mean they're benign. I also now know that "no proof of harm" doesn't necessarily mean something is safe.

As I read reports and scientific studies, I was surprised by how many precautionary measures I could incorporate daily. I went from being helpless to being empowered. I also have more trust than ever in common sense, and I believe in continually improving it with new information.

The American College of Obstetricians and Gynecologists issued a statement in October 2013 urging their members to inform patients of precautionary measures that they can take to protect their unborn or future children. In part, it said:

> Robust scientific evidence has emerged over the past 15 years, demonstrating that preconception and prenatal exposure to toxic environmental agents can have a profound and lasting effect on reproductive health across the life course. Exposure to toxic environmental agents also is implicated in increases in adverse reproductive health outcomes that emerged since World War II; these changes have occurred at a rapid rate that cannot be explained by changes in genetics alone, which occur at a slower pace. (American College of OB/GYN 2013)

KEY POINTS

01. Be mindful of whom you are getting advice from. Consider how broad and informed their perspective is. Even excellent physicians can be unaware of important factors that shape our health.

02. The factors that influence wellness and disease are complex and not fully understood. However, leading authorities are increasingly recognizing the value of reducing one's exposure to toxicants.

Chapter I.3
The Unique Vulnerability of Children

My husband and I recently started watching *Mad Men*, the hit television series about an advertising company in 1960s Manhattan. It's amazing to see how much we, as a country, have learned. For example, I am struck by the amount of smoking and drinking, especially among pregnant women!

It reminds us of what we didn't know back then: Fetuses and young children are especially vulnerable. We now know that a fetus exposed to too much alcohol can develop fetal alcohol syndrome and that exposure to cigarette smoke is linked to numerous adverse health effects.

When pregnant with my first child, I sought out the best books I could find that would teach me all the ways to give her the healthiest start. I was fascinated by how she was growing and changing, and I was diligent in doing whatever I could to support and protect that development. My plan for a healthy pregnancy focused on four main goals: getting good rest, exercising, eating healthfully, and drinking lots of water.

Despite these good intentions and hard work, I missed an important area of concern: I never considered the threat of toxicants in my foods and beverages, everyday purchases, outdoor and indoor air, and even the dust in my home. While they were mentioned in books, I didn't have the background to appreciate the warnings so I didn't worry about it. However, if I could do things differently, I would have incorporated a fifth goal: minimizing unnecessary exposures to toxicants.

Even while ignorant on the topic, however, my instincts cautioned me against some exposures. For example, when I was pregnant with my first child, my husband and I had taken our car to an auto repair shop. After a few minutes in the waiting room, I felt compelled to run out of the building to vomit. My body's strong reaction wouldn't dissipate until I was far enough from the building that I could no longer sense the fumes from the shop. Years later, I learned about the highly toxic effects of benzene (found in auto products and gasoline): It's a carcinogen and can damage chromosomes (McGinn 2000). Immediately, I wondered if my body knew that the baby's well-being was at risk.

My protective instincts peaked during the prenatal period with each of my three children and remained high through their first year of life. Although I remain concerned and diligent about their health and safety, I've relaxed more each year after the initial one. Interestingly, this timing is perfectly in sync with their most biologically vulnerable stages.

This chapter spotlights the unique vulnerability of children given their biology and their behavior.

THE BIOLOGICAL REALITY OF CHILDREN

Children are not little adults. From conception until about 20 years of age, the foundation of one's body—the central nervous system, respiratory system, immune system, reproductive system, and so on—is developing under the direction of countless hormonal, neural, and genetic messages. Therefore, this stage of development is an important one to protect.

Given the rapid and dynamic changes during development, the potential for errors to occur is high. The developing brain, for example, triples in weight during the first year of infancy and "doubles to 200 billion cells by the age of two," according to Devra Davis PhD MPH (2010), an award-winning scientist and writer, in her book *Disconnect*. During this stage of intense growth and development, "low levels of exposure" that would not materially harm the adult brain can permanently damage the developing brain (Grandjean and Landrigan 2014).

Children's brains are more vulnerable than those of adults for many reasons. First, the natural protective and detoxification mechanisms that protect adults are immature in children. For example, in infants, the blood–brain barrier (BBB), which protects the brain from unwanted molecules in the

Life in Utero

The prenatal period is a time of rapid development as a response to a variety of biological signals determined by genetics, hormones, and environmental factors. Therefore, it is a period that is vulnerable to disruption.

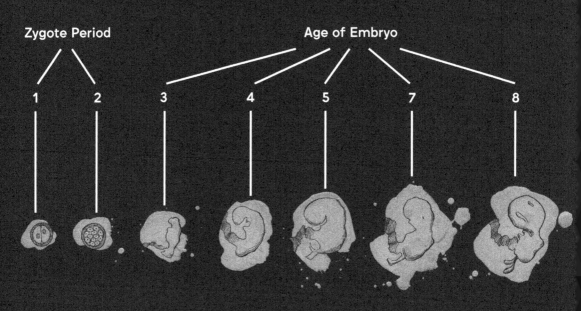

Zygote Period | Age of Embryo

1   2   3   4   5   7   8

central nervous system

heart

upper limbs

eyes

lower limbs

teeth

palate

ears

Fetal Period

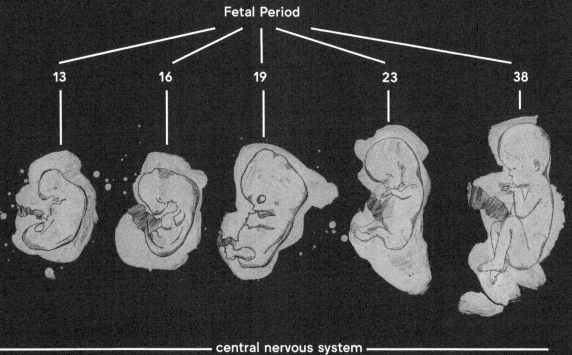

13   16   19   23   38

central nervous system

eyes

teeth

external genitalia

ears

(Source: CDC 2014a)

FIGURE #04

bloodstream (Bunim 2012), has been frequently cited in the scientific literature as being "immature" or "leaky" (Saunders, Liddelow, and Dziegielewska 2012). Estimates on when this barrier fully develops vary—anywhere from before birth (Daneman et al. 2010) to six months after birth (Schettler et al. 2000). While the BBB is still not fully understood (Saunders, Liddelow, and Dziegielewska 2012), it is widely believed to be more porous in infants and children than in adults, allowing greater amounts of unwanted molecules to reach the developing brain. Further, various toxicants and conditions (such as radiation from microwaves and other sources, infections, high blood pressure, and brain injuries) may weaken or open the BBB (Chudler 2014).

Second, the skull of a child is thinner than that of an adult, and a child's brain has a relatively higher fluid content (Davis 2010). As chapter I.14 spotlights, this renders them more vulnerable to radiation exposure from wireless technologies and medical imaging. How these characteristics may increase the brain's vulnerability to other exposures is unknown, but an international community of scientists—including the WHO (2014e), foreign governments (WiFi in Schools Australia 2014), and the BioInitiative Working Group (2014b)—are actively researching the adverse effects of wireless technologies. The brain could be the most vulnerable organ since it is still developing until a person is 20 years old (NIMH 2011).

CHILDREN ARE EXPOSED TO TOXICANTS EVEN BEFORE THEY ARE BORN

Exposure to toxicants begins in the womb. With improved biomonitoring technology, scientists have learned that newborns carry a substantial chemical burden. One of the few studies to look at a very broad range of chemicals—and one that is referenced often—was conducted in 2005. The American Red Cross collected and examined umbilical cord blood from 10 American newborns to check for 413 industrial chemicals. The study, led by the Environmental Working Group (EWG), found a total of 287 chemicals and an average of approximately 200 industrial compounds, pollutants, and other chemicals in these newborn babies. Pollutants detected in umbilical cord blood included chemicals used in fast-food packaging, pesticides, and flame retardants used on clothing and textiles. More specifically, of the 287 chemicals found in newborn umbilical cord blood:

— 180 cause cancer in humans or animals
— 217 are toxic to the brain and nervous system
— and 208 cause developmental problems

The scientists involved believed that the more chemicals they tested for, the more they would have found (EWG 2005a).

CHILDREN'S BODIES ABSORB RELATIVELY MORE TOXICANTS FROM OUR ENVIRONMENT

After they are born, children come in contact with toxicants through normal daily things: diet, toys, personal care products, medications, and the overall indoor and outdoor environments in and around their homes, schools, daycare centers, and even vehicles. However, due to children's faster metabolic rate and smaller size, their relative exposure is larger than that of adults. In proportion to body weight, "children drink 2.5 times more water, eat 3 to 4 times more food, and breathe 2 times more air" than do adults. Consequently, on a per pound basis, children are also exposed to more toxicants than are adults (Steingraber 2010).

Their behavior also increases their exposure to environmental toxins further: crawling on floors, hiding in dusty places such as under beds and behind furniture, and putting their fingers (and many other things) in their mouths. Moreover, children tend to have less diverse diets, and they favor dairy and packaged foods that are more likely to have higher concentrations of certain toxicants.

TOXICANTS STAY INSIDE CHILDREN'S BODIES FOR LONGER

Once inside children's bodies, toxicants may be metabolized and excreted more slowly than in adults because children's metabolic pathways are immature, especially during the prenatal and postnatal periods. Also, the levels of chemical-binding proteins arc lower in children than in adults, which permits higher concentrations of unbound, biologically active agents to reach organs throughout children's bodies, including the brain. Therefore, toxicants can stay in their bodies for longer. Furthermore, children have many more years of life ahead than do adults—more time in which toxicants can impair their biology, they can be exposed to additional environmental stressors, and to develop diseases (Reuben 2010).

CHILDREN CAN BE MORE VULNERABLE TO TOXICANTS

While children are generally resilient to common physical injury and illness, when their developing systems are damaged by toxicants, the damage doesn't necessarily have time to repair. Instead, the damage can be incorporated into the growth plan, altering the foundation from which the body develops (This idea is revisited in chapter I.15).

Children's unique vulnerability is not fully understood. However, according to the EWG's report *Body Burden: The Pollution in Newborns*, the Environmental Protection Agency (EPA) reviewed the research and concluded that carcinogens are, on average, 10 times more potent in babies than in adults, with certain chemicals being up to 65 times more powerful (EWG 2005b). Subsequently, the EPA updated its cancer risk guidelines in 2005 to incorporate better protection against childhood exposures, including exposure assessment, dose-response assessment, hazard assessment, and risk characterization (EPA 2005).

In September 2008 Leonardo Trasande MD MPP, a pediatrician and assistant professor at the Mount Sinai School of Medicine at the time, testified before the US Senate Environment and Public Works Committee. He told its members:

> The heroic work of decoding the human genome has shown that only about 10 to 20 percent of disease in children is purely the result of genetic inheritance. The rest is the consequence of interplay between environmental exposures and genetically determined variations in individual susceptibility. Moreover, genetic inheritance by itself cannot account for the sharp recent increases that we have seen in incidence of pediatric disease. (Trasande 2008)

WHAT YOU CAN DO

Informed parents, caregivers, school administrators, teachers, and physicians can help protect children. Seemingly small choices can decrease exposure to toxicants, as you will see in parts III and IV.

Mothers have a unique influence, for several reasons. Their bodies are the first homes of their children, and they usually buy the family's food and household products. Furthermore, mothers have unique protective instincts, which are sharpened with information and with greater understanding of how toxicants may challenge the biology of children. Mothers, and fathers, should never doubt their instincts.

KEY POINTS

01. Children are uniquely vulnerable to toxicants, and the younger they are, the more vulnerable they are.

02. Parents, caregivers, teachers, school administrators, healthcare providers, and other authorities can protect children by making informed choices.

03. Even informed instincts are helpful.

Chapter I.4
Our Invisible Reality

"But I grew up not worrying about these things, and I turned out okay..."

Years ago, in a taxi cab in New York City, my mother-in-law said something to the effect of: "It's so interesting how nowadays people are so interested in eating organic foods and avoiding plastic. When I was growing up, no one worried about this sort of stuff—and we turned out okay."

I hear those comments often. In reality, a lot has changed. The environment in which we grew up—not to mention the one our parents and grandparents once knew—is drastically different from the one in which today's children live.

OUR CHEMICAL EXPLOSION
The change in our environment from our chemical production is invisible to most of us. Yet, it has been profound.

Although the synthetic chemical industry began in the second half of the 19th century, it wasn't until after World War II that synthetic chemicals began to infiltrate our lives through our household products. They first appeared in the innovative products required by the war effort, such as low-cost, durable materials and foods to clothe and feed our soldiers. After the war ended, mainstream practical applications were found for these chemicals in consumer products such as pesticides, plastic products, fabrics, fire retardants, water and stain repellents, pharmaceuticals, processed foods, and more. The popular demand for convenience and inexpensive pleasure fueled research to discover tens of thousands of additional chemicals and their applications. Production of synthetic materials was approximately 350 times higher in 1982 than in 1940, according to data presented in the book *Our Stolen Future* (Colborn, Dumanoski, and Myers 1997).

In other words, since World War II, an overwhelming *number* of chemicals have been introduced into the environment. The exact number is unknown, but approximately 84,000 of them are registered in the US (WHO and UNEP 2013).

In addition, the *rate* at which new chemicals are introduced into the environment and into consumer products is robust. Estimates for how many are introduced each year vary widely. For example:
— In 1962, Rachel Carson estimated in *Silent Spring* that almost 500 new chemicals were introduced annually (Carson [1962] 2002).
— In 2009, the US Government Accounting Office estimated that an average of 700 new chemicals are introduced annually (GAO 2009a).
— The 2010 PCP report estimated that "1,000–2,000 new chemicals are created and introduced into the environment each year" (Reuben 2010).
— In March 2012, as reported in the *New York Times*, Leonardo Trasande MD MPP, an associate professor of pediatrics, environmental medicine, and population health at New York University, estimated that "1,000 to 3,000 new chemicals were introduced into our environment each year over the past 30 years" (Tortorello 2012).
— In September 2014, the editor in chief of *Environmental Science & Technology*, Jerald L. Schnoor (2014), described the growing list of chemicals in the Chemical Abstracts Service Registry, the most comprehensive national database of disclosed chemicals, as "eye-popping, with approximately 15,000 new chemicals and biological sequences [identified] each day." The registry contains "more than 90 million organic and inorganic substances and 65 million sequences" (CAS 2014). While not all of these are necessarily in commercial use, no one knows all of the ones that are in use and what health risks they pose (Blum 2014).

While the rate at which the unique number of chemicals has infiltrated our environment is staggering, the production *volume* is also provocative. In its 2008–2009 report, the PCP indicated that approximately 42 billion pounds of chemicals are produced in or imported into the US *daily* (Reuben 2010). This figure was based on data collected during the 2002 Inventory Update conducted by the EPA under a requirement of the Toxic Substances Control Act (Wilson and Schwarzman 2009; BIWG and NPPTAC 2005).

By the 2005 reporting period, this number had risen to about *74 billion pounds per day*. These estimates "include substances used in industrial processes and products and do not include fuels, pesticide products, pharmaceuticals, or food products" (Wilson and Schwarzman 2009).

Established by Congress in 1986 through the Emergency Planning and Community Right-to-Know Act, the EPA Toxics Release Inventory (TRI) is a database of nearly 700 toxic chemicals emitted from thousands of US facilities (EPA 2014i). In 2012, approximately 3.6 billion pounds of TRI chemicals were released into the environment. However, the database provides only a minimum estimate of toxic chemical releases: it does not include all toxic compounds or involve all sectors of the US economy (EPA 2014a).

Moreover, too many of these chemicals are known to be harmful to our Homes. As of August 2010, nearly 3,000 chemicals used in the US were high-production-volume (HPV) chemicals, meaning that annual production or importation exceeds 1 million pounds (EPA 2010). HPV chemicals are used throughout our homes, schools, and communities, and are dispersed in air, water, soil, and waste sites. Almost half of the 214 known human neurotoxicants for adults are HPV chemicals, with pesticides being the largest group (Grandjean and Landrigan 2014; Landrigan 2010). According to the CEHC, "of the top 20 chemicals discharged to the environment, nearly 75 percent are known or suspected to be toxic to the developing human brain" (CEHC 2014a).

UNINTENTIONAL BY-PRODUCTS AND UNINTENTIONAL TOXICANTS ARE A CONCERN

Aside from the compounds that are deliberately manufactured, "Unintentional By-products" may be created in manufacturing, combustion, and breakdown through metabolism or natural biodegradation. For example, a group of chemicals collectively known as dioxins can be created as by-products of waste incineration, chemical manufacturing, vinyl production, paper bleaching, and other processes. Dioxins have been described as the most toxic man-made chemicals based on experiments in laboratory animals. These studies have demonstrated biological changes in doses as low as parts per trillion (Cone 2012a). The EPA (2012a) recently concluded that current exposures to dioxins, which occur mainly through dietary intake of animal fat, do not pose a significant health risk. However, the unique risks to vulnerable populations, such as fetuses and young children, remain unknown.

Unintentional By-products can combine with other Unintentional By-products or parent compounds to create additional unintentional compounds. Collectively, I refer to these unintentional compounds later in this book as "Unintentional Toxicants."

KEY POINTS

01. We have an unprecedented number of different types of chemicals in our Homes. Since World War II, approximately 84,000 new chemicals have been introduced into American commerce, and the rate at which new chemicals are being introduced is estimated at 1,000 to 3,000 per year.

02. The volume of chemicals in our environment is also unprecedented. According to the US EPA, several billion pounds of toxic chemicals are released into the environment each year (EPA 2014c).

03. Unintentional By-products and Unintentional Toxicants are a concern. They further complicate tracking the compounds that are in our environments.

Chapter I.5
Our Chemical Explosion at Home

I like living with scarcity. You would never suspect this from visiting my home because we have too much *stuff*. But I do prefer owning the minimum number of things possible. I like the things I own to be multifunctional, high-quality, and beautiful. I don't like clutter.

Children invite—almost seem to require—clutter.

THE "BENEFITS" OF OUR CHEMICAL EXPLOSION

When I was nine months pregnant with my eldest daughter, my husband and I attempted to prepare for her arrival by visiting a major retailer that carried everything one might want for a baby. Not knowing what a baby needs, I was overwhelmed by the abundant options. Not only did this mega-store contain floor-to-ceiling shelves with uncountable varieties of baby products—pacifiers, clothes, lotions, shampoos, conditioners, balms, powders, creams, toys, infant formulas, car seats, high chairs, cribs, nursing pillows, and seemingly thousands more, but also *each product category* also offered many options.

I was so overwhelmed that I developed a headache within minutes. My husband and I left the store empty-handed soon after arriving, having decided to buy essentials on an as-needed basis, which is easy to do in Manhattan.

However, I left the store with the impression that the brands and products that I had seen were safe. After all, this retailer was an "expert" in what babies need. Safety was at the top of the list.

Once our daughter was born in 2007, as I prepared to leave the maternity ward, I was given a bag of products to help me: diapers, creams, infant formula, and so forth. Since the hospital gave me the products, I assumed they too were safe.

As I used the baby body wash, shampoo, wipes, and diaper cream, and then slathered the fragranced lotions over my daughter's delicate body to remain until her next bath,

I wondered what was in these products. Eventually I learned that many ingredients in children's personal care products threaten their biology. Many of those same ingredients were in products carried by the major retailer—and in the hospital gift bag. This experience was the first among many that would raise my concern as they highlighted how frequently I assume product safety.

MUCH IS UNKNOWN ABOUT OUR CONSUMER PRODUCTS

I was shocked to learn how little is known about the ingredients in, and therefore the safety of, our consumer products. First, manufacturers of many household goods—cleaning products, personal care products, interior furnishings, and children's items—are not required to disclose the ingredients in their products. A lot of information is protected as confidential and proprietary.

After reading about this, I went to a local drugstore to double-check what I had learned. I found that cleaning product labels had very little information. Manufacturers vaguely list "active" and "inactive" ingredients. Personal care products reveal more, but the average consumer isn't equipped to assess their safety—the complex chemical names of the ingredients are essentially meaningless to anyone who isn't well grounded in chemistry. Considering this complexity, I assumed that someone else—per the law—was knowledgeably regulating the ingredients and that safety measures were in place. My research later debunked that assumption.

Except for pesticides and food, which are treated with greater caution, manufacturers are not required to test for safety. There is also no unbiased third party reviewing the safety of products. According to the EWG, manufacturers of cleaning products can use nearly any ingredient—even those known to cause adverse effects (EWG 2014b)—with no legally binding upper limits (EWG 2014c). In personal care products, only 11 chemicals are restricted in the US (Campaign for Safe

Cosmetics 2014a), compared with 1,373 that are banned from cosmetics in the EU (European Commission 2014).

As researchers identify gaps in our knowledge about our chemical production and use, their concerns grow regarding the effects of most chemicals under real-world circumstances. More specifically, most chemicals are not tested for carcinogenicity, neurotoxicity, endocrine disruption, developmental and reproductive toxicity, immune system toxicity, and harm to developing fetuses and children.

— *Cancer*: Less than 2 percent of chemicals on the market have been tested for their ability to cause cancer (Mishamandani 2014).

— *Developmental neurotoxicity:* Epidemiological studies have established that 11 industrial chemicals are developmental neurotoxicants. It is likely that many other neurotoxicants remain undiscovered (Grandjean and Landrigan 2014).

— *Endocrine disruption*: While there have been great advances in understanding endocrine-disrupting chemicals over the past 10 years, the EPA has noted, "substantial endocrine effects data [are] lacking for most chemical substances" (EPA 2011b).

THE CHEMICALS IN OUR HOMES
The chemical explosion discussed in chapter I.4 appears in our homes as desirable and often useful products. Many of these enticing products also contain hidden hazards that are not disclosed or fully understood.

The growing concern about the toxicants in household products is another reason to fight *clutter*.

KEY POINTS
01. The chemical explosion shows up in our homes through products we buy as well as through air, soil, and water.
02. We should reevaluate our assumption that most things are safe. Generally, we do not have enough information to assess the safety of most chemicals that create our consumer products.
03. The best way to reduce the chemical contamination throughout our Homes is to consume less and more mindfully.

Chapter I.6
The Trails of Contamination throughout Our Homes

My grandmother, who lived into her mid-70s, suffered from asthma. When I think of her, I always remember her compromised breathing. I can still almost hear it now.

She believed that the air pollution in her hometown in Taiwan was a major cause of her respiratory challenges. Whenever I heard that, I always thought, Phew… Thank God I live in upstate New York!

OUR INVISIBLE POLLUTION

At one time, the word *pollution* brought to my mind images of industrial contamination and smog hovering over cities. Now I'm aware of the invisible pollution—toxicants—in our built environments, our bodies, and our planet.

We inadvertently contribute to this invisible pollution in various ways. One significant way is through our consumption, as chapter I.5 introduced.

This chapter explains how our possessions pollute our Homes by taking a closer look at a popular material, vinyl. However, vinyl is only one representative example of many other popular materials of concern.

Generally made of petroleum-based ingredients and other toxicants, popular materials of concern not only pollute the environment during their manufacturing, but also release toxicants during their use and disposal, and in some cases for many years after they were discarded or destroyed. Later in this book, I refer to this as the "Trails of Contamination."

Popular materials of concern each leave their own Trails of Contamination; they are profiled in chapter II.3 and I refer to them as "Household Materials of Concern." Ultimately, their trails end in us.

THE TRAILS OF CONTAMINATION FROM OUR VINYL PRODUCTS
Contamination during manufacturing

Vinyl, also known as polyvinyl chloride (PVC), is one of the most widely used materials as well as one of the most toxic. Manufacturing vinyl requires a complex chemical formula that usually includes toxic ingredients, such as those in the following paragraphs.

— *Mercury*: The PVC industry is the second-largest consumer of mercury, a potent neurological and reproductive toxin, according to the report *Pass Up the Poison Plastic: The PVC-Free Guide for Your Family & Home* (Liu, Schade, and Simpson 2008) from the Center for Health, Environment and Justice (CHEJ). Another report, *Environmental Impacts of Polyvinyl Chloride Building Materials* (Thornton 2002) from the Healthy Building Network, estimates that the vinyl life cycle is associated with the release of "many tons of mercury" into the environment each year.

— *Chlorine*: The PVC industry is the largest single user of chlorine. The adverse effects of this chemical on human health depend on the exposure, but they can include damage to the respiratory, neurologic, and reproductive systems as well as cancer, developmental issues, and death (ATSDR 2010). In the environment, low levels can cause harm, especially to organisms living in water and soil (EPA 1994). An article in the *Western Journal of Emergency Medicine*, "Chlorine Gas: An Evolving Hazardous Material Threat and Unconventional Weapon," warns of the hazards of chlorine gas in the case of industrial accidents and raises the idea that it could be used as a terrorist weapon (Jones, Wills, and Kang 2010). Further, since chlorine is highly reactive, it's likely to form Unintentional Toxicants.

— *Ethylene dichloride:* Created from chlorine gas, ethylene dichloride is a key ingredient in manufacturing vinyl (CHEJ 2014b). It is a probable human carcinogen that may also affect the central nervous system and internal organs, such as the liver (EPA 2006).

— *Vinyl chloride:* This is another key component of vinyl, and there is no threshold below which it does not increase cancer risk (Thornton 2002; CHEJ 2014a).

— *Heavy metals:* Heavy metals are sometimes used as stabilizers and can be released from vinyl products. Ones commonly reported include lead, a neurotoxin that harms the developing brain at all detectable levels, and cadmium, a recognized human carcinogen (Thornton 2002).

— *Phthalates*: This class of compounds, known to be hormone disruptors and reproductive and developmental toxicants, is used to soften hard plastic. Phthalates pose "considerable health and environmental hazards" and can leach from vinyl products (Thornton 2002).

— *Dioxins:* An unintentional by-product, dioxins can be created and released into the environment when manufacturing and incinerating vinyl. In doses as low as parts per trillion, dioxin has been found to damage development, reproduction, and the immune and endocrine systems. In fact, there hasn't been a detected dose that doesn't cause biological harm (Thornton 2002). The US Green Building Council's Technical Science Advisory Committee reported that "dioxin emissions put PVC consistently among the worst materials for human health impacts" (Lent 2007).

Contamination during our use

At home, vinyl is found in our mattresses, floors, bench cushions, shower curtains, place mats, and more. In children's products, vinyl can be found in playpens, high chairs, children's watches, backpacks, pencil cases, raincoats, rain boots, toy dolls, and many more toys.

Several reports (such as OECD 2009; Liu, Schade, and Simpson 2008; and Thornton 2002) warn that consumers may be exposed to hazards during a product's use since toxic chemicals are not necessarily bound to their products. For example, toxicants such as phthalates, lead, and cadmium have been found to migrate from their products.

Parents, prospective parents, and caregivers should take precautionary measures. Some phthalates have been associated with reproductive problems like shorter pregnancy duration (Latini et al. 2003), premature breast development in girls (Colon et al. 2000), sperm damage (Duty et al. 2003), and impaired reproductive development in males (Liu, Schade, and Simpson 2008; Swan et al. 2005). While some phthalates have been banned from children's toys in the US since February 2009 (Liu, Schade, and Simpson 2008; Layton 2008), we don't know if replacement formulas are safer and other toxicants can be present. For example, lead, used as a stabilizer, is still found in many different PVC products even though it's hazardous, especially for children (Liu, Schade, and Simpson 2008; Thornton 2002).

Heat and humidity facilitate the release of chemicals into the air (Liu, Schade, and Simpson 2008; CA EPA 1999; Rudel 2000; Uhde et al. 2001), conditions that are common for a vinyl shower curtain. Particles in toxic fumes can settle in dust and on surfaces, from which they can be inhaled, ingested (through children's hand–mouth behavior), or absorbed through the skin. Since Americans spend approximately 90 percent of their time indoors, according to EPA estimates (EPA 2009a), indoor air and household dust are two major sources of exposure to a wide range of toxicants.

Contamination during disposal

Upon disposal, vinyl products can continue to contaminate our planet and us. During incineration, or as vinyl rest in landfills and oceans (since vinyl is not biodegradable), vinyl can lead to Unintentional By-products and Unintentional Toxicants.

Contamination after a product's useful life

My father *loves* vinyl-sided homes. He says with enthusiastic advocacy, "They're cheap, durable, and you never have to repair them!"

Those are valid benefits. However, the durability that makes vinyl so popular during its useful life also makes it a growing problem at the end of the product's life cycle: It never fully biodegrades. Scientists say that in the world's oceans, there are at least five "garbage patches" made mostly of plastics that are caught in giant gyres, which are large spirals of ocean currents and wind.

For example, the Pacific Garbage Patch, which has grown a hundredfold during the past 40 years, is estimated to be twice the size of Texas; it is 90 feet deep at some points and is expected to double in size every decade (Peralta 2012; Hoshaw 2009). It contains plastic that is half a century old, and it is causing profound changes to marine life. It is also a huge breeding ground, allowing insects to reproduce as never before (Johnston 2012).

In December 2014, scientists estimated that the world's oceans contain more than 5 trillion plastic pieces that weigh over 250,000 tons (Eriksen et al. 2014).

KARMA?

Vinyl and many other plastic products continue to contaminate the environment beyond the end of their useful life. On land, sunlight can degrade chemicals from plastic into dust, which we then inhale, absorb, and ingest. Moreover, in the oceans, plastic can both leach chemicals, like BPA (Barry 2009), and absorb others, such as PCBs and the pesticide DDT (both of which cannot dissolve in water).

Some of this plastic may be consumed by marine life. One analysis found that in the intermediate depths of the North Pacific, fish ingest plastic at a rate of roughly 12,000 to 24,000 tons per year. That same study estimated that 9 percent of captured fish had plastic in their stomachs (Davidson and Asch 2011; Peralta 2012). The plastic consumed by fish leaches chemicals into their tissues.

As the vinyl and other plastic products that we produce, buy, and throw away contaminate water and wildlife, they also contaminate the animals that drink the water and eat the wildlife. Higher up the food chain, we continue the process and contaminate ourselves. Seems like karma to me.

WHAT'S GOING ON WITH WILDLIFE?

The WHO, UNEP, and EPA call wildlife an "important sentinel for humans" (WHO and UNEP 2013; van der Schalie et al. 1999); wildlife patterns can provide advance warning for humans on environmental hazards. For example, in the early 1900s, coal miners would send canaries into coal mines first to "test" for toxic gases, mainly carbon dioxide, since birds are more sensitive to it than humans are.

So what's going on with wildlife?

Health trends in wildlife are similar to those found among humans: reproductive dysfunction, abnormal behaviors, cancer, immune dysfunction, endocrine disruption, and population declines (WHO and UNEP 2013).

The bodies of wildlife accumulate various toxicants, such as persistent organic pollutants (POPs), and other ingredients from our consumer products and pharmaceuticals. This has been associated with certain health disorders. For example, among beluga whales in the St. Lawrence River in Canada, POPs are suspected of causing skeletal disorders, ulcers, pneumonia, bacterial and viral infections, and thyroid abnormalities—afflictions

rarely seen in belugas living in less contaminated waters (UNEP 2010).

Very concerning has been the drastic decline in the honeybee population, the result of a syndrome referred to as Colony Collapse Disorder (CCD). In the past, average annual bee losses ranged from 5 to 10 percent (Haberman 2014). Since 2007, however, they have been disappearing in the US at around 30 percent per winter, according to an article published in the *Journal of Agricultural Research* (Steinhauer et al. 2014). Honeybees, as well as other bee species, are dying in other countries as well (Spivak 2015).

While health trends in wildlife continue to be studied, the declining bee population has attracted special interest since bees are integral to our food supply. They pollinate an estimated 30 percent of what Americans eat (Haberman 2014); worldwide, they affect crops valued at $30 billion per year that feed 90 percent of the population (*BBC* 2014).

Increasingly, experts believe that the disappearing bees are resulting from a perfect storm of multiple factors, mainly those in figure #05. Collectively, they, and perhaps other factors, are most likely weakening the bees' immune systems, contributing to their alarming decline.

The good news is that we have reversed undesirable trends in the past. Regulation has proved helpful in this regard. After certain chemicals (like PCBs, organochlorine pesticides, dioxins, and other hormone-disrupting chemicals) were restricted, some populations of wildlife species that were declining began to recover (WHO and UNEP 2013). Regarding the bees, experts recommend that we plant more bee-friendly flowers, do not spray them with pesticides, and support eco-friendly farming practices.

OUR BODY BURDEN

"Body burden" is the accumulated chemical load we all carry around in our bodies. It's a concept that I've incorporated into my everyday choices.

The US CDC currently monitors more than 300 environmental chemicals or their metabolites that have been found in our bodies (CDC 2012c). In North America, body burdens were found to be at least 10 times higher than those of Europeans and others (Lorber 2008). Ken Cook, president and founder of the Environmental Working Group, testified

What's Going On With Honeybees?

Since 2007 they have been vanishing at about 30 percent per winter. Current thinking believes that their declining population is a result of a perfect storm of several factors, including those below.

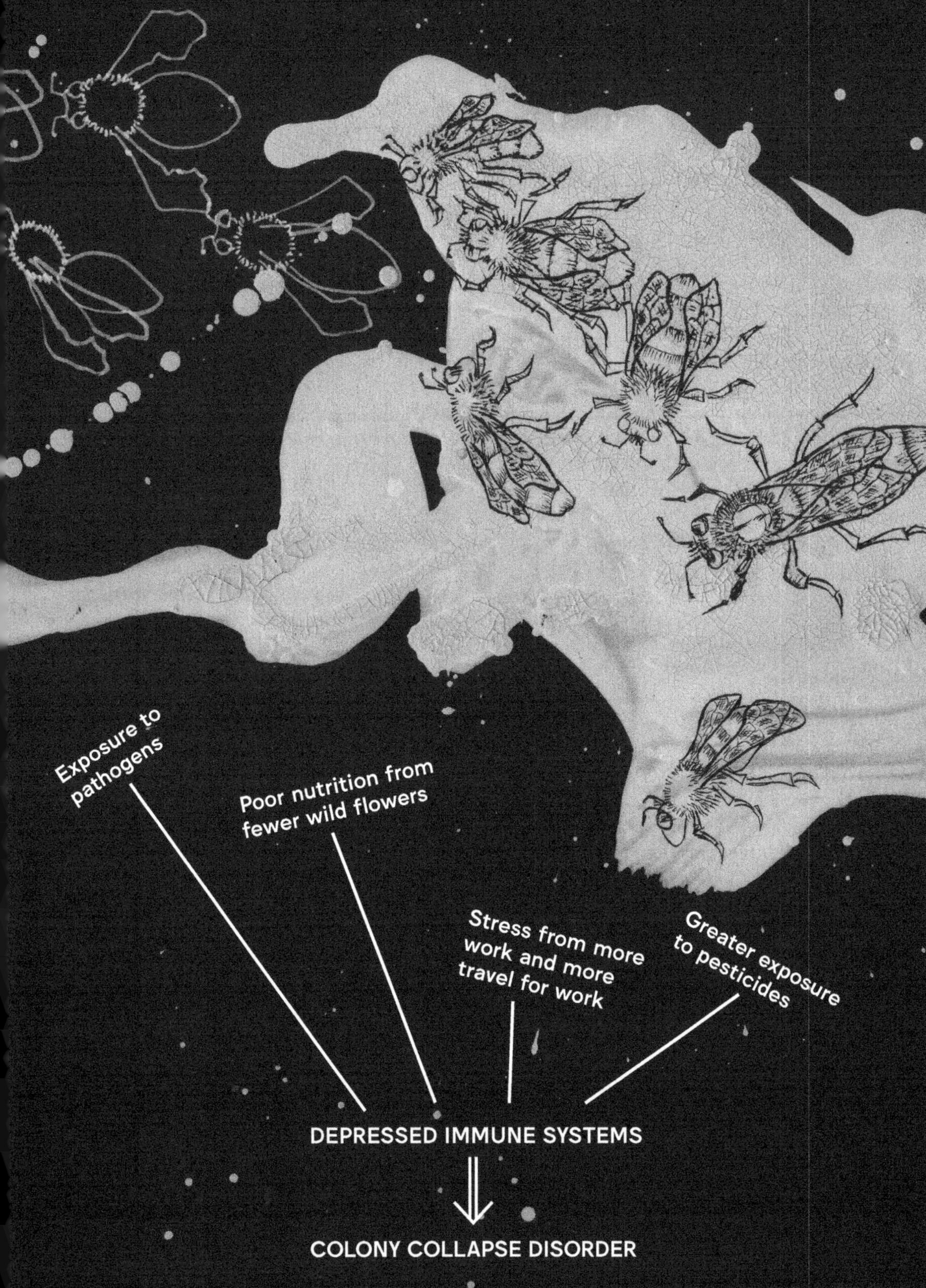

(Sources: Spivak 2014, Haberman 2014)

Exposure to pathogens

Poor nutrition from fewer wild flowers

Stress from more work and more travel for work

Greater exposure to pesticides

DEPRESSED IMMUNE SYSTEMS

⇓

COLONY COLLAPSE DISORDER

FIGURE #05

on July 29, 2010 before a subcommittee of the House of Representatives that over the previous 15 years, EWG had tested more than 200 people for 540 chemicals and detected up to 482 of them (EWG 2010b).

The WHO and UNEP (2013) report that "it is now virtually impossible to identify an unexposed population around the globe."

Women often have more toxic and hormone-disrupting substances in their bodies than do men (Reuben 2010). This is especially concerning because a proportion of a woman's chemical burden is passed on to her children during pregnancy through maternal blood and placental tissue, when a fetus's organs and various biological systems are developing. She may also pass on chemicals through breast milk (EWG 2005b).

The toxic body burdens of men may also affect their children's health. While this hasn't received as much attention, there may be reasons for concern. Below are the findings of a few studies.

— *Birth Defects*: Higher among veterans exposed to Agent Orange or other herbicides during their service in Vietnam or Korea (Department of Veteran Affairs 2013).

— *More girls than boys*: Twice as many girls as boys are fathered by men whose blood levels of dioxin reach the equivalent of 1 drop in 7,400 bathtubs (Chemical Industry Archives 2009).

— *Childhood Cancer*: Studies have found increased incidences of cancer among children whose parents were exposed to pesticides. For example, paternal occupational exposure may cause increased risk of brain tumors (Vinson et al. 2011; Shim, Mlynarek, and van Wijngaarden 2009; Runkle 2014). Children exposed to household use of pesticides during critical stages of development are also at higher risk of adverse health effects (Ma et al. 2002).

Children can have higher body burdens than do adults, especially for certain toxicants, such as those below.

— *Chemical flame retardants*: An average American baby is born with the highest concentrations of flame retardants among infants anywhere in the world (Callahan and Hawthorne 2012).

— *PBDEs*: One study in Australia found PBDEs in blood to be greatest for children ages 2-5 compared with those of older children and adults (Axelrad et al. 2013; Toms et al. 2009). Another study of people from throughout the US found that PBDE blood levels were about three times higher in children ages 1.5-4 than those of their mother (Axelrad et al. 2013; Lunder et al. 2010).

— *PFCs*: Among people living near a manufacturing facility that used PFCs in chemical formulas for resistance to stains and sticking, concentrations of two popular PFCs—C8 and PFOS—tended to be higher in children than in adults. For example, children under age 5 had an average of 44 percent more C8 in their blood than did their mothers, and differences persisted until they were about 12 years old. Blood concentrations of PFOS tended to be 42 percent higher in children than in their mothers, and this difference persisted until they were at least 19 years old (Mondal et al. 2012; Cone and *Environmental Health News* 2012).

WHAT IS THE THREAT OF TOXICANTS IN OUR BODY?

While not completely understood, our body burden can reach a tipping point—via accumulation or coupled with other stressors—and cause illness, if not immediately, then at some future point. For example, a few studies have found that stored toxicants may be released from our fat reserves as we lose weight or breastfeed (WHO and UNEP 2013; Carson [1962] 2002; Glass 1975; Steingraber 2001; Gever 2010). This can introduce chemicals into the blood, which may cause adverse effects (WHO and UNEP 2013). Chapter I.8 discusses the potential biological effects of these toxicants in greater detail.

KEY POINTS

01. Certain materials are known to create a toxic trail throughout their life cycle, and sometimes beyond their intended useful life. Their Trails of Contamination leave behind the Unintentional By-products and Unintentional Toxicants that are of concern. Ultimately, they reside in us.

02. We can minimize contamination of our Homes by selecting less-toxic materials and buying only what we need: We must be conscious of the manufacturing that we support and the amount of waste we create.

Chapter I.7
Do Toxicants Ever Die?
The Threats of Immortality

My husband lured me into the world of vampires through the HBO series *True Blood*. As I watched the vampires suffer through, and feel cursed by, their immortality, I couldn't help but think of plastics and other persistent materials and compounds!

Chapter I.6 described the contamination that occurs through the key milestones in the life of a single material, vinyl. This chapter begins by zooming in on a particular toxicant that has a life of immortality: PFOA (perfluorooctanoic acid), also known as C8 because it has eight carbons.

This chapter then transitions into how highly persistent toxicants, like C8, enter our bodies. Some of these chemicals were banned decades ago but are still detected in us. Their longevity continues to haunt us.

THE POSSIBILITIES IN THE AFTERLIFE

When I think about the lives of some toxicants, I can't help but think of reincarnation. They begin with specific intentions for their use. After they are created, they are merged with other components to create a product. For example, toxicants may become part of a chemical formulation (e.g., for nonstick or stain-resistant coatings) or a component of an intermediate product (like vinyl). Eventually they are incorporated into an end product, such as a vinyl shower curtain or nonstick pots and pans.

At the end of a product's useful life, it is discarded. However, disposal doesn't mean the end of existence for the product's components, as was discussed in the case of vinyl in chapter I.6.

Throughout the life of a product, toxicants are released into the environment. Some will biodegrade quickly. Others will exist for a longer time. The biological consequences of some materials—their Unintentional By-products and Unintentional Toxicants—may be eternal. Collectively, I refer to this sequence of design, manufacture, useful life, disposal, and immortality/reincarnation as the "Life Cycle," illustrated in figure #06.

Toxicants can persist for much longer than their designed use

Like plastics, some toxicants can persist in the environment for decades: Some will break down into other compounds and will have endless opportunities to resurface; others will persist unchanged for a long time before finally breaking down; the most chemically stable will live a life of virtual immortality.

Toxicants' activities in the afterlife are relatively unstudied, but what we do know is disturbing. Pesticides, for example, are dangerous because they are designed to kill by chemically interfering with biological processes. And some are so persistent that they are detected throughout our environment even decades after their use has ended.

DDT, a popular pesticide that was banned in 1972, is still detected in fish, crops, and breast milk (EPA 2011a). The "afterlife" effects of DDT and its breakdown compound, DDE (dichlorodiphenyldichloroethylene), continue to be examined.

The human body metabolizes DDT into DDE, a chemical that acts like estrogen, and several studies have found higher levels of DDE in women with breast cancer. Biochemist Mary Wolff and her colleagues conducted the first major study on the relationship between DDE and breast cancer. Out of the 14,290 women studied, Wolff found that the blood of breast cancer patients contained 35 percent more DDE on average than that of healthy women. Furthermore, the women with the highest DDE levels in their blood were four times more likely to have breast cancer than those with the lowest levels. While Wolff concluded that "breast cancer was strongly associated with DDE" (Wolff et al. 1993), later studies did not confirm this. However, the design of those studies did not necessarily consider factors that scientists now accept as relevant, such as exposures during critical stages of development.

Another example of a persistent toxicant is C8. It was particularly useful in

The Life Cycle of a Toxicant
A closer look at the path of C8 (or PFOA)

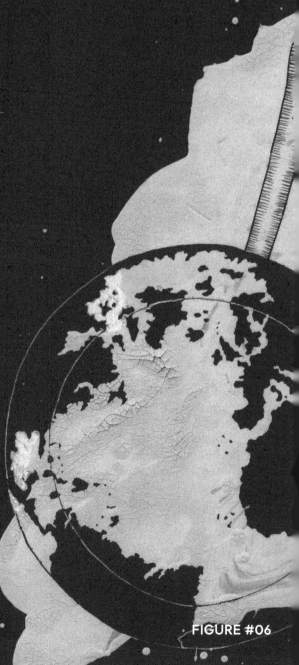

CONCEPTION
Toxicants are created for specific desirable traits. For example, PFCs are a family of compounds of which C8 is a member. They are popular for their key role in nonstick chemical formulas.

PRODUCT'S USEFUL LIFE
Later, the toxicant is developed further into an ingredient, material, or "end product."

Intermediate Products
C8 can become part of a chemical formula to impart nonstick qualities to end products (EPA 2014d; Naidenko et al. 2008).

End Products
As part of an intermediate product, C8 contributes to the performance of helpful end products: Nonstick pots and pans, inner coatings of takeout/delivery food containers and wrappers, and products made of treated textiles, such as carpets, sofas, and clothes (EPA 2014d; Naidenko et al. 2008).

END OF THE PRODUCT'S USEFUL LIFE
The end product's useful life stops when the consumer discards it into the trash.

THE AFTERLIFE OF THE END PRODUCT
Immortality or Reincarnation
However, PFCs can survive the end product's useful life. In fact, C8 is thought to persist forever (EWG 2003b), accumulating in our environment and in our bodies.

UNINTENTIONAL BY-PRODUCTS AND UNINTENTIONAL TOXICANTS
Other PFCs can break down into C8.

FIGURE #06

chemical formulas as coatings of nonstick pans, inner linings of takeout/delivery food containers, and treatments of textiles (EPA 2014d; Naidenko et al. 2008).

C8 is one of the few chemicals that have been examined relatively thoroughly. Due to its contamination of drinking water, class action lawsuits by more than 70,000 residents of Ohio and West Virginia (Gersowitz, Libo, and Korek, PC 2014), as well as a lawsuit by the EPA, were filed against DuPont, a manufacturer of C8. This forced the disclosure of internal company toxicity data, which revealed that DuPont had suspected a health threat from C8 as early as 1961 (Hawthorne 2005).

In 2004, DuPont agreed to a settlement that included, among other things, the company's commitment to rid the area's water supply of C8 and to pay for the medical monitoring of residents. In addition, a court-appointed panel of epidemiologists, the C8 Science Panel, was formed to study the health effects of exposure to C8. Conclusions of the panel would determine what additional medical care DuPont would pay for.

In November 2012, the panel announced a "probable link" between C8 and high cholesterol, ulcerative colitis, thyroid disease, kidney cancer, testicular cancer, pregnancy-induced hypertension, and pre-eclampsia (C8 Science Panel 2012). As a result of the findings, DuPont's settlement will total approximately $343 million to include residents' medical costs associated with C8. The settlement also allows residents with a disease or health problem associated with C8 to seek compensation beyond the $343 million settlement (Clapp et al. 2014).

While the EPA has been working with manufacturers to reduce or, preferably, phase out their use or production of C8, this chemical is expected to persist in our environment indefinitely. As C8 settles into the deep waters of the ocean, they are expected to persist "for many centuries" (WHO and UNEP 2013).

Tragically, manufacturers knew for decades that C8 does not biodegrade (EWG 2003b), while the EPA was unaware of this. The EPA began discovering the threat of C8 only in the 1990s, after investigating a chemical, PFOS, in another popular formula. C8 and PFOS are part of a larger class of chemicals called PFCs (perfluorinated compounds), which serve similar purposes. And they can be created both intentionally and unintentionally: C8, for example, can be created from the breakdown of various PFCs (EPA 2014d).

The *Canadian Arctic Contaminants Assessment Report on Persistent Organic Pollutants* stated, "The total mass (and average concentration) of [C8] and PFOS in the marine environment is expected to increase for the next 10 to 20 years" (Muir, Kurt-Karakus, and Stow 2013). Nearly everyone in the world has traces of PFCs in their bodies.

Toxicants hang out at home or travel the world

Depending on the chemical characteristics of the toxicants, some remain close to home, while others travel the world. Above water, those with a low vapor pressure tend to stay low to the ground as they disperse from the point of their original release. Given their short stature, children can have greater exposure to these low-hanging toxicants than adults.

Toxicants with high vapor pressures evaporate more easily. According to the report "Monitoring and Reducing Exposure of Infants to Pollutants in House Dust" by Roberts et al. (2009), "Pesticides with higher vapor pressures may condense closer to the point of application in the winter and translocate to cooler climates in the summer." This process has been referred to as the grasshopper effect (Riseborough 1990; Lioy 2006).

Sandra Steingraber PhD, a leading ecologist, environmental activist, and popular author, explains the grasshopper effect on POPs in her book *Living Downstream*. In warmer climates, winds and dust carry POPs to cooler areas, where they condense and are deposited on the ground or onto bodies of water. Should that area warm, the POPs again vaporize and move as before (Steingraber 2010). Ultimately, these toxicants move away from the equator and settle in polar and mountain areas, where the cooler temperatures mean less evaporation and little chance for further transport (UNEP 2005).

Steingraber (2010) adds that the grasshopper effect explains why the Arctic, which would seem to be the most pristine region of the world, has become one of the most chemically contaminated. The contamination is from pesticides and industrial chemicals that have traveled hundreds or thousands of miles (UNEP 2005).

Historically, the Arctic ice provided the rest of the world some protection by isolating a portion of these synthetic chemicals. Global warming, however, is releasing increasing levels of toxicants into the larger environment. Therefore, a larger population is experiencing a higher load of chemicals in air, water, soil, and food.

Toxicants reside and accumulate in our food supply

Once in the body, some chemicals are excreted or metabolized into less harmful compounds. However, others—the fat-loving ones—are not so readily degraded, and they accumulate in fatty tissues throughout the body. With repeated exposures, concentrations within an organism can become far greater than the concentration in the surrounding environment. This buildup over time is called bioaccumulation.

Furthermore, a substance present at a minuscule level in an organism at the base of the food chain can increase by a hundred-fold (up to many thousands of times higher than background levels) in an organism at or near the top of the food chain. This increasing concentration of chemicals with the ascension through the food chain is called biomagnification or bioamplification (NRDC 2005). Methylmercury (a neurotoxin that is high in predator fish like shark and tuna) and POPs are examples of persistent chemicals that biomagnify. Consuming contaminated fish is a primary source of exposure to certain chemicals for wildlife and humans (WHO and UNEP 2013).

At the top of the chain are humans. This is why the indigenous peoples of the Arctic, whose traditional diets rely on animal foods, have some of the highest recorded levels of the most toxic chemicals of the 20th century. This is because fish, birds, and mammals in this cold region have more body fat for natural insulation against freezing temperatures. Through bioaccumulation and biomagnification, toxicants grow to even higher levels in these organisms—and in the people who eat them (UNEP 2005).

Moreover, while some fat-soluble toxicants are found in higher concentrations in the fats of animals, their concentrations can be even higher in animal by-products, like cheese and butter. The clearest example of this that I came across in my research was in Rachel Carson's ([1962] 2002) historic book, *Silent Spring*. In it, she discusses the concentration of DDT in milk versus the concentration in butter made from that milk. In one analysis, DDT increased more than twentyfold—from 3 parts per million in milk to 65 parts per million in butter created from that milk. DDT is just one example of how a very small dose of a synthetic chemical may end as a heavy concentration.

Other toxicants work similarly. They include flame retardants (American Chemical Society 2004), PFCs (WHO and UNEP 2013; Safer Chemicals 2014), and pesticides. Therefore, diet is a major source of exposure to certain toxic chemicals (WHO and UNEP 2013). In May 2012, the *Chicago Tribune* reported that the blood levels of popular flame retardants had doubled in adults every two to five years between 1970 and 2004. Studies have shown that even after certain flame retardants were banned, levels of those flame retardants did not decline in the US (Callahan and Roe 2012c).

As they reside in our body fat, mothers share their lifetime accumulation of toxicants with their children through pregnancy and breast milk, as chapter I.6 explained.

Seems to me like a life of immortality.

KEY POINTS

01. The intentional creation of useful chemicals may result in parent compounds that persist well beyond their intended life, as well as Unintentional By-products and Unintentional Toxicants.

02. The contamination of the Earth's poles epitomizes the tragedy of how business activities in one location can harm innocent populations who live far away.

03. Since humans are at the top of the food chain, we are especially vulnerable to POPs and other fat-soluble toxins that bioaccumulate as they ascend the food chain.

Chapter I.8
The Threat of Unknown Consequences

Occasionally as I worked on this book project, I remembered a particular moment from childhood: I was about nine years old, in the kitchen with my mother and six-year-old brother. My mother and I were chatting about something as my brother sat on the countertop. I opened a kitchen cabinet for a glass for a drink of water.

I was excited to see new, colorful plastic cups. I grabbed one and proceeded to fill it up with water. My mother urged, "Please wash the cup first! It's probably dirty and has leftover chemicals in it."

I don't remember if I followed her urging, but I do remember rolling my eyes inside, thinking, "You're *sooooo* paranoid… A little dirt and chemicals aren't going to kill me."

TWO "TEACHERS"

Before becoming a mother, I often dismissed concerns about synthetic chemicals and other environmental issues. However, learning about two major classes of chemicals—POPs and endocrine disrupting chemicals (EDCs)—changed my perspective profoundly.

Both POPs and EDCs have attracted international study and are among the most thoroughly researched of all toxicants. Studies of these chemicals have revealed a lot about their complex behaviors and potential consequences, and about toxicants in general. And these studies continue because of their highly complex threats.

The Stockholm Convention on POPs

The most persistent, toxic, and threatening synthetic chemicals that are officially recognized as such are POPs. Even those that were banned decades ago are still relevant and threaten us today because they remain in our air, soil, and water. For example, PCBs and DDT, two POPs, which have been regulated or banned in most countries for several decades, are still detected in humans worldwide (EPA 2014e).

Adopted in 2001 and becoming international law in 2004, the United Nations' Stockholm Convention on Persistent Organic Pollutants is a commitment among countries to reduce and eventually eliminate the use and production of the worst POPs (EPA 2014e). This collaboration has more than 170 participating countries (Stockholm Convention 2014d).

Initially, the Stockholm Convention targeted 12 POPs, sometimes referred to as the "dirty dozen." Since May 2009, more chemicals have been added to the target list for worldwide reduction and eventual elimination, bringing the total to at least 22 (Stockholm Convention 2014a; 2014b; 2014c). In general, the Convention addresses pesticides, industrial chemicals, and unintentional by-products (Stockholm Convention 2014c). However, it is almost certain that many thousands of POPs remain to be discovered.

Endocrine Disrupting Chemicals

EDCs are a class of chemicals that you will be hearing a lot more about. Not only are they mentioned throughout this book, but they also will be in the news for years to come as more studies uncover their influences on our bodies.

Anywhere from 800 (WHO and UNEP 2013) to nearly 1,000 (TEDX 2014c) EDCs have been identified. Chemically diverse, EDCs are primarily man-made, mostly derived from oil and natural gas. They pose the key threats highlighted in this chapter: They interfere with biological processes at low doses; have boundless potential for various effects; travel the world; and bioaccumulate. They can interfere with metabolism, fat storage, bone development, and the immune system, which suggests the potential susceptibility of all endocrine systems.

Within our homes, they are found in common products that the average person uses routinely: toothpaste, soap, shampoo, conditioner, lotions, cosmetics, fragrance, and other personal care products. They are found in our food and drinks and in their packaging. They further infiltrate our homes as pesticides, flame retardants, plastic additives, electronics, pharmaceuticals, clothing, and other products (WHO and UNEP 2013). Products for babies and children are not exempt either. EDCs are in baby formula, baby lotions, baby shampoo, baby conditioners, crib mattresses, toys, and much more, as parts II and III detail.

EDCs can be released from products that contain them. They can also be made as breakdown products from various chemicals in the environment, humans, wildlife, and plants (WHO and UNEP 2013).

Just as the international scientific community was galvanized to study and regulate POPs, it has been researching EDCs. Reports from the WHO, the UNEP, the Endocrine Society (Diamanti-Kandarakis et al. 2009), the European Commission (Kortenkamp et al. 2011), and the European Environment Agency (EEA 2012) view EDCs as a "concern to public and wildlife health" (WHO and UNEP 2013).

Leading organizations have been calling for decreased exposure to EDCs. In 2009 the Endocrine Society, an organization of more than 14,000 research scientists and physicians from more than 100 countries, announced:

> The evidence for adverse reproductive outcomes (infertility, cancers, malformations) from exposure to endocrine disrupting chemicals is strong, and there is mounting evidence for effects on other endocrine systems, including thyroid, neuroendocrine, obesity and metabolism, and insulin and glucose homeostasis (Diamanti-Kandarakis et al. 2009).

In 2009 the American Medical Association announced steps to support the Endocrine Society's call for decreased public exposure to EDCs (Endocrine Society 2014a).

The ideas I examine in this chapter illuminate the complexity of the possible biological and chemical effects of toxicants, which scientists have learned largely from our two enlightening teachers, POPs and EDCs. Effects vary by dosage and timing of exposure. Individuals and certain demographic groups have unique vulnerabilities to toxicants. Both inside and outside the body, there are various types of effects: additive, synergistic, potentiating, and perhaps other, unknown effects. I refer to these collectively as "Unintentional Potential Effects" because they were not considered in the toxicants' or products' original design and are not fully understood.

This chapter ends with a spotlight on the threat of the unknown, raising questions that are difficult to answer. Collectively, the threats and unknowns that are discussed in this chapter motivate me to be more selective about what I put on my skin, ingest, inhale, store in my home, and dispose of. Now, I constantly refine which purchases and possessions are *necessary*.

THE THREAT OF LOW DOSES

Traditional thinking is that the dose makes the poison. One of the fundamental principles of modern toxicology is that almost any substance is harmful at a high enough dose and, at the same time, is harmless at a very low dose.

Current thinking, however, recognizes that there are effects created at low doses that are not seen at higher doses. For example, the breast cancer drug tamoxifen stimulates breast cancer growth at low doses but inhibits it at higher ones (Cone 2012b). Below are low doses at which popular pharmaceutical drugs are designed to have therapeutic activity (Cook 2008):
— Cialis, used to treat erectile dysfunction: 30 parts per billion (ppb)
— Paxil, an antidepressant: 30 ppb
— Albuterol, a popular ingredient in asthma inhalants: 2.1 ppb
— Nuva Ring, a popular birth control: 0.035 ppb

Moreover, certain demographic groups have unique vulnerabilities. For the developing brain, there is no safe exposure to lead. For some chemicals, such as asbestos, there is no safe dose for anyone.

So, exposures to even low doses matter.

THE THREAT OF UNKNOWN INTERACTIVE EFFECTS

Toxicology usually examines one substance at a time. In reality, we are exposed to hundreds of chemicals every day through multiple sources: air, water, diet, cleaning products, personal care products, and much more.

This situation raises questions about the conventional approach used in

Low Doses

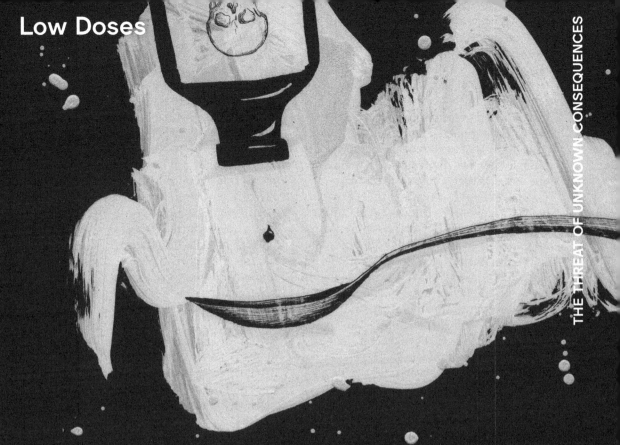

In our daily lives, we intentionally use small doses of pharmaceuticals to control things like reproduction (birth control pills) or addictions (nicotine patches). In the book *Our Stolen Future*, Frederick vom Saal PhD, a leading researcher on the effects of BPA, is cited as discovering that "as little as one-tenth of a part per trillion" of free estrogen is "capable of altering the course of development in the womb" (Colborn, Dumanoski, and Myers 1997). *One part per trillion is equivalent to "about one-twentieth of a drop of water in an Olympic-size swimming pool"* (Walsh 2010). Below are other examples that provide perspective on the potential effects of exposures to "low doses."

— According to the Chemical Industry Archives, a project of the EWG, "at just [five] parts per billion" in human maternal blood, the presence of PCBs during fetal development "can cause adverse brain development, and attention and IQ deficits that appear to be permanent" (Chemical Industry Archives 2009; Schettler et al. 2000). "Five parts per billion is equivalent to *one drop of water in 118 bathtubs*" (Chemical Industry Archives 2009).

— In the case of lead, low doses can impact the immature developing brain while having no effect on adults. For example, two-year-olds with 100 parts per billion in their blood have been found to have significantly lower IQ during adolescence and adulthood. One hundred parts per billion is "the equivalent of *one drop in six bathtubs*" (Chemical Industry Archives 2009).

— Scott Belcher PhD, led a team of researchers at the University of Cincinnati studying effects from various doses of BPA and estradiol, an important type of estrogen for females. According to "Endocrine Disruptors: Bisphenol A and the Brain," an article in *Environmental Health Perspectives* (Barrett 2006), Belcher and his team caused effects at "very low doses"—below one part per trillion—and at "higher doses." However, they weren't seen at intermediate doses (Barrett 2006; Zsarnovsky et al. 2005).

toxicology research, which is discussed more in chapter I.11. Historically, few studies have attempted the very complex task of examining the health effects of *combinations* of chemicals (Cone 2009b). Since 2002, however, greater attention has been focused on simultaneous exposure to multiple compounds. Results have raised concern over not just repeated exposures to a single chemical, but exposures to mixtures of chemicals that create an unknown "cocktail effect." For example, in the Belcher research (Zsarnovsky et al. 2005) mentioned earlier, Barrett (2006) reported in *Environmental Health Perspectives* that when BPA was injected alone, "it mimicked estradiol," but when BPA was injected with estradiol, "it blocked estradiol action."

Moreover, from laboratory studies, we know that mixtures of chemicals can create synergistic effects that are greater than the sum of the individual effects. For instance, researchers have discovered that PCBs and mercury—which are commonly found in fish—can "interact to cause harm at lower thresholds than either substance acting alone" (Schettler et al. 2000). In humans and wildlife, however, synergistic effects are poorly understood, mostly because they have been insufficiently studied, if at all (HESIS and LOHP 2008; Reuben 2010; WHO and UNEP 2013). In addition, other stressors, like obesity and poverty, may contribute to interactive effects.

While the cocktail effects from pharmaceuticals and personal care products have historically been unstudied, they are now a major area of research (EEA 2013).

THE THREAT FROM REPEATED EXPOSURES

Arsenic is a naturally occurring element found in water and soil. However, human activities such as burning fuel, mining, and using pesticides have increased arsenic levels in the environment. It is now so abundant that it pervades our food supply.

As I learned about the cancer-causing form of arsenic in drinking water, rice and rice by-products, and juice boxes (all discussed later in this chapter), I became uncomfortable with exposing my children to any source that could reasonably be avoided. After all, who is monitoring how safe their *cumulative* exposure is?

For example, young children are offered juice boxes frequently. At first, I wondered if children's repeated exposures to this one toxin (arsenic) from this *single* source (juice boxes) was safe. Later, however, I realized that children are being exposed to arsenic from *multiple* sources: rice, rice cereal, rice cakes, rice milk, other rice by-products, and more.

Similarly, as I learned about endocrine disrupting chemicals and how pervasive they are, my commitment to monitoring the purity of what I buy for my children and our home was reaffirmed. Over the past decade, it has been established that low levels of endocrine disruptors that may not be harmful individually can work together—additively or synergistically—to generate adverse effects (WHO and UNEP 2013).

For example, researchers at the Institute of Environmental and Human Health at Texas Tech found cancer risks doubled when two carcinogens, arsenic and estrogen, were present at "safe" levels. At certain very low levels, each poses little threat to human health. In combination, however, the two are almost twice as likely to create cancer in prostate cells (Davis 2013). Remember: Arsenic and EDCs, some of which can mimic estrogen, are found in a wide range of consumer products.

THE THREAT OF POTENTIATING EFFECTS

As I continued my research, I learned about potentiation, the ability of one compound to increase the harm arising from subsequent exposure to another compound, even if the latter would not cause the harm by itself (HESIS and LOHP 2008). For example, certain chemicals can make you more vulnerable to carcinogens. Below are more examples:

— Results from a 2010 study (Melkonian et al. 2010) suggest that certain environmental factors, such as sun exposure or a history of smoking and high fertilizer use, may potentiate the effects of arsenic exposure.

— In the 1970s, methoxychlor was considered a safer replacement for DDT (banned in 1972), despite being chemically similar to DDT, because it doesn't generally accumulate in the body. Later, however, we learned that if the liver has been damaged by another agent (another toxin or a disease), then the body can store methoxychlor at 100 times its normal rate. Under these circumstances, the chemical can then have long-lasting DDT-like effects on the nervous system (Vandenberg 2008). Although methoxychlor was phased out by the end of 2004, this example illustrates why it is necessary to be conservative with exposures to synthetic chemicals, especially pesticides. The effects of multiple compounds are unknown and potentially dangerous.

IN THE BODY, THE EFFECTS ARE VARIED AND COMPLEX

The following two subsections provide additional insight into the complexities of understanding the effects of toxic exposures. The information was reported by the state of California, *Understanding Toxic Substances: An Introduction to Chemical Hazards in the Workplace* (HESIS and LOHP 2008), unless specified otherwise.

Immediate versus delayed effects

The amount of time it takes for disease or other harm from toxicant exposure to appear is called the latency period. If effects manifest immediately or within days of one or a few exposures, then they are described as "acute" effects with short latency. If effects appear years or decades after repeated exposures to low doses, then they are described as "chronic" effects with long latency (Carson [1962] 2002).

Acute effects are usually reversible, whereas chronic effects are usually irreversible. The long latency period of some diseases—such as cancer, for example—complicates the study of cause and effect.

Moreover, just because symptoms appear to resolve doesn't necessarily mean that the exposed person is recovered or safe. For example, a person exposed to high levels of solvents at work may experience immediate effects, such as headaches and dizziness that disappear at the end of the day, once the worker has been home for a while. Over months, however, the worker can show latent effects, such as liver and kidney damage.

Chronic exposures are threatening for three main reasons. First, someone may be exposed repeatedly to doses that are not high enough to trigger overt reactions but are still high enough to harm the body. Second, the body can accumulate exposures un-til the burden reaches a tipping point. Last, any adverse effects created from chronic exposures may not resolve even after exposure ends, possibly creating serious effects such as inflammation and scarring in organs like the lungs or kidneys.

Among fat-soluble toxicants, many may have little, if any, short-term toxicity at low doses but substantial toxicity as concentrations accumulate. Consequences may not be noticeable to us while still occurring: Some of these toxicants may interfere with the immune system, while others may affect organ development, promote cancer, and so on.

Local versus systemic effects

Effects of toxicants may be "local," appearing at the point of exposure—commonly the skin, eyes, nose, throat, and lungs. Alternatively, if the toxicant penetrates the skin or lungs and enters the bloodstream, then its effects may be "systemic" as it harms internal organs throughout the body. Affected organs may include the liver, kidneys, heart, the nervous system (including the brain), and the reproductive system.

Both local and systemic effects may occur. For example, someone exposed to a liquid toxicant can show immediate skin irritation at the point of contact. The liquid can also penetrate the skin and eventually damage the liver and kidneys.

More threatening, however, is that systemic harm may occur without any local effect or warning. For example, a toxic solvent can pass through the skin, enter the bloodstream, and cause significant internal damage without causing any symptoms on the skin (HESIS and LOHP 2008).

TIMING MATTERS

At infinitesimal amounts, hormones—estrogen, testosterone, thyroid hormones, and others—guide the development of organs and a wide range of biological processes. While always important, exposures to toxicants during critical stages of development— such as in utero, in early childhood, during puberty, and in menopause—should be especially conservative because toxicants can mimic signals that shouldn't be present, or block the signals that should be.

Therefore, the *timing* of exposure to certain toxicants, especially EDCs, is an important determinant of their effects (WHO and UNEP 2013). During some stages, there may be no safe dose for hormone-mimicking chemicals (Bienkowski 2012; Cone 2012b) since EDCs may undermine tissue and organ development and function and, consequently, alter susceptibility to various diseases throughout life (WHO and UNEP 2013). They have been linked to the health trends highlighted in figure #02.

A study titled "DDT and Breast Cancer in Young Women: New Data on the Significance of Age at Exposure" (Cohn et al. 2007) found that women exposed to high levels of DDT at or before age 14 (before puberty) in 1945, when wide use of DDT began, were five times more likely to be diagnosed with breast cancer by age 50 than those with the lowest levels of exposure (Steingraber 2010). However, in women exposed to DDT after age 14, no association existed between that exposure and breast cancer (Cohn et al. 2007; Steingraber 2010).

While fetuses and young children are uniquely vulnerable to toxic chemicals, people of all ages have vulnerability. The mechanisms by which our bodies operate throughout our lives are not completely understood, but we know that they're highly complex and sophisticated. Additionally, we know that hormones are active throughout our life span; among these are thyroid hormones, which regulate many biological functions including metabolism (WHO and UNEP 2013).

FORM AND EXPOSURE ROUTE MATTER
Rachel Carson ([1962] 2002) explains in *Silent Spring* that the form of a toxicant influences its toxicity. For example, as a powder, DDT is not readily absorbed through the skin. However, dissolved in oil, as it usually was, DDT enters the body more easily. If it is ingested, the digestive tract absorbs it slowly. It can also be absorbed through the lungs. The body then stores it in fatty tissues such as the adrenals, testes, thyroid, liver, kidneys, and intestines.

UNIQUE VULNERABILITIES
Some individuals are more sensitive to toxicants than are others, such as those with genetic predispositions or significant prior exposures. According to the Environmental Working Group, "EPA-funded research [Hattis et al. 2001] documented a 10,000-fold variability in human response to certain airborne particles." The EWG explains that this is why people who breathe the same air do not all have asthma (EWG 2014d).

Children have unique vulnerabilities, as chapter I.3 discusses. Other populations with unique vulnerabilities include those with compromised detoxification mechanisms, such as those with certain diseases (e.g., HIV); and the elderly, whose detoxifying mechanisms are less efficient (Steingraber 2010).

Everyone, however, should learn more about the threat of toxicants to our health. Those who should take special interest include men and women (especially women) who plan to become parents, and parents whose children are undergoing stages of rapid development (i.e., fetuses, infants, preschool children, and adolescents).

THE THREAT OF THE UNINTENTIONALS
The Unintentional Potential Effects that have been discussed so far may result not just from parent compounds, but also from Unintentional By-products and Unintentional Toxicants. In some cases, Unintentional By-products—including breakdown products from biodegradation and metabolism—may be more toxic or more persistent (or both) than the parent compound (Letcher, Klasson-Wehler, and Bergman 2000). For example, metabolites of several EDCs (e.g., PCBs and PBDEs) can have a stronger potential for endocrine disruption than can their parent compounds (WHO and UNEP 2013; Dingemans et al. 2008; Hamers et al. 2008; Meerts et al. 2004).

THE THREAT OF THE UNKNOWN
Going back to when I was nine years old, I probably quickly rinsed the new plastic cup that my mother told me to wash because I wasn't a rebellious child. However, knowing my attitude back then, I probably barely rinsed it. I had an innocent sense of safety, a trust that persisted until my husband and I decided to start a family.

Throughout all my pregnancies, labors, and childbirths and while breastfeeding and caring for my young children, I became increasingly humbled by the mysteries of life and health. There is still so much that is not understood about conception, labor, breastfeeding, and wellness. For example, even though our scientific advances have been impressive, we still don't fully understand something as basic as how labor starts in a pregnant woman. However, the pregnant body knows exactly what to do. My point is that our bodies—and Mother Nature—have a wise intelligence and resiliency, much of which remains mysterious to us.

With greater awe for nature's complex brilliancy, I have also grown to appreciate the threats from the unknown consequences of introducing toxicants into our bodies. While synthetic intervention is very helpful and can even be lifesaving, unnecessary exposure can interfere with what Mother Nature is supposed to do.

Whatever chemicals I may have drunk when I was nine years old, most likely a single experience wouldn't have steered my health down a suboptimal path. It is my *pattern of behavior* that really influences my family's evolving body burdens and contributes to the Unintentional Potential Effects of our various exposures.

While the study of POPs and EDCs has taught us so much, it has also spotlighted the risks of the unknown. One of my biggest lessons learned is that lack of proof of harm should not be assumed to be proof of safety. Lack of proof of harm can often mean that studies haven't been done: For most chemicals, we haven't sufficiently studied neurotoxicity, reproductive toxicity, fetotoxicity, carcinogenicity, immunotoxicity, developmental toxicity, and the Unintentional Potential Effects from parent compounds, Unintentional By-products, and Unintentional Toxicants. According to Dr. Philip Landrigan at the Mount Sinai Hospital, toxicity testing has not kept pace with knowledge about diseases. As a result, "We are conducting a vast toxicological experiment on our children which will affect generations to come" (Schettler et al. 2000).

All the issues examined in this chapter are still active areas of research. However, as I learned about the unknowns, I became motivated to think more critically about exposures to avoid. Since diet can be a major source of exposure, toxicants should be considered at least as often as are calories, carbohydrates, protein, and fat content.

In the following pages, I share my personal heartache over my children's exposures to extraordinarily high levels of the cancer-causing form of arsenic in popular foods.

KEY POINTS

01. Cause-effect dynamics between toxicants and our bodies are constant and complex. Many of these synthetic chemicals are persistent, bioaccumulative, threatening, and they travel the world. The Unintentional Potential Effects from parent compounds, Unintentional By-products, and Unintentional Toxicants are seemingly incalculable. Biological and chemical effects are complicated: Timing matters, effects vary by dose, people have unique vulnerabilities, effects can be seen immediately after exposure or much later, and the severity of reactions varies greatly.

02. Exposures to low doses matter. Historically, low doses were not considered harmful. However, we now know that they can create effects that are different from those created at high doses. And effects from low doses can be serious.

03. The forms and routes of exposure matter. They may vary in the risks they pose.

04. The "cocktail effects" of exposures to multiple toxicants are not well understood. This is a major area of research, however, because in real life we are exposed to myriad combinations of chemicals.

05. POPs have been linked to harmful effects seen in wildlife and humans. Dietary intake of animal fat and seafood is the main route of exposure to these compounds, the first major class of chemicals to attract international attention.

06. EDCs are attracting concern as studies highlight their Unintentional Potential Effects.

07. Our recurring exposures to toxicants from our patterns of behavior can be more important than occasional exposures to toxicants.

Arsenic in a Few Packaged Foods

Much is unknown about the parameters within which toxicants are safe, such as at what dosage harm is caused, and the Unintentional Potential Effects from parent compounds, Unintentional By-products, and Unintentional Toxicants. Therefore, how can anyone know what is a safe dose in any single product?

ARSENIC IN JUICE BOXES

In recent years the cancer-causing type of arsenic, inorganic arsenic (as opposed to organic arsenic), has been detected in juice boxes and brown rice syrup. In September 2011 on *The Dr. Oz Show*, it was reported that arsenic levels above the EPA's drinking water standards of 10 parts per billion were detected in boxed apple and grape juices, including organic products, after tests on dozens of samples from three cities in America. An uproar ensued among consumers, the Food and Drug Administration (FDA), and the juice industry. Follow-up tests were conducted by the FDA and *Consumer Reports* magazine.

How was arsenic getting into juice boxes? First, arsenic is a naturally occurring substance that exists throughout our environment. However, its presence has increased in step with developments in farming practices and industrialization. In the US, arsenic-based pesticides were banned in 1970. However, most juice is made from concentrate that comes from all over the world. It is likely that some concentrates are contaminated from apples grown in contaminated soil or from pesticides used in other countries (FDA 2014).

Uncertainty and debate over the arsenic in juice boxes continued for a couple of years. Mehmet Oz MD was accused of making misleading statements and needlessly worrying consumers. Critics pointed out that only a minority of the juices tested contained the inorganic arsenic at levels that exceeded permissible levels in drinking water, and that Dr. Oz had reported *all* arsenic, not just the inorganic kind. Experts also debated whether it was fair to compare arsenic standards for drinking water, which is consumed regularly, with arsenic levels in juices, which are consumed much less regularly.

Regardless, I was grateful to know about even the inconclusive data. While most juice boxes tested "safe," keeping track of which ones passed the test was not realistic, and, based on the studies' results, it would be hard for me to trust that every batch of a "safe" brand was indeed safe.

I tried my best to have my children avoid juice completely. That turned out to be impossible because juice boxes are so popular. They are offered to children many times each week by family, friends, and caregivers in schools, at camps, and at parties. Instead, I reduce their consumption of processed juices whenever it will not put a damper on a great time, and I discuss my concerns with my children in age-appropriate ways.

Updated FDA guidelines

Prompted by the controversy and subsequent investigations, in July 2013 the FDA set the permitted level of inorganic arsenic in apple juice at 10 ppb, which is the same as the standard for arsenic in public drinking water and bottled water (FDA 2014). I'm grateful for this. However, the controversy also led me to wonder how anyone can determine a safe level of arsenic in processed juice when it enters our body through multiple ways and in various forms.

All the test results and additional information can be found on the website of the FDA and at www.doctoroz.com.

ARSENIC IN RICE AND RICE BY-PRODUCTS

When I was evaluating organic formula for my daughter, I had two serious candidates. One contained high-fructose corn syrup, which I wanted to avoid. The other was sweetened with brown rice syrup, which seemed like a healthier choice.

A SPOTLIGHT

Later I noticed that brown rice syrup was the main sweetener in many other organic products that we used: cereals, snack bars, crackers, hemp milk, and much more. I interpreted this prevalence among seemingly healthier products as reassurance that it was a wholesome ingredient. Needless to say, I was devastated when I learned that higher-than-normal levels of arsenic were detected in brown rice and therefore brown rice syrup.

The FDA announced in September 2013 that it would investigate arsenic in rice and rice by-products to assess whether it poses a public health threat. According to *Consumer Reports* (2014a), which conducted its own investigation of 200 samples in 2012 (*Consumer Reports* 2012), the FDA's testing of more than 1,300 samples of rice and rice products indicated that these products provide significant exposures to inorganic arsenic. High levels were found in parboiled white rice (an average of 114 ppb), instant rice (59 ppb), and beer (15 to 26 ppb). The magazine also reported, "The [FDA] study noted that more than 10 percent of the rice in China, Pakistan, and Bangladesh is estimated to have arsenic concentrations exceeding 200 ppb, while in the US, more than 50 percent of the rice is estimated to contain arsenic at those elevated levels." (How to approach this issue in your diet is discussed in chapter III.4.)

As I learned about the FDA's findings, again I wondered how it could determine a safe dose in an individual product when diets may offer several exposures to small doses that accumulate in the body.

These stories are just a couple of examples among many that convinced me to minimize consumption of processed foods and rely on a plant-based, whole foods, *diverse* diet with ingredients that are organically farmed. While they are contaminated too, the chemical burdens are less and the nutrient density is higher.

ARSENIC IN A FEW PACKAGED FOODS

Chapter I.9
We Are Interconnected

I *love* Oprah Winfrey. Her show *Super Soul Sunday* has inspired me through the years to persist toward this book's completion amid great sacrifice and uncertainty.

As a regular viewer of this show on spirituality, I have been struck by the consistent message that all people are interconnected. Guests of varied backgrounds and expertise have incorporated this theme while sharing their unique experiences. I was impressed to hear the same message from several physicians, such as Jill Bolte Taylor PhD, a Harvard-trained neuroscientist who survived a stroke and shared her enlightening story in her book, *My Stroke of Insight*, and Deepak Chopra MD, an alternative medicine advocate and a spiritual guru.

It was coincidental to hear this message while working on this book. In my pursuit of learning how to protect human health, I now know that our body's inner ecosystem is a microcosm of the chemistry not only of our indoor built environments but also of our planet at large.

In his books *The Universe Within: Discovering the Common History of Rocks, Planets, and People* and *Your Inner Fish: A Journey Into the 3.5-Billion-Year History of the Human Body*, paleontologist Neil Shubin PhD explains that we are connected not just with all animal bodies that ever existed on Earth but also with the solar system and the universe beyond. The evolutionary histories of all life-forms and environments reside within us, he explains (Shubin 2009; 2013).

In this chapter, I take a closer look at how our bodies are interconnected, and why individual choices matter.

THE CONTAMINATION OF OUR COLLECTIVE HOME: EARTH

In China, "every 30 seconds a baby is born with physical defects due to chemical waste pollution," according to an official of the National Population and Family Planning Commission (Stockholm Convention and UNEP 2012).

While it's easy to think that news headlines about pollution in other parts of the world are irrelevant to us, we are interconnected in several ways. The grasshopper effect, introduced in chapter I.7, distributes toxicants around the world through the key constituents of Earth—air, water, soil, and climate. And those basic elements of Earth are deteriorating from our planet's increasing load of toxicants. In addition, we are further interconnected through our increasingly international economies, including our international food supply.

We share polluted air

From 1978 through the 1990s, Deng Xiaoping led the People's Republic of China through major transformation, opening China to the rest of the world. As a result, China's share of the world GDP has grown from approximately 5 percent in 1978 to over 15 percent in 2012 (Hu 2001; *Economist* 2012). While this evolution has benefited many, it has created serious threats to the health of all life-forms and our environment.

Air pollution in China, for example, is a serious concern. One measure of air pollution is the size of the particulate matter. If small enough, these toxicants can penetrate deep into the lungs and enter the bloodstream. Exposure to airborne particles less than 2.5 microns in diameter (called PM 2.5) in concentrations greater than 25 micrograms per cubic meter over a 24-hour period is considered hazardous by the WHO (WHO 2014b). Certain cities in China have PM 2.5 levels that can range from 350 to north of 600 micrograms per cubic meter; one northeastern city, Harbin, has reached 1,000 micrograms (Associated Press 2014). As a comparison, one study found the US city with the worst air pollution to be Bakersfield, California, which has a PM 2.5 level of 18.2 (McCarthy 2015).

China is not alone in its struggles with air pollution, however. In a report released by the WHO in March 2014, air pollution was named "the world's largest single environmental health risk" (WHO 2014a). Air pollution is estimated to have "claimed seven million lives around the world in 2012" (Jacobs and Johnson 2014), accounting for one out of every eight deaths (Jacobs and Johnson 2014; WHO 2014a).

Just as natural forces—such as wind, temperature changes, and precipitation—drive the grasshopper effect, they also make air pollution, regardless of its location of origin, a worldwide threat. China's air pollution, for instance, has traveled over the Pacific Ocean to settle in the western US through strong winds called Westerlies (Than 2014).

Moreover, while air pollution is commonly understood to impair our biology, it is not as widely seen as contaminating other things, such as our food supply. But it does.

Air pollution can damage agricultural crops, reduce their yields (Tai, Val Martin, and Heald 2014), and taint food. Contamination can even occur with packaged foods on store shelves. For example, Joe Thornton PhD, a professor in the department of human genetics and the department of ecology and evolution at the University of Chicago, notes that perc, a common dry cleaning solvent, is a volatile compound that vaporizes easily into the air. In his book, *Pandora's Poison: Chlorine, Health, and a New Environmental Strategy*, he gives an example of how this may affect us in our daily lives: "Butter sold from grocery stores near dry cleaning establishments, for example, [were] found to contain extremely high concentrations of perc, in some cases greater than 1,000 parts per billion—hundreds of times higher than in butter sold in stores not located near dry cleaners" (Thornton 2000).

While many factors influence the health effects of perc, the New York State Department of Health notes that it "may affect the central nervous system, the liver, kidneys, blood, immune system, and perhaps the reproductive system." Its effect on the development of infants and children is not known (NY DOH 2013).

The choices of others affect our drinking water

Not only does water contain and globally distribute the persistent toxicants mentioned in this book, but it also contains remnants of what others eat, drink, put onto their skin, and use as pharmaceuticals and recreational drugs. These products and their ingredients are released into the environment as we excrete them, discard them down the drain, and throw them into our landfills (Kluger 2010). Many of them find their way into our water supply.

John Spatz, former commissioner of Chicago's Department of Water Management, explained to *Time* magazine in 2010 that, in the US, we use about 3,000 prescription pharmaceuticals and thousands more over-the-counter drugs (Kluger 2010). The Campaign for Safe Cosmetics (2014b) says that "of the more than 10,000 chemical ingredients in our personal care products, 89 percent have not undergone safety testing." Among all our consumer products, there are more than 80,000 potential combinations of chemicals that could end up in our drinking water (Kluger 2010).

The EPA, the WHO, and the US Geological Survey have been investigating this impact on our drinking water. According to a 2010 article, "Occurrence and Fate of Human Pharmaceuticals in the Environment," published in *Reviews of Environmental Contamination and Toxicology*, only in recent decades have analytical methods existed to detect the low doses of pharmaceuticals that pervade our environment. Since then, more than 100 drugs have been detected in aquatic environments, including antibiotics, analgesics, anti-inflammatories, hormones, and lipid regulators (Monteiro and Boxall 2010).

These compounds, in addition to some chemicals used as ingredients in personal care products, are found in the bodies of wildlife. These include parabens, triclosan, antidepressants, and human contraceptives. Some chemicals—such as triclosan, PFOS, and BPA—that are found either as parent compounds or as breakdown products can be converted into more or less potent forms in the environment (WHO and UNEP 2013).

Our water treatment systems are not necessarily equipped to remove these consumer products, pharmaceuticals, and related by-products from water (WHO 2011c; WHO and UNEP 2013). Tests have found municipal wastewater to be an important source of pharmaceuticals in the global environment (Monteiro and Boxall 2010; WHO 2012; WHO and UNEP 2013). Since the risks from exposures even at very low concentrations are not known, authorities, including the WHO (2012), are investigating further.

Our soil quality is depleted

Industrial activities have a long history of polluting the environment and disrupting ecosystems, including our soil quality. Consumers, however, play a role too. Our decisions regarding what we buy and who we buy from support industrial, business, and farming practices. For example, buying groceries from local farmers who practice organic farming is better for our environment than buying foods produced on conventional industrial farms.

In December 2012, the World Economic Forum's Risk Response Network reported that "40 percent of soil used for agriculture around the world is classed as either degraded or seriously degraded" (World Economic Forum 2012). While factors that determine soil quality are dynamic and highly complex, urbanization, industrial farming methods, climate change, and our increasingly toxic environment are among the key factors exacerbating the degradation.

Deteriorating soil quality has been found to impair food production as well as the nutritional value of the harvested foods. Donald R. Davis PhD, a former researcher at the Biochemical Institute of the University of Texas at Austin, has published several studies on the declining nutritional content of fruits and vegetables (Davis, Epp, and Riordan 2004; Davis 2009). *Scientific American* described his 2004 research, which examined USDA nutritional data from 1950 and 1990 for 43 vegetables and fruits, as a "landmark study on the topic." The researchers found "reliable declines" in the amounts of a variety of nutrients (Scheer and Moss 2011). While Davis notes that these studies, like all studies, have their limitations, his 2009 research estimated "declines of 5 percent to 40 percent or more in some minerals in groups of vegetables and perhaps fruits" (Davis 2009).

A 2006 study from Cornell University found that "the [US] is losing soil 10 times faster—and China and India are losing soil 30 to 40 times faster—than the natural replenishment rate" (Lang 2006). Given current rates of soil degradation, rough estimates forecast that we have approximately 60 years remaining of usable topsoil, the layer that allows plants to grow (World Economic Forum 2012).

OUR INCREASINGLY INTERNATIONAL ECONOMY

Shopping at my regular grocery store, I find organic bananas from Mexico and organic avocados from Costa Rica. Packaged foods are often from international sources as well, as the story of apple juice concentrate in chapter I.8 exemplifies.

Of course, it's not only our food chain that has become more international; the manufacture of our consumer products has as well. It is becoming increasingly hard to find toys, books, and furniture without components from China and other countries.

While our increasingly international economy has created great efficiencies, it further connects us on the issue of the environment: Products (including food) are made of components drawn from all over the world, which exposes us to the manner in which foreign manufacturers produce and use toxic materials. What we buy can pollute our Homes with toxicants—including those, like lead, that were phased out in the US and whose imports are regulated.

The varying national policies toward toxic and potentially toxic chemicals challenge our understanding of chemicals that are used in commerce and that circulate throughout our environment. They further challenge our ability to evaluate the potential effects from Unintentional By-products and Unintentional Toxicants. This is why we all benefit from spreading awareness and taking sensible precautionary measures when we can.

The environments of other countries matter to us.

THE CHEMICAL PRODUCTION AND POLICIES OF ALL COUNTRIES AFFECT OUR BODIES

As I learned about the phase-out or regulation of certain toxic chemicals, I felt relieved that they were no longer a current threat. Later, I learned that this was a false sense of security: As toxic chemicals were banned or regulated in the US, some had new opportunities abroad (Peeples 2013).

For example, as domestic production of PFOS, the key ingredient in a popular

Worldwide Chemical Production

In complying with European REACH requirements (Registration, Evaluation, Authorisation and Restriction of Chemicals), governments around the world were prompted to track chemical substances used in their products in order to be able to sell to European markets (Stockholm Convention and UNEP 2012). In 2007, an organization in China set up an online effort to aggregate lists of chemical substances registered in China, the EU, the US, Canada, Japan, Korea, Taiwan, the Philippines, Australia, and New Zealand (CIRS 2011).

While the lists of chemical substances reported by nations are imperfect (reporting requirements vary by country, and compliance with reporting varies as well), the attempt to track this information from a global perspective is unprecedented. The sample list below most likely underestimates the true chemical burden on our Homes. The registered chemicals don't reflect our reality.

Location	Number of Registered Chemicals	Information Source
European Union	143,000 preregistered under REACH	WHO and UNEP 2013; Tortorello 2012
United States	84,000	WHO and UNEP 2013; CIRS 2014h
Taiwan	79,000	CIRS 2014f
China	45,612	CIRS 2014c
Korea	42,652	CIRS 2014e
Australia	+38,000	CIRS 2014a
Philippines	24,000	CIRS 2014g
Canada	23,000	CIRS 2014b
Japan	20,600	CIRS 2014d

chemical formula for stain repellents (introduced in chapter I.7), was phased out in the US in 2001 and 2002, production increased in China during that same time frame. The limited data on the health effects of PFOS indicate that it lowers female reproductive capacity, alters menstrual cycles, and reduces fetal growth. Moreover, since this chemical may remain in our oceans for *centuries*, our exposure will likely continue over generations (WHO and UNEP 2013). So even though China's environmental pollution may not seem relevant, it is. It also signals that the manufacture, production, use, and disposal of chemicals by other countries affect our body burdens.

As we know from chapter I.4, there's a lot that the US doesn't know about chemicals in our commerce: the number of existing chemicals, the rate of new chemical introductions, and the production volume of toxic and potentially toxic chemicals. The US is not alone, however. The next section details the released estimates from other countries. The true numbers are unknown.

CLIMATE CHANGE

While former vice president Al Gore's 2006 Academy Award–winning documentary, *An Inconvenient Truth*, generated more mainstream debate over global warming, experts now recognize that global warming is only one aspect of a broader, more dynamic change in overall climate patterns.

By 2014, environmental authorities were in nearly unanimous agreement that climate change is no longer a future concern: It is happening now. Established by a presidential initiative in 1989 and mandated by Congress in 1990, the US Global Change Research Program is a federal program that assesses the global environment and its impact on society. It is legally required to complete a review, a National Climate Assessment, every four years. In its third report, produced by a team of more than 300 experts and released in May 2014, the *National Climate Assessment* states, "Over recent decades, climate science has advanced significantly. Increased scrutiny has led to increased certainty that we are now seeing impacts associated with human-induced climate change" (National Climate Assessment 2014).

According to the EPA (2014b), climate change refers to "major changes in temperature, precipitation, or wind patterns, among other effects, that occur over several decades or longer." According to the National Aeronautics and Space Administration (NASA), the global warming trends are "proceeding at a rate that is unprecedented in the past 1,300 years." While Earth has been warming since 1880, "most of this warming has occurred since the 1970s, with the 20 warmest years having occurred since 1981 and with all 10 of the warmest years occurring in the past 12 years" (NASA 2014). The evidence also points to fewer colder days, warming oceans, rising sea levels, melting ice sheets and Arctic sea ice, retreating glaciers, and increasing acidification of the ocean.

Climate change also manifests as more extreme weather events—such as more frequent heat waves, extraordinary droughts, intense precipitation, mudslides, and cyclones (also known as hurricanes and typhoons). In fact, air pollution in Asia is being linked to more intense cyclones over the Pacific and greater overall precipitation in the Pacific Northwest of the US (by 7 percent over what it would be otherwise) and is said to be contributing "significantly" to climate change (Stromberg 2014).

What are the risks of climate change?

Established by the UNEP and the World Meteorological Organization in 1988, the Intergovernmental Panel on Climate Change (IPCC) consists of more than 1,300 scientists from the US and other countries. In March 2014, the IPCC released a report, *Climate Change 2014: Impacts, Adaptation, and Vulnerability*, which identifies global risks (IPCC 2014). A *New York Times* headline on March 31, 2014, summarized the IPCC's views most succinctly: "Panel's Warning on Climate Risk: Worst Is Yet to Come" (Gillis 2014). Other agencies that are in agreement include the EPA, NASA, WHO, and the CNA Military Advisory Board (MAB).

Risks include threats to our food, water, and energy supplies; other "systemic risks," such as threats to "infrastructure networks and critical services" for health and emergency services (IPCC 2014); "displacement of people and potential mass migrations" (Gillis 2014); changing patterns of infectious diseases (WHO 2003); and the disturbance of terrestrial and marine ecosystems from a loss of biodiversity (WHO 2003; IPCC 2014).

In a May 2014 report, the MAB, which includes an elite group of retired generals and admirals from the US Army, Navy, Air Force, and Marine Corps, warned that the risks identified in its first report in 2007 "are advancing noticeably faster than we anticipated" (MAB 2014). In fact, journalist Elizabeth Kolbert argues in her Pulitzer Prize-winning book *The Sixth Extinction* that we are in the midst of a mass extinction (dinosaurs were killed in the fifth one), having already rapidly lost a variety of species due to human activities.

YOUR CHOICES MATTER

The health of our Homes is in jeopardy. Experts agree, however, that it's not too late to make a difference.

According to Global Climate Change (2015), a division of NASA, 97 percent of climate scientists agree that climate change has been caused largely by human activities. Yet, 52 percent of Americans do not believe that human activities have been responsible for climate change (Yale Project on Climate Change Communication 2015). In a global survey, "Americans were among the least concerned about climate change threatening their country," according to PewResearchCenter (Motel 2014).

The National Climate Assessment (2014) reports that "global climate is projected to continue to change over this century and beyond, but there is still time to act to limit the amount of change and the extent of damaging impacts." The US and even China have made great progress in attempting to curb harmful emissions. In November 2014, Secretary of State John Kerry announced that the two countries had agreed to reduce carbon emissions. They reached agreement ahead of a deadline created by the international community in hopes of inspiring other nations to pursue ambitious steps to do the same. While this commitment by the world's two largest economies, who also consume the most energy and emit the most greenhouse gases, is extraordinary, Kerry also told the *New York Times*, "There is no question that all of us will need to do more to push

toward the de-carbonization of the global economy" (Kerry 2014).

Therefore, there is a lot that we can do individually to help change the trends. To begin, engaging in productive change and spreading awareness are key.

The MAB writes, "Each citizen must ask what he or she can do individually to mitigate climate change, and collectively what his or her local, state, and national leaders are doing to ensure that the world is sustained for future generations" (MAB 2014). In May 2015, Pope Francis joined the public dialogue through a letter known as the encyclical. Acknowledging human-induced climate change and noting that our "habit of wasting and discarding has reached unprecedented levels," he urged us to change our current patterns of production and consumption.

Hence, consuming consciously will take on growing importance. What (and how much) we consume supports all the manufacturers and manufacturing processes involved in creating every chemical, ingredient, and material involved in our purchases. We need to consider what Trails of Contamination our purchases support. For example, a meaningful portion of China's toxic emissions result from the production of exports. In 2006 alone, approximately 20 to 30 percent of China's air pollutants were associated with export production, and approximately 20 percent of that was associated with exports to the US (Than 2014).

Our consumer activity has contributed to the high demand for fossil fuels, deforestation, and harmful agricultural practices. This has caused the accumulation of unprecedented amounts of greenhouse gases in the atmosphere, including carbon dioxide, methane, nitrous oxides, and fluorinated gases. From 1990 to 2010 alone, net emissions of greenhouse gases produced from human activities increased 35 percent worldwide; carbon dioxide, which makes up three-fourths of total emissions, rose 42 percent (EPA 2014f).

As I developed the remaining parts of this book, I realized that most of what I call "Household Repeat Offenders" are petroleum-based substances. These substances threaten our bodies in the ways described in chapters I.3 and I.8; leave Trails of Contamination throughout their Life Cycle as described in chapter I.6; and contribute to climate change, which threatens all of us.

This means that the strategies and tips that are best for our bodies are also best for our planet.

KEY POINTS

01. Our planet is our collective home. The quality of Earth's air, water, and soil affects all life-forms. Pollution within any borders seeps into other territories, including our bodies.

02. The environment and nations' chemical policies are global issues that require worldwide, interdisciplinary cooperation with a holistic perspective. Such a perspective integrates environmental health, human health, wildlife health, the latest in science and medicine, awareness of what we do not yet know, practical solutions, business and economics, and impacts over the short and long term. The current body of evidence makes a strong argument for a prompt, precautionary approach to preserving the health of our Homes.

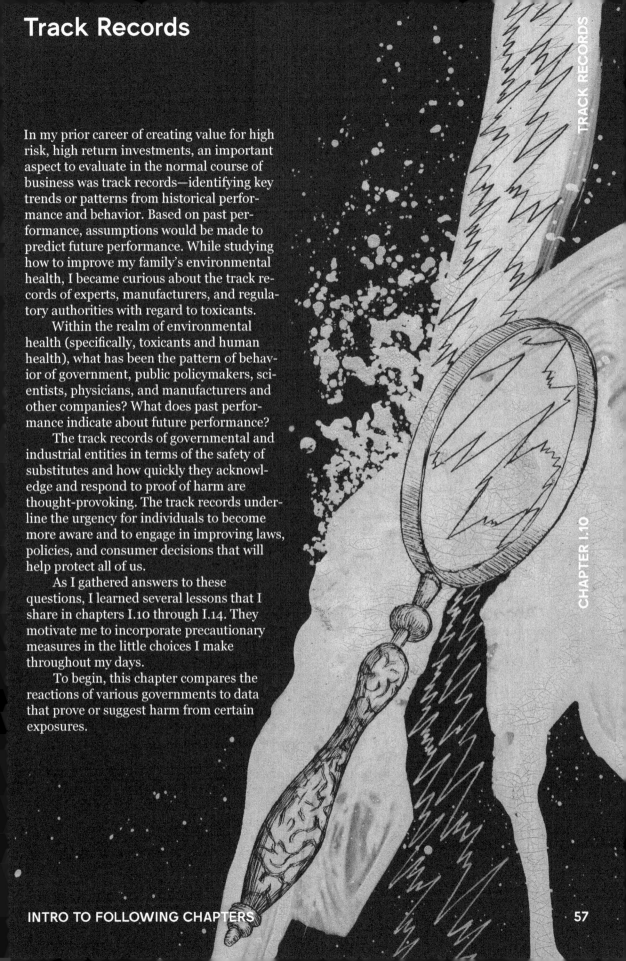

Track Records

In my prior career of creating value for high risk, high return investments, an important aspect to evaluate in the normal course of business was track records—identifying key trends or patterns from historical performance and behavior. Based on past performance, assumptions would be made to predict future performance. While studying how to improve my family's environmental health, I became curious about the track records of experts, manufacturers, and regulatory authorities with regard to toxicants.

Within the realm of environmental health (specifically, toxicants and human health), what has been the pattern of behavior of government, public policymakers, scientists, physicians, and manufacturers and other companies? What does past performance indicate about future performance?

The track records of governmental and industrial entities in terms of the safety of substitutes and how quickly they acknowledge and respond to proof of harm are thought-provoking. The track records underline the urgency for individuals to become more aware and to engage in improving laws, policies, and consumer decisions that will help protect all of us.

As I gathered answers to these questions, I learned several lessons that I share in chapters I.10 through I.14. They motivate me to incorporate precautionary measures in the little choices I make throughout my days.

To begin, this chapter compares the reactions of various governments to data that prove or suggest harm from certain exposures.

Chapter I.10
Government Responses to Public and Environmental Health Threats

When I had a newborn in 2007, there was controversy and alarm surrounding BPA in consumer products, especially as it related to infants and children. Since the experts couldn't agree on whether common exposures were safe, I was thoroughly confused.

In response to media headlines, I began researching BPA in late 2007. I was surprised at how difficult it was to make sense of its health risks. There were more than 800 published studies on the health effects of BPA. Authoritative groups—such as the PCP, the EWG, the CEHC, the International Endocrine Society, and the American Medical Association—publicly acknowledged concern about children's exposure to this potential hormone-disrupting chemical. For instance, the PCP wrote:

> Over the past decade, more than 130 studies have linked BPA to breast cancer, obesity, and other disorders. In 2007, a group of 38 independent [National Institute of Health]-funded investigators concluded there was strong cause for concern that exposure could result in cancer and early puberty. A 2008 study found that adults with higher urinary BPA levels had elevated rates of heart disease, diabetes, and liver abnormalities. Studies also suggest that BPA may interfere with cancer treatments. (Reuben 2010)

And the US Department of Health and Human Services noted this about children's exposure:

> The highest estimated daily intakes of [BPA] in the general population occur in infants and children.... Infants and children have higher intakes of many widely detected environmental chemicals because they eat, drink, and breathe more than adults on a pound for pound basis.... The [National Toxicology Program] has some concern for effects on the brain, behavior, and prostate gland in fetuses, infants, and children at current human exposures to [BPA]. (NTP 2008)

Yet the FDA maintained that the chemical was safe.

I was further baffled by a lawsuit filed in 2010 by the Natural Resources Defense Council (NRDC), an international nonprofit environmental organization that has been described by the *New York Times* as "one of the nation's most powerful environmental groups" (Zeller 2008). In 2008, the NRDC had petitioned the FDA to prohibit the use of BPA in food packaging, food containers, and other materials that will likely come into contact with food. The FDA had three choices: It could agree to ban BPA, reject the petition, or accept some parts of it and not others. Whatever its decision, the FDA was legally required to respond. However, it failed to do so, according to a press release from NRDC (2011).

To force the FDA to respond, the NRDC filed a lawsuit in US District Court for the Southern District of New York against the FDA in June 2010 (NRDC 2010). The court gave the FDA until March 31, 2012, to answer. The FDA finally responded, on March 30, stating that the science presented in the petition did not prove that currently approved uses of BPA are unsafe (*Reuters* 2012; NRDC 2012).

However, the FDA indicated that it would continue to review the safety of BPA. In the meantime, consumer concerns led some major manufacturers to voluntarily phase out BPA in certain products, while retailers promoted presumably safer alternatives on their shelves (Mui 2008). According to CBS News, "In 2008, Wal-Mart Stores Inc. and Toys 'R' Us said they began phasing out bottles, sippy cups, and other children's items containing BPA. By the end of 2009, the six leading makers of baby bottles in the [US] went BPA-free" (CBS News Staff 2012).

Ultimately, in July 2012, the FDA banned BPA from baby bottles and children's drinking cups. However, the official rule just formalized behavior that had already been implemented (CBS News Staff 2012).

Later, the FDA reiterated its earlier position that current exposure levels to BPA appeared safe, based on its review of the data. In an August 2013 update the agency wrote, "The Food and Drug Administration's assessment is that the scientific evidence at this time does not suggest that the very low levels of human exposure to BPA through the diet are unsafe." It also specifically addressed children's exposure: "FDA scientists have also recently determined that exposure to BPA through foods for infants is much less than had been previously believed and that the trace amounts of the chemical that enter the body, whether it's an adult or a child, are rapidly metabolized and eliminated" (FDA 2013a).

GOVERNMENTS HAVE DIFFERENT RESPONSES TO THE SCIENCE

As I tried to gauge an appropriate level of concern about my family's exposure to BPA, I searched for authoritative opinions outside the US I learned that at least a dozen foreign governments—such as the EU, Canada, Malaysia, China, and the United Arab Emirates—had banned BPA from certain products. I also discovered that at least 11 states in America, including New York and California, had banned BPA from certain products too, even while the FDA was maintaining that BPA in consumer products was safe (Feinstein 2011; Lee 2011; Houlihan, Lunder, and Jacob 2008).

This piqued my curiosity about how governments around the world were responding to the emerging science on toxicants in general. The following paragraphs provide just a few examples of the many governments that follow a precautionary approach—that is, they choose to regulate potential threats to human and environmental health even in the absence of scientific certainty. (In other words, they do not interpret "no proof of harm" as being proof of safety.) Learning about these authoritative actions made me feel less extreme in my desire to be more cautious than some US agencies suggested was necessary.

A PRECAUTIONARY APPROACH
The European Union

In 1998, the member governments of the EU renounced the union's established policy on chemicals for its ineffectiveness in protecting people and the environment. In 2006 the EU adopted a new policy known as REACH: Registration, Evaluation, Authorization, and Restriction of Chemicals (EU OSHA 2014). The policy, which entered into force on June 1, 2007, shifts the burden of proof of safety from regulators to manufacturers. Companies have more responsibility than ever for knowing about the substances in their products, and must prove that their products are safe. REACH generally takes the position "no data, no market" (European Commission 2015).

While controversy surrounds the cost and animal testing involved in proving safety, the undertaking will provide greater understanding of the toxicants that already pervade our Homes. REACH requires the same rules for new and old chemicals alike, including 62,000 chemicals that are exempt from Toxic Substances Control Act regulation under US law, which is explained later in this chapter (Steingraber 2010).

A PROACTIVE APPROACH
Canada

Canada has been proactive toward certain synthetic chemicals. For example, in 2008, Canada was the first country to ban BPA in baby bottles (Kim 2011). And many local governments have pursued proactive measures to reduce the public's exposure to unnecessary pesticides—specifically, those used "cosmetically" to improve the appearance of lawns and gardens.

Perhaps some localities were responding to research done by the Ontario College of Family Physicians, which conducted a systematic review of the scientific literature on pesticides. It found "consistent links to serious illnesses, such as cancer, reproductive problems, and neurological diseases" with long-term exposure to pesticides, which were even found in kitchens of residents who did not actively use them (Ontario College of Family Physicians 2004).

So far, seven Canadian provinces have banned the sale and use of pesticides used purely for cosmetic reasons. And more than 170 provinces and municipalities across

Canada have restricted the use of cosmetic pesticides (Pesticide Free BC 2013).

The Stockholm Convention on POPs

The Stockholm Convention on POPs, introduced in chapter I.8, is a collaboration among countries to reduce and eventually eliminate the use and production of the most toxic, pervasive, and persistent synthetic chemicals in the world. As of 2014, there were 179 parties to the Convention (178 nations and the EU; Stockholm Convention 2014d).

While the US participated in negotiating the treaty and signed it in 2001, it is not a party to the Convention because the treaty has not yet been ratified in the Senate, as the US Constitution requires. Parties to the Convention commit to implementing certain obligations that serve to eliminate or restrict the "production and use or import of POPs" (EPA 2014e).

A REACTIONARY APPROACH
The United States

Unlike the many governments that follow precautionary or proactive approaches, the US generally takes a *reactionary* approach toward toxic, or potentially toxic, chemicals in consumer products. In essence, the law assumes chemicals to be innocent (and therefore produced and used) until proven guilty. For example, according to the 2010 President's Cancer Report, "Atrazine, a widely used herbicide believed to have endocrine-disrupting and possible carcinogenic properties, was banned by the EU in October 2003 because of its ubiquitous and unpreventable water contamination. The same month, the [US] EPA approved the continued use of atrazine in the [US]." (Reuben 2010).

Even when there has been a dedicated effort to regulate a toxic substance, the required proof of harm is so high that the EPA couldn't even ban a known carcinogen: asbestos (EWG 2004a). The Toxic Substances Control Act, the main law governing industrial chemicals, was a major impediment.

The Toxic Substances Control Act

In 1976, Congress passed the Toxic Substances Control Act (TSCA), which put the EPA in charge of reviewing new chemicals used in industry. It is our country's main law aimed at regulating chemicals that are

components of many everyday products. Among those familiar with the TSCA, there's consensus—even by the American Chemistry Council (2014), a chemical industry trade association—that it's outdated.

In November 2013, James Jones, then assistant administrator for the EPA, explained the need for TSCA reform in testimony before a subcommittee of the House of Representatives. Jones confirmed that of the more than 84,000 chemicals listed on the TSCA Inventory, the "EPA has only been able to require testing on just a little more than 200" (EPA 2013b).

Lisa P. Jackson, former head of the EPA, also fought "to bring TSCA into the 21st century." In December 2009, Jackson testified before the Senate that the EPA had "only issued regulations to control five existing chemicals determined to present an unreasonable risk under Section 6 of TSCA. Five, from a total universe of more than 80,000 existing chemicals listed on the TSCA inventory. Though many of these chemicals likely pose little or no risk, the story is clear—we've only been able to effectively regulate a handful of chemicals, and we know very little about the rest" (Senate Committee on Environment and Public Works 2014b).

In general, TSCA impedes adequate regulation in three major ways: authorizing a data gap to exist for thousands of chemicals, setting impractical thresholds for the EPA to meet in regulating toxicants, and allowing a conflict to persist between business interests and public/environmental health (Wilson and Schwarzman 2009).

TSCA creates a data gap

— Some 62,000 chemicals are exempt: When TSCA was enacted in 1976, approximately 62,000 chemicals were already used in commerce. These chemicals were grandfathered in, and they have never been required to undergo testing for safety (Rosenberg 2014).

— TSCA does not require that toxicity data be submitted for approval of a new chemical: Those looking to produce or import a new chemical must provide the EPA with at least 90 days' notice commonly in the form of a Premanufacture Notification (PMN). The PMN, according to a report by Richard

Denison PhD, a lead senior scientist at the Environmental Defense Fund, provides basic information on "anticipated use, production volume, exposure, and release—to the extent such information is known or reasonably foreseeable by the submitter at the premanufacture stage." However, chemical manufacturers are not required to provide toxicity data on new chemicals (Denison 2009).

— TSCA does not require chemical companies to prove the safety of chemicals (GAO 2009b): Manufacturers do not voluntarily test their products' safety for our Homes. After all, such testing requires time and quite a bit of money—about $200,000 per chemical (EPA 2010). It also exposes their businesses to extra risk, because any knowledge of harm creates responsibility and potential liability. Manufacturers are better off choosing ignorance. In fact, according to oral testimony from Heather White JD, executive director of the EWG and a nationally recognized expert on federal environmental law and policy, before the House of Representatives in July 2013, "85 percent of the premanufacture submissions have zero information about the toxicity of those new chemicals" (EWG 2013b). The EPA found that of the nearly 3,000 high-production-volume (HPV) chemicals that the US produces or imports, 43 percent lack testing data on basic toxicity and just 7 percent have a "full set" of basic test data. Obviously, there are many chemicals in the US for which data gaps exist, and as the EPA points out, "it is clear that companies need to do more to address this problem" (EPA 2010).

— Claims of confidentiality protect the identities of chemicals: TSCA allows companies to omit identifying ingredients in their products on the grounds that such details are confidential business information (CBI). EPA officials estimate that approximately 95 percent of the notices to the EPA on new chemicals contain claims of confidential information, leaving the agency in the dark almost as much as the public (GAO 2005; EWG 2013d; GAO 2009b).

According to the EWG (2013d) and the WHO and UNEP (2013), of the more than 84,000 chemicals on the EPA's inventory list, the identities of 17,000 are protected by the CBI provision. The public has no access to any of this information (EWG 2013d).

Of the 151 confidential chemical compounds produced or imported in amounts greater than 300,000 pounds a year, at least 10 are used in products that are specifically intended for children ages 14 and under (EWG 2010a).

TSCA makes it difficult for the EPA to regulate harmful chemicals

TSCA creates two key challenges for the EPA: It creates an impractical burden of proof for the agency to meet, and it limits the time within which the EPA can realistically reject new chemicals. Collectively, I refer to these later as "Impractical Thresholds for the EPA."

— An impractically high burden is placed on the EPA: Before the EPA can regulate a chemical, it must demonstrate, in spite of data gaps, that the subject chemical may pose "unreasonable risk," among other things. Only then can it obtain additional information from the manufacturers to assess risk or require companies to test their chemicals further themselves. The EPA must also establish that the advantages of regulation outweigh the costs and that it "has chosen the least burdensome means of addressing the source of unreasonable risk; and that no other statute could adequately address the risk" (Wilson and Schwarzman 2009). The agency is left having to prove harm—on a chemical-by-chemical basis—through its own reviews of academic or industry data or by using computer modeling to estimate risk. This helps explain why, as Heather White included in her testimony, "EPA attempts to restrict less than 10 percent of new chemicals" (EWG 2013b).

— The EPA has as little as 90 days to begin denial of permission to use a new chemical: As mentioned above, for new chemicals introduced after 1976, companies have to alert the EPA at least 90 days before producing or importing them. If the EPA does not take steps to reject the application within 90 days—"extendable to 180 days under certain conditions" (EPA 1997)—the chemical is given a green light by default (Urbina 2013). In practice, 80 percent of chemicals are approved in three weeks (EWG 2014e).

An Example of TSCA's Inadequacy: The Case of Asbestos

Asbestos, a naturally occurring substance, has been mined for more than 4,000 years (Powell 2014), and perhaps as long as 5,000 (Ross and Nolan 2003). In the US, use of asbestos as an industrial product began in 1858. Asbestos was considered a miracle mineral for its capacity to withstand high temperatures. Consequently, it was widely used as a fireproofing and insulating material in ships, buildings, and a variety of consumer products, including wallboard, roofing, flooring, cement, insulation, drinking water pipes, automobiles, clothing, paper, hair dryers, garden products, home appliances, artificial fire logs, and children's toys (White 2004).

Millions of Americans have been exposed to asbestos. Estimates vary from 27 million for the 1940–1979 period (Carroll et al. 2002) to 100 million for the 20th century (Biggs et al. 2001).

According to the EEA, as early as 1898, a UK factory inspector warned of the harmful and "evil" effects of asbestos dust. In 1906 in France, 50 factory worker deaths from asbestos were reported. Between 1935 and 1949, asbestos manufacturing workers in the US and elsewhere experienced lung cancer, asbestosis, mesothelioma, and other asbestos-related illnesses. By the 1920s, as physicians began to recognize that asbestos exposure caused disease, British medical journals published information regarding asbestosis, causing US and Canadian insurance companies to deny life insurance coverage to asbestos workers (EEA 2001).

It wasn't until the 1970s, however, as evidence of asbestos-related health hazards strengthened, that both the Occupational Safety and Health Administration and the EPA issued safety standards and regulations for this dangerous fiber (EPA 1989). After reviewing more than 100 studies on the health hazards of asbestos, as well as public comments on a proposed rule, the EPA determined in 1989 that there is no known safe exposure level to asbestos (GAO 2009a).

Symptoms of the health effects of asbestos may take 10 to 50 years to develop following exposure, and smoking increases the risk of developing illness from exposure (EEA 2001; EWG 2014a). According to the EPA, "Asbestos fibers are not broken down to other compounds in the environment and, therefore, can remain in the environment for decades or longer" (EPA 2014g).

TSCA COULD NOT EMPOWER THE EPA TO BAN ASBESTOS

The EPA's attempt to ban asbestos, one of the most potent carcinogens known, is the best example of the Impractical Thresholds for the EPA to ban a toxic substance. Following some restrictive regulatory steps in the 1970s, the EPA invested $10 million and more than 10 years to develop the Asbestos Ban and Phaseout Rule of 1989. The rule would have affected 94 percent of all asbestos consumption at that time. The asbestos industry fought back fiercely, citing job losses and potential economic ruin. It filed a lawsuit to challenge the ban under TSCA, claiming that alternative materials were neither more effective nor safer than asbestos. The EPA maintained that a ban was needed (EWG 2004a).

In 1991 the industry won. The federal Fifth Circuit Court of Appeals largely vacated the 1989 ban, even as it acknowledged asbestos as a recognized human carcinogen with the ability to contribute to additional diseases if inhaled. Even more disturbing, according to the EWG, was the first Bush administration's decision to not appeal the case (EWG 2004a).

LITIGATION HAS BEEN A TOOL FOR JUSTICE

Although TSCA wasn't effective in banning asbestos, the American legal system empowered citizens to effectively halt the asbestos industry by bankrupting it. According to Michelle J. White PhD, a professor of economics at the University of California, San Diego,

"Legal claims for injuries from asbestos involve more plaintiffs, more defendants, and higher costs than any other type of personal injury litigation in [US] history." The pressure of litigation caused US producers to eliminate asbestos from many products by the late 1970s, resulting in a sharp decline of overall US consumption (White 2004).

As a result of the litigation, at least 85 corporations filed for bankruptcy, and many insurance companies either failed or are—yes, still—in financial distress (White 2004). In 2012, Forbes reported, "It is estimated that the total costs of asbestos litigation in the [US] alone total over $250 billion already" (Baldwin 2012). The *Wall Street Journal* reported on the state of asbestos litigation in a March 2013 article, "As Asbestos Claims Rise, So Do Worries About Fraud." The newspaper "reviewed trust claims and court cases of roughly 850,000 people filed since the late 1980s until as recently as 2012" and estimated that "personal-injury claims continue to pile up at a rate of 85 per day" (Searcey and Barry 2013).

OTHER COUNTRIES BANNED IT

In the US, asbestos is now banned from a short list of products and uses under the Clean Air Act and TSCA. However, the EPA has no ban on many asbestos-containing products or uses. For example, it may still be used in cement shingles, disc brake pads, automatic transmission components, roof coatings, and vinyl floor tiles (EWG 1999). According to EWG, asbestos can still be found in approximately 35 million homes, schools, buildings and even in products on consumer shelves. Further, asbestos can occur in unexpected places: "In 2007, ADAO [Asbestos Disease Awareness Organization] identified five consumer products, including a child's toy, that were contaminated with asbestos" (EWG 2013c).

In contrast, more than 50 countries have banned asbestos and asbestos-containing products (International Ban Asbestos

Secretariat 2014). The International Commission on Occupational Health supports a global ban on asbestos mining and the sale and use of all forms of asbestos in order to eliminate asbestos-related diseases (ICOH 2014). Other organizations have taken similar stands, and scientists too continue to fight for an international ban, noting that no exposure level is known to be safe, including those associated with "controlled use" (Collegium Ramazzini 2010).

In September 2009, the administrator of the US EPA at that time, Lisa P. Jackson (2009–2013), shared in a speech, "In 1989, after years of study, EPA issued rules phasing out most uses of asbestos, an exhaustively studied substance that has taken an enormous toll on the health of Americans. Yet, a court overturned EPA's rules because it had failed to clear the many hurdles for action under TSCA" (EPA 2009b).

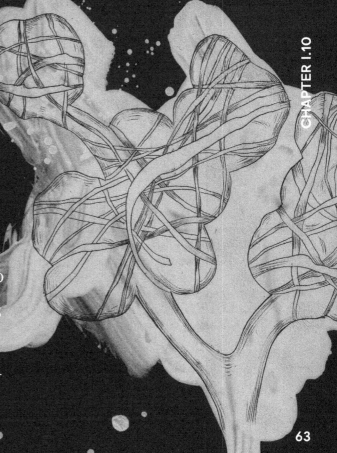

THE CASE OF ASBESTOS

TSCA allows a misalignment between manufacturers' interests and public/environmental health

Since known hazards must be reported and there is no penalty for ignorance, manufacturers have mainly risks to incur if they investigate the possible dangers of their products (Wilson and Schwarzman 2009). As a result, no proof of harm means a chemical is treated, and is often marketed, as safe. And that's not illegal. "No evidence of harm" often is true only because no one has tested for it, not necessarily because the chemical is safe. For reasons of statistical power, safety tests in animals are frequently conducted at high doses (Bienkowski and *Environmental Health News* 2013). Historically, when researchers have said that low doses have no effects in animals, it has often been because they have not looked (Chemical Industry Archives 2009).

In recent years, there has been bipartisan efforts in Congress to modernize TSCA (Senate Committee on Environment and Public Works 2014a). While this is a positive milestone, given the various interest groups involved in drafting and approving a new law, compromises will inevitably have to be made. For example, the chemical industry has been integrally involved in the process of trying to update TSCA. They benefit from current TSCA loopholes in a number of ways (GAO 2009b) and lobby to manage TSCA changes so that their business interests are protected. From 2012 to 2015, major chemical companies spent $190 million in lobbying efforts as updating TSCA intensified (Foley 2015). To stay current on this actively evolving issue, visit SaferChemicals.org and EWG.org.

KEY POINTS

01. When looking for informed guidance on controversial health claims, it's worthwhile to look outside American borders. The factors that determine official policies are complex, so considering a variety of them can provide better insight.
02. Our main law regulating chemicals, TSCA, fails to protect us adequately. It could not even empower the EPA to broadly ban asbestos, a known carcinogen. TSCA is in urgent need of reform.
03. While our laws are imperfect and can be abused (when litigation claims are unwarranted, for example), in the case of the asbestos industry, litigation was not only a tool for compensating victims, but a means of protecting public health by nearly bankrupting an industry that was creating highly toxic products.

Chapter I.11
Track Records with Proof of Harm

Just recently retired, my father was an effective obstetrician gynecologist, beloved by his patients and community. He is wise and extremely open-minded and curious, especially considering his generation and cultural background.

However, when I started discussing various environmental dangers with my father, early in my research, he would at times shut down further consideration of an idea with the response "But there's no proof." At these times, his open-mindedness became blocked by the assumption that truths are proven: If a health factor is legitimate (i.e., if there is enough proof), then he would have learned about it in medical school or read about it in his medical journals. Furthermore, if something is not yet proven, then it is not really worth worrying about. Until recently, I also operated under this mode of thinking.

My father, and others who share a similar mindset, inspired this chapter. While chapter I.10 examined the impractical legal challenges of proving harm, this chapter spotlights additional challenges—practical and political.

ESTABLISHING PROOF OF HARM
In the US, for a chemical to be regulated, the EPA must prove harm (EWG 2013b). While the complexities of scientifically proving harm cannot be properly addressed in this book, the topic merits some discussion. The following paragraphs spotlight six main challenges. The main objective of this section, however, is to spotlight why we should not interpret a lack of proof of harm as proof of safety. Establishing proof of harm involves a lot of time, resources, and luck.

Challenges in studying toxicology
The more we learn about toxicants, the more we appreciate how little we understand their Unintentional Potential Effects. We have already looked at a few key areas of active research: the various effects (when they appear, their location in the body, and their type) at various dosage levels (low, high, and levels with no observable adverse effects) while considering various vulnerabilities (age, ethnicity, and sex).

Great uncertainty exists about how toxicants will impact our health, food supply, and future outlook. In fact, according to the most current review of the science on EDCs by the WHO and UNEP, we have so far discovered only the "tip of the iceberg" (WHO and UNEP 2013).

Studying the effects of real-life exposures to chemicals poses some tough practical challenges. To get a complete picture, scientists would have to identify and monitor all individual substances to which an individual might be exposed and determine which ones are stored in the body, and to what degree. They would also have to assess interactions among the substances, the dosage of each substance, and the timing of exposure in the womb and during an individual's lifetime. In addition, genetic predisposition, lifestyle, and health factors (like obesity and stress) would have to be considered (Reuben 2010). Thus, regardless of changes in business practices and regulation, establishing proof of harm will always be difficult.

Figure #07 summarizes the key toxicology challenges that have already been mentioned, as well as additional difficulties. Its main message is that acquiring irrefutable proof of harm is complex.

Conflicts of interest
In addition, some industries have dynamic webs of influence that shape opinions and decision makers in a variety of fields. This will be discussed in the next chapter.

Studying the impact of environmental factors on human health has been a low priority
Research on the effects of common toxicant exposures has been a relatively low priority among government agencies, the general academic and scientific community, and the public. Consequently, the study of environ-

Toxicology Challenges

REVIEW FROM PRIOR SECTIONS

1. Chemical traits are complex
Toxicants have various traits: Some are attracted to fat, water, bones, or blood; their toxicity varies by their form (liquid, gas or solid); their persistence and toxicity can change as they break down in the environment and in our bodies; and they can combine with other toxicants to create different effects. For example, some chemicals can affect the endocrine system in its original form, while others are more endocrine active after they are transformed in the body or environment (WHO and UNEP 2013).

2. We have unique vulnerabilities
Critical stages of development should be considered (EWG 2005a), and women, men, and various ethnicities have different vulnerabilities (Adler and Rehkopf 2008).

3. What is the influence of fetal origins?
In recent decades, scientists have realized that prenatal and early childhood exposures affect our susceptibilities (EWG 2005a).

4. Our body burdens evolve
We inherit a body burden from our parents, and it evolves over our lifetime (EWG 2005a). There are unknown consequences from stored toxins in the body that may be released during weight loss, pregnancy, or some other major physical stress (WHO and UNEP 2013; Steingraber 2001).

5. What is a safe dose?
What is a safe dose if we experience repeated exposures to small doses? What is a safe dose if we don't understand the cocktail effects with parent compounds and Unintentional By-products? What dosage levels cause no effect in various life stages, especially in fetuses and infants?

6. There is insufficient disclosure of what's in our products
Manufacturers are not required to disclose all product ingredients and potential health risks, which challenges further the identification and testing of common exposures (WHO and UNEP 2013).

7. The unintentionals are not fully understood
We don't know of all parent compounds produced and their Unintentional By-products, Unintentional Toxicants, and Unintentional Potential Effects (WHO and UNEP 2013).

8. We have weak laws
Our federal laws have not kept up with our chemical explosion (Reuben 2010).

ADDITIONAL CHALLENGES

1. Animal studies are limited

The relevance of animal studies to humans is complex. Historically, laboratory animal studies missed the impact of exposures before birth and in childhood. Increasingly, exposures at various life stages are being considered (Reuben 2010). Also, humans can be more sensitive to toxicants than test animals. We learned from our experience with lead, mercury, and PCBs that animal tests grossly underestimate risks to human neurological development (Schettler et al. 2000). Generally, "bad news for a lab rat is bad news for all other mammals," including humans (Michaels 2008).

— According to the Chemical Industry Archives (2009), we learned that "animal tests missed the toxic dose of PCBs by 10,000 times."

— In a survey, "humans were shown to be up to 200 times more sensitive than animals to 21 chemicals known to cause birth defects" (Chemical Industry Archives 2009).

2. Other challenges: Information gaps?

Public health advocates have been challenged by limited resources, lack of public interest, insufficient information, low priority given to scientific study of this issue, a dearth of experts in the field, and political obstacles. There can also be conflicts of interest among those involved in studies.

THE UNKNOWN

There is still so much more to discover. As the WHO and UNEP 2013 report explained:

> Right now only a narrow spectrum of chemicals and a few classes of EDCs are measured, making up the tip of the iceberg. More comprehensive assessments of human and wildlife exposures to diverse mixtures of EDCs are needed. It should be a global priority to develop the abilities to measure any potential EDCs.

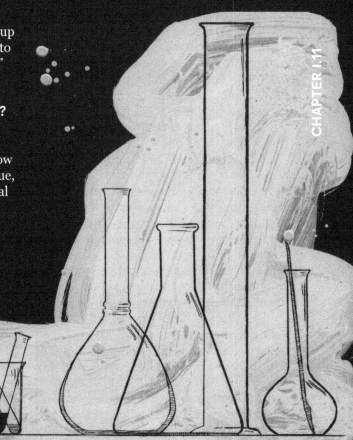

FIGURE #07

67

mental toxicology and oncology, especially in preventing chronic illnesses, has attracted inadequate funding and has developed relatively few experts (Reuben 2010). Therefore, finding answers to important questions will take longer.

Lack of public support

Lack of public awareness has led to lack of public pressure on government to improve laws and policies that protect the public from toxic exposures. In the spring of 2013, an activist told me there was bipartisan support for the first time to update TSCA and said that the biggest obstacle was actually "the apathy of the American public."

Concern is growing, however, as evidenced by consumers' increasing demand for more healthful products. Some retailers and manufacturers are responding to this by taking proactive measures before laws require them, as in the case of major retailers refusing to sell baby bottles that contain BPA (CBS News Staff 2012).

Information gaps

No matter how well managed, all large organizations have communication gaps and consequently information gaps. It's inevitable because nothing is perfect.

Similarly, there are gaps in communication and information between the scientific community and the medical, political, and public communities. Additional gaps form as the number of people involved increases and interest groups become engaged. Along with this come increasing complexities in decision making.

While politicians and health advocates work hard toward filling the gaps, all of us can participate in protecting ourselves as well. Toward that end, increased awareness of weaknesses within our "operating system" is necessary, as is curiosity about what we do not know, as individuals and collectively as a society. In waiting for irrefutable proof of harm, it helps to understand the complexities of establishing that proof.

Political obstacles

Inevitably, lack of public awareness and support challenges the intentions of public and environmental health advocates. Furthermore, the information gap and demand for irrefutable proof of harm hinder policymaking, which requires reaching a consensus despite scientific and medical uncertainty. In the meantime, as is discussed in chapter I.12, manufacturers sometimes use effective strategies to delay and prevent regulation.

As I've said, it was my confusion over the FDA's position on the safety of BPA that inspired the research that led to this book. My confusion dissipated as I began to see a pattern of behavior by regulatory agencies. In short, politics is complicated, and it influences decision making.

ACKNOWLEDGING AND RESPONDING TO PROOF OF HARM

Even when information gaps have been narrowed, it takes time for individuals to learn about the threats of harm, and then even longer for them to change habits and behavior.

In December 1971, President Richard Nixon launched the "war on cancer." Since then, organizations like the National Cancer Institute and the American Cancer Society have received billions of dollars a year from both private and federal sources. Clifton Leaf, who wrote the book *The Truth in Small Doses: Why We're Losing the War on Cancer—and How to Win It*, estimated that the US funds cancer research to the tune of about $16 billion annually (Nazaryan 2013).

Yet, despite the good intentions and ample resources, cancer is still a leading cause of death worldwide (WHO 2014d). And although we now know that certain lifestyle choices—such as smoking, excessive alcohol intake, and physical inactivity—increase cancer risk, such choices remain common.

In an article titled "WHO: Imminent Global Cancer 'Disaster' Reflects Aging, Lifestyle Factors," the World Cancer Report (produced by an arm of the WHO) estimated that cancer cases will increase 57 percent in the next 20 years (Hume and Christensen 2014).

Proof of harm of an exposure doesn't necessarily cease its use

Used for centuries, lead provides an example—one among many—of how long it takes for governments, scientists, manufacturers, and the public to establish, understand, acknowledge, and then respond to proof of harm.

The toxic effects of lead have been known from as early as 2000 BC but it took centuries to appreciate its potent effects. While lead poisoning was first recognized as a pediatric disease in 1892 (WHO 2010), it wasn't until recent decades that we realized that there is no safe level of exposure for the developing brain. In 1960, "safe" blood lead levels were revised to 60 µg/dl, and then to 10 µg/dl in 1990 (Schettler et al. 2000). In 2012, the CDC revised its reference level of blood further to 5 µg/dl (CDC 2013a).

As science proved harm at increasingly low levels in the blood, lead was gradually phased out of certain products, such as gasoline (phased out in the 1970s and banned in 1995) and paint (banned in 1978 in the US; WHO 2010).

Despite the known hazards of lead, global consumption is *increasing* (WHO 2010). Worldwide demand for lead is anticipated to grow 5 to 6 percent annually to 16 million metric tons per year by 2025 (Doe Run Company 2013). It can be found in common household products, such as cosmetics, toys, toy jewelry, vinyl, hair dyes, ceramic glazes, and pipes.

Each year, lead poisoning in children leads to an estimated $43 billion in medical and societal costs in the US alone (WHO 2010).

KEY POINTS

01. Besides weak laws and regulation, several other obstacles impede proving harm:
— Lack of information
— Practical challenges of studying real-life exposures at various developmental stages of life
— Low priority, funding, and interest in prevention
— Limited numbers of trained experts in the relevant fields
— Inadequate resources to support toxicology testing to prove harm quickly enough
— Challenges in assessing additive or synergistic effects
— Inability to extrapolate from animal studies all effects on humans
— Inconsistencies between factors such as politics and economics and the best interests of public health
— Confusion, complexity, and doubt generated by industry-funded research and other efforts

02. The WHO/UNEP report (2013) called for interdisciplinary efforts that integrate knowledge from wildlife, experimental animal, and human studies. A more well-rounded approach is needed to determine which chemicals contribute to the increasing prevalence of disease and health challenges.

03. Even after proof of harm is established, policymakers, physicians, and the public are slow to respond accordingly.

04. Given the complexities of proving harm, regardless of changes to laws and business practices, consumers still need to be proactive, and they should not assume that no proof of harm means proof of safety.

05. Chemicals—such as lead—that have been proved harmful are still found in common household products, including children's products.

Chapter I.12
Track Records of Manipulative Business Strategies

I am a first-generation immigrant. Born in Taipei, Taiwan, I moved here with my family when I was nine months old.

Throughout my childhood, I heard about why my parents moved to the US. My father often reminded me that simply being an American citizen and living in America placed my quality of life in the top one percent of the world. Given this context, I have a deep gratitude and appreciation for what it means to be American.

Given my love for, and deep loyalty to, America, when I used to hear comments or stories about government or corporate dysfunction, I immediately blocked them out. I didn't want to hear about America's imperfections. I didn't care that it wasn't perfect. It was perfect enough to me.

Now that I'm a mom, my concern for my children's health has pushed me to learn about difficult aspects of America's history: the track record of influential companies' disregard for public health and the environment and the sometimes baffling behavior of regulatory agencies.

In my research, I have tried to focus on credible, dispassionate reviews of the facts, many of which came from the discovery process associated with litigation, which centers on gathering information from relevant plaintiffs and defendants. From the release of millions of pages of internal company documents, a pattern of behavior—and sometimes actual business strategies—from companies in a wide range of industries emerged.

I read roughly a dozen stories, written and researched by different authors, with nearly the same plot. All that differed were the settings: the tobacco, asbestos, chemical, pharmaceuticals, food, oil, and telecommunications industries. All of these stories had a lot of depth and dimension and were full of complex webs of important details that are beyond the scope of this chapter. Instead, I will take a broad view here, using specific examples to illustrate common business strategies.

The detailed accounts of the practical applications of these strategies inspired me to spread awareness. These tactics effectively influence not only most of our consumer beliefs, behaviors, and preferences, but also government regulation and official, authoritative opinions. Further, the impacts of these strategies extend beyond borders. They pollute our food, water, air, and soil. They are disrupting our biological processes, our climate, and our ecosystems. They jeopardize the quality of our children's future.

As I learned about repeated uses of business strategies that manipulate demand for products that directly or indirectly threaten the health of our Homes, I got mad at the American system for not incorporating the same precautionary or proactive measures that other countries have. My immediate reaction was a desire for more government intervention. But my entrepreneurial side then became concerned about the potential for too much government involvement.

While updated laws and regulations are needed to create more transparency and proof of safety, I still prefer the American tendency toward *minimal* government intervention. I believe that allowing supply and demand to settle into their natural equilibrium creates the best setting to foster the innovation and efficiencies that are uniquely American.

The goal of this chapter is to help level the playing field between consumers and businesses by informing individuals of influential business strategies that don't always serve the best interests of human and environmental health. I spotlight six manipulative business strategies that have been used by a wide variety of industries: 1) Establish a web of influence; 2) deny with deception; 3) manufacture doubt and confusion as proof of harm emerges; 4) divert attention; 5) fight transparency; and 6) delay leveling the playing field in order to maximize sales. I will refer to them collectively as "Manipulative Business Strategies."

Generally, these Manipulative Business Strategies have greatly influenced our perspective, preferences, purchases, and behaviors. These strategies are important to know because they are still used today by some companies. Once we become aware of the playing field that we're on, however, we can form individual strategies to protect ourselves.

A RECURRING THEME

My search for clarity on the BPA issue in 2007, discussed in chapter I.10, led me to excellent reports by various authors published by the EEA. One of these, "Tobacco Industry Manipulation of Research," enlightened me as to the highly effective strategies that the tobacco industry used to protect cigarette sales despite mounting evidence of their health risks. The goal was to delay regulation of cigarettes and smoking—as well as victim compensation—for as long as possible (Bero 2013). I refer to this mission of delaying regulation of products that threaten human and environmental health as "Corporate Interests."

The strategies that Big Tobacco pioneered were so effective that other industries adopted them too. From the Bero report (2013), I learned that the chemical, asbestos, and lead industries used the same Manipulative Business Strategies that the tobacco industry established. I then wondered how prevalent these strategies were. I proceeded to read about them in accounts of other industries, from sources such as those below, which you may prefer to skim. I will refer to them, collectively, as "Sources":

— Two different reports by Lisa A. Bero PhD, a professor at the University of California San Francisco: Each are titled "Tobacco Industry Manipulation of Research," and they chronicle the clever manipulation tactics of the tobacco industry. One was published by the EEA in 2013 as part of its *Late Lessons from Early Warnings* series. The other was published in 2005 by the peer-reviewed journal *Public Health Reports*.

— A report by the Union of Concerned Scientists, a nonprofit organization founded in 1969 by faculty and students of the Massachusetts Institute of Technology: "*Smoke, Mirrors & Hot Air: How ExxonMobil Uses Big Tobacco's Tactics to Manufacture Uncertainty on Climate Science*" provides a detailed overview of how the oil giant successfully employed the same Manipulative Business Strategies to delay regulation by attacking the science on climate change, denying—somewhat illogically—both that it was occurring and that it was human-induced (Union of Concerned Scientists 2007).

— A leaked 2002 memo from political consultant Frank Luntz to the Bush White House: "The Environment: A Cleaner Safer, Healthier America" recommends talking points on various environmental issues. The section on climate change advises on how to continue to challenge the science that proves it is occurring (Luntz Memorandum to Bush White House 2002).

— The book *Disconnect: The Truth About Cell Phone Radiation, What the Industry Has Done to Hide It, and How to Protect Your Family* by Devra Davis PhD MPH, who, among a long list of accomplishments, was once appointed by President Clinton to the Chemical Safety and Hazard Investigation Board and was former Senior Advisor to the Assistant Secretary for Health in the Department of Health and Human Services: It mentions Manipulative Business Strategies in the telecommunications industry (Davis 2010).

— The book *The World According to Monsanto*, which earned the author, Marie-Monique Robin, the 2009 Rachel Carson award for her contributions to raising awareness of concerns over genetically modified seeds (Rachel Carson–Prisen 2014): It describes Manipulative Business Strategies by the agrochemical giant Monsanto in its history with PCBs, dioxins, DDT, artificial growth hormones for dairy cows, and genetically modified seeds (Robin 2010).

— The book *Doubt Is Their Product* by David Michaels PhD MPH, an epidemiologist and the assistant secretary of labor for the Occupational Safety and Health Administration: It describes Manipulative Business Strategies among a number of industries. The case studies—involving tobacco, asbestos, lead, plastics, diacetyl (an ingredient in some formulas for artificial butter flavor), beryllium, chromium, and others—were based on materials revealed during legal proceedings. They included "documents that prove industry campaigns to manufacture uncertainty; others that prove corporate knowledge of significant health hazards for years, if not decades, before they were acknowledged; and vital scientific studies that should have been in the literature but were hidden by their corporate sponsors" (Michaels 2008).

— The book *Pandora's Poison* by Joseph Thornton PhD, a professor in the department of human genetics and the department of ecology and evolution at the University of Chicago: It provides a more in-depth look at the chemical industry, including the use of Manipulative Business Strategies (Thornton 2000).

— The book *The China Study* by T. Colin Campbell MS PhD, professor emeritus of nutritional biochemistry at Cornell University, and his son, Thomas M. Campbell II MD: It provides a comprehensive overview of the science examining the link between nutrition and a wide range of diseases. The authors mention Manipulative Business Strategies that have been used in the food industry (Campbell and Campbell 2006).

— "The Perils of Ignoring History: Big Tobacco Played Dirty and Millions Died. How Similar Is Big Food?" by Kelly D. Brownell PhD, dean of the Sanford School of Public Policy at Duke University, and Kenneth E. Warner, dean of the University of Michigan School of Public Health: The article draws parallels between the defensive actions taken by the food and tobacco industries in response to concerns that their products may cause harm (Brownell and Warner 2009).

— Two books by Gerald Markowitz PhD, a professor at the John Jay College of Criminal Justice and the Graduate Center, and David Rosner PhD MPH, a professor at Columbia University: *Deceit and Denial: The Deadly Politics of Industrial Pollution* is about manipulations by the chemical and lead industries (Markowitz and Rosner 2002); and *Lead Wars: The Politics of Science and the Fate of America's Children* takes a closer, updated look at the lead industry (Markowitz and Rosner 2013).

STRATEGY 1: ESTABLISH A WEB OF INFLUENCE

A vital component to the success of Manipulative Business Strategies has been a diversified and international web of influence. The Sources recount several instances of powerful companies that successfully established support for Corporate Interests from people in science, academia, and government as well as regulatory agencies, advisory panels, the media, lawyers, consultants, research organizations, and nonprofit organizations. I refer to this network of parties from a variety of fields that support Corporate Interests as a company's or industry's "Web of Influence."

As proof of harm emerges, some companies finance sophisticated, international efforts "to keep the debate alive" (Bero 2013) in order to delay potential, or manage actual, regulation. Those companies then feed those in their Web of Influence with information that serve Corporate Interests, such as with Pro-industry Research, explained later in this chapter.

In the tobacco industry, as evidence accumulated that secondhand smoke (also known as environmental tobacco smoke, or ETS), posed health risks, Philip Morris grew its Web of Influence by establishing an international research network to stimulate controversy. The effort was chronicled in the notes of a meeting of the UK Industry on Environmental Tobacco Smoke in London on February 17, 1988:

> In every major international area (USA, Europe, Australia, Far East, South America, Central America and Spain) they are proposing, in key countries, to set up a team of scientists organized by one national coordinating scientist and American lawyers, to review scientific literature or carry out work on ETS to keep the controversy alive. They are spending vast sums of money to do so… Because of the heavy financial burden, Philip Morris are inviting other companies to join them in these activities […] (Drope and Chapman 2001)

The international scope and sophistication of Big Tobacco's network "to keep the controversy alive" was surprising, and I was further dismayed to read about ties to influential government officials—specifically, those who influence regulation and standard setting. As the EEA (2013) wrote, "Regulators have in the past not always judged and decided objectively and independently with respect to corporate interests. In several cases, regulatory agencies and committees included experts with a conflict of interest, who could shape policy recommendations by interpreting scientific evidence in the interests of the industry."

These dynamics have been described not just for the tobacco industry, but also for the telecommunications (Davis 2010), food (Campbell and Campbell 2006; Brownell and Warner 2009), and chemical industries (Robin 2010; Michaels 2008).

And these types of conflicts of interest between public health and the private sector have occurred under various presidential administrations both Democratic and Republican (Union of Concerned Scientists 2007; Robin, 2010).

STRATEGY 2: DENY WITH DECEPTION

There's denying with innocence, denying with ignorance, and then there's denying with deception. Among the accounts given in the Sources were stories of companies or industries that had data indicating potential, or even unquestionable, toxicity but didn't report it to the regulatory authorities and didn't investigate it further.

Worse, as evidence of harm mounted and concerns increased, companies denied with deception. In the tobacco industry, internal documents "revealed the extent to which the effects of nicotine were known and intentionally blurred for consumers by creating doubt about the health risk" (EEA 2013; Hurt and Robertson 1998). In the petroleum industry, as concerns grew over global warming and climate change, Exxon (now ExxonMobil) publicly denied the existence of the problem by contesting the science, even though, according to the EEA, climate change had been "privately identified" (EEA 2013).

The Global Climate Coalition—formed in 1989 by energy, automotive, and petroleum companies—tried to delay regulation by pursuing Manipulative Business Strategies. Its Web of Influence helped to confuse and deny with deception. The Union of Concerned Scientists (2007) reported, "Drawing on a handful of scientific spokespeople during the early and mid-1990s, the Global Climate Coalition emphasized the remaining uncertainties in climate science. Exxon and other members of the coalition challenged the need for action on global warming by denying its existence as well as characterizing global warming as a natural phenomenon."

STRATEGY 3: MANUFACTURE DOUBT AND UNCERTAINTY AS PROOF OF HARM EMERGES

Used for millennia by Native Americans for ceremonial and health reasons, tobacco was introduced to Europe in the early 1500s. It became increasingly popular and accepted worldwide. The invention of the cigarette-making machine in the 1880s made smoking even more accessible.

Starting in the late 1930s, however, an unhealthy pattern among smokers began to emerge: increased death rates, most likely from lung cancer caused by smoking cigarettes (EEA 2013). As proof of harm was established and the Surgeon General ordered that a warning label appear on cigarette packages from 1966 onward, the tobacco industry used obfuscating tactics to protect its revenues (Michaels 2008).

One key strategy was to manufacture doubt, confusion, and uncertainty, as clearly shown in a 1969 memo from Brown and Williamson, a former American tobacco company. Prepared to guide the responses of the company's employees to strengthening proof of the health risks of tobacco, it stated, "Doubt is our product since it is the best means of competing with the 'body of fact' that exists in the mind of the general public. It is also the means of establishing a controversy" (Bero 2005).

Eleven years later, the tobacco industry would implement the same strategies to undermine evidence and concerns over the hazards of secondhand smoke. And as the tobacco industry strategies have remained notably constant—and effective—since the early 1950s (Bero 2005), other industries have adopted them as well. Documents like the 2007 report by the Union for Concerned Scientists and the memorandum written by GOP consultant Frank Luntz to the Bush White House describe how well ExxonMobil deployed Manipulative Business Strategies. For example, in the Luntz Memorandum to the Bush White House (2002), Luntz wrote:

> Voters believe that there is *no consensus* about global warming within the scientific community. Should the public come to believe that the scientific issues are settled, their views about global warming will change accordingly. Therefore, *you*

The Asbestos Industry: Denied with Deception

While the first documented asbestos-related death occurred in 1906 and the first diagnosis of asbestosis was made in the UK in 1924, some believe that the hazards of asbestos were known from "ancient times," as David Michaels writes. The author writes that by 1918, anyone in the industry who wanted to know about asbestos-related disease could, and should, have known. By the 1930s, "the evidence was simply overwhelming" (Michaels 2008). Court documents involving the US asbestos industry show that officials knew of health risks starting in the 1930s and "went to extraordinary lengths to conceal the truth about asbestos from workers, the public, and the press" (EWG 2004b).

According to "Asbestos: Think Again," a 2004 report by the EWG, the asbestos industry withheld important information on the link between asbestos exposure and adverse health effects. In one of many examples in the EWG report, a medical doctor employed by an asbestos company clearly communicated the known link between asbestos and cancer in a 1964 report to his employer:

> There is an irrefutable association between asbestos and cancer. This association has been established for cancer of the lung and for mesothelioma. There is suggestive evidence . . . for cancer of the stomach, colon and rectum also. There is substantial evidence that cancer and mesothelioma have developed in environmentally exposed groups, i.e., due to air pollution for groups living near asbestos plants and mines. Evidence has been established for cancer developing among members of the household. Mesotheliomas have developed among wives, laundering the work clothes of asbestos workers. Substantial evidence has been presented that slight and intermittent exposures may be sufficient to produce lung cancer and mesothelioma. There should be no delusion that the problem will disappear or that the consumer or working population will not become aware of the problem and the compensation and legal liability involved. (EWG 2004b; Bowker 2003)

According to the EWG report, the company fired the doctor soon after he submitted his report. In another example, a 1973 Asbestos Textile Institute memo stated:

> Our prediction is that approximately 25,000 past and present employees in the asbestos industry have died or will eventually die of asbestos-related disease . . . and the good news is that despite all the negative articles on asbestos health that have appeared in the press over the past half-dozen years, very few people have been paying attention (EWG 2004b).

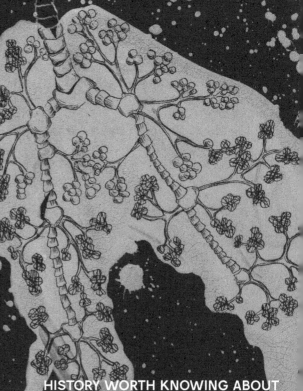

need to continue to make the lack of scientific certainty a primary issue in the debate [emphasis in original], and defer to scientists and other experts in the field.

How do companies manufacture doubt, confusion, and uncertainty about emerging evidence of harm? The effective strategy has been multipronged and focuses on debating and attacking the science. Michaels (2008) explains that "debating the *science* is much easier and more effective than debating the *policy* [emphasis in original]."

Attack the limitations and uncertainties in the studies

Science inherently contains limitations in its studies, and the causes of human diseases are highly complex, as we have seen. For example, lung cancer caused by asbestos can be hard to distinguish from lung cancer caused by tobacco or other factors (Michaels 2008).

Another trait that makes science vulnerable to debate and attack is that science works well studying one thing at a time. Controlling variables is important in understanding the effects of a specific toxicant. The strategy of attacking science with science provides ample opportunities to confuse the public and policymakers. Manipulative Business Strategies capitalize on the fact that nonscientists are not usually qualified to distinguish good science from bad science (Michaels 2008).

For example, the tobacco industry dissected every study that threatened its Corporate Interests, challenging study design, methodology, and conclusions and even the scientists themselves. The industry looked at other causes of lung disease, smokers who didn't have the disease, and any new associations that would divert attention from cigarettes. Bero explains that the tobacco industry also worked with the chemical, petroleum, plastics, and chlorine industries to develop a campaign that criticized the risk assessment techniques used for low doses of toxins (Bero 2005). In short, it attempted to delay regulation through "paralysis by analysis" (EEA 2013). The aforementioned Sources and others, including an article in *Washington Monthly*, "Paralysis by Analysis: Jim Tozzi's Regulation to End All Regula-

tion" (Mooney 2004), discuss how it still occurs today.

Regardless of the imperfect proof from epidemiological and other scientific studies, conclusions can be deduced from the weight of the evidence after considering the strengths and weaknesses of each individual study (Michaels 2008). However, since policymaking is facilitated by consensus (Bero 2005), the strategy of debating and attacking the science is effective in confusing stakeholders and delaying change.

Luntz included in his 2002 memo about climate change, *"The scientific debate is closing [against us] but not yet closed. There is still a window of opportunity to challenge the science* [emphasis in original]." (Luntz Memorandum to Bush White House 2002).

Use strategic rhetoric to attack the science

Popular sound bites to attack science include accusations of "junk science," used to ridicule research that threatens Corporate Interests, regardless of the merit of that research. Other popular sound bites are "Let's not rush to judgment," "More research is needed," and "Let's pursue good epidemiological practices." Statements made to attack threatening science may suggest that animal data are irrelevant, human data are unrepresentative, or exposure data are unreliable. They may imply recall bias among test subjects, cite other causes for disease, and highlight exceptions to conclusions (Michaels 2008). They cultivate a "pro-science" image, recognizing that the best way to attack scientific evidence of harm is with conflicting science.

Create Pro-industry Research and obscure industry involvement

Another strategy used to attack and debate the science has been to create "Pro-industry Research"—that is, science that benefits Corporate Interests—and not disclose unbiased involvement in doing so.

Companies or industries can be involved in scientific studies by various means, such as funding, designing, conducting, and interpreting research and editing reports and conclusions. Sometimes, as in the case of the tobacco industry, business executives and industry lawyers—

rather than scientists—were involved. For example, after an influential 1981 Japanese study linked lung cancer to passive smoking, the tobacco industry pursued its own study, the Japanese Spousal Smoking Study, to create confusion about the 1981 results (Hong and Bero 2002). Big Tobacco also hid its involvement in the design, conduct, and dissemination of this study.

Bero (2005) explains that a law firm for the tobacco industry, Covington and Burling, was the project manager; a tobacco industry scientist supervised the research; and a tobacco industry consultant helped review the study design and interpreting data. "The goal of the study was to produce a credible, peer-reviewed article that could be used as a public relations tool," wrote Hong and Bero in a 2002 article, "How the Tobacco Industry Responded to an Influential Study of the Health Effects of Secondhand Smoke," that was published in *The BMJ* (formerly the *British Medical Journal*), one of the world's oldest medical journals.

While it may seem obvious that results of studies can be influenced by industry funding, Michaels corroborates that investigations have found a close correlation between the results desired by a study's funders and the results reported by its researchers, which he describes as the "funding effect." When firms fund research, "the likelihood that the result of that study will be favorable to that firm is dramatically increased" (Michaels 2008). Bero describes how this has been executed by the tobacco industry:

> Lawyers selected which projects would be funded, including reviews of the scientific literature on topics ranging from addiction to lung retention of particulate matter. These law firms also funded research on potential confounding factors for the adverse health effects associated with smoking. For example, projects were funded that examined genetic factors associated with lung disease or the influence of stress and low-protein diets on health. These deflected attention from tobacco as a health hazard and protect[ed] tobacco companies from litigation. (Bero 2005)

Other industries have been found to use this strategy as well. For example, Michaels (2008) notes that documentation linking pharmaceutical industry sponsorship with studies that reached pro-industry conclusions began to appear in the 1990s. Bero (2005) notes that the food, chemical, asbestos, and lead industries have done this as well.

Davis gives an example of how it's carried out today. Her book discusses Manipulative Business Strategies in the telecommunications industry, in which studies are designed to create confusion and scientists are hired to show that results that threaten Corporate Interests can't be replicated. Allan H. Frey is an American neuroscientist who began publishing pioneering work in the 1960s showing that "microwave radiation like that used in cell phones today could weaken the membranes surrounding our hearts, brains, eyes, and lungs." In Davis's book, Frey explains that small changes in the design of scientific studies can be critical. "Studies are done not to clarify the problem, but to confuse people," he says. "We've got quite a history of that in this field" (Davis 2010).

Manipulate science through the design of the studies

Earlier chapters spotlight nuances that influence toxicant effects: timing of exposure, unique vulnerabilities, dosage effects, and so on. Some of the Sources discuss how science can be manipulated through the design of the study, including *which* questions are examined, and which are not. For example, Davis (2010) explains that studies on how cell phone radiation affects the brain fail to consider the unique characteristics of children's brains. Robin (2010) provides another example: In the case of one popular pesticide, its active ingredient is harmless, but the overall formula, the combination of active and inactive ingredients, poses risks. The registration of this pesticide, however, included tests for only the active ingredient and not the overall formula.

The *form* of the toxicant exposure—such as ingested (solid) or inhaled (gas)—also matters, as chapter I.8 introduced. Michaels (2008) explains that diacetyl was a common ingredient in artificial flavoring for microwave popcorn. When scientists examined the literature in 1980, they found no danger in consuming diacetyl in the small quantities used to flavor food. Diacetyl was, and still is, included on the list of "generally recognized as safe" food additives (FDA 2013b), and is used in some formulas for butter-flavored popcorn. However, the effects of *inhaling* the chemical hadn't been assessed, although the National Institute for Occupational Safety and Health (NIOSH) did learn of risks to workers who inhaled diacetyl in workplaces.

Michaels spoke to the FDA, which is in charge of ensuring the safety and security of our nation's food supply, about this; he says in his book that the agency chose not to explore the issue further since NIOSH studies showed risks only to certain workers. According to Michaels, from the FDA's perspective, there was no evidence of harm to consumers in inhaling fumes from diacetyl so there was also no reason to investigate further (Michaels 2008).

In August 2012, the *Chicago Tribune* reported that most manufacturers of butter-flavored popcorn had voluntarily phased out diacetyl. However, several manufacturers chose 2,3-pentanedione as the replacement chemical, which was found by government researchers to pose similar respiratory health risks. According to the article, further testing has not been pursued (Eng 2012).

Disseminate science that supports Corporate Interests

Once created, Pro-industry Research is disseminated throughout the industry's Web of Influence, such as to policymakers and the consumer press. This helps to influence popular opinion and forestall regulation (Bero 2005).

According to the Union of Concerned Scientists (2007), ExxonMobil was so active in confusing the public on global warming that the scientific community tried to intervene:

> In September 2006, the Royal Society, Britain's premier scientific academy, sent a letter to ExxonMobil urging the company to stop funding the dozens of groups spreading disinformation on global warming and also strongly criticized the company's "inaccurate and misleading" public statements on global warming. The unprecedented letter from the British Royal Society demonstrates the level of frustration among scientists about EM's efforts to manufacture uncertainty about global warming.

STRATEGY 4: DIVERT ATTENTION

As proof of harm emerges, an industry or company may divert attention with help from front organizations. Front organizations appear to have one purpose but really serve Corporate Interests. They pursue a few goals, of which three key ones are discussed in this section.

One goal of some front organizations is to enhance the corporate image of sponsors through philanthropic efforts and research that appears to serve public and environmental health. In 1954, US tobacco companies formed the Tobacco Industry Research Committee (TIRC). While industry representatives claimed that the TIRC was formed to help evaluate a possible association between smoking and lung cancer, internal documents show that it "was actually formed for public relations purposes, to convince the public that the hazards of smoking had not been proven" (Bero 2005).

Another goal of some front organizations is to produce, disseminate, and publish Pro-industry Research designed to contradict and divert attention from emerging health concerns. For example, the Foundation for Clean Air Progress, run by the PR firm Burson-Marsteller and partially funded by the petroleum, trucking, and other industries, "issues regular reports showing how pristine our environment is, questioning why anyone would want to strengthen the laws responsible for such excellent air" (Michaels 2008).

In another example, Philip Morris, R.J. Reynolds, and Lorillard formed the Center for Indoor Air Research (CIAR) in 1988. To divert attention from increasing concerns over the hazards of secondhand smoke, CIAR emphasized research on other indoor air pollutants (Bero 2005).

The EEA (2013) points out that flooding the scientific debate with Pro-industry Research can undermine confidence in the nonbiased scientific findings. ExxonMobil, for instance, was reported to have published and republished the "non-peer-reviewed works of a small group of scientific spokespeople" (Union of Concerned Scientists 2007).

Robin (2010) writes about the review of published articles on the safety of recombinant bovine growth hormone (rBGH), which is used to enhance milk production in dairy cows. After a call from a farmer who was upset about how sick his cows were from rBGH, Samuel Epstein MD, emeritus professor of environmental and occupational medicine at the University of Illinois School of Public Health, investigated the underlying science for the product. In 1987 and 1988 issues of the *Journal of Dairy Science*, Epstein found many "promotional articles" by American and European researchers who had tested rBGH for Monsanto. These articles claimed that rBGH posed no major health problems, but the conclusions were supported by little serious data (Robin 2010).

Finally, another key goal of front organizations is to recruit spokespeople who will attack emerging proof of harm. This presents the appearance of different and more numerous "voices" that are in agreement with messages that serve Corporate Interests. Michaels writes that the food and restaurant industries fund the Center for Consumer Freedom "to attack studies that link fat consumption to obesity. The same group started FishScam to promote the idea that mercury in fish does not pose a danger to pregnant women" (Michaels 2008). The Union of Concerned Scientists (2007) writes that ExxonMobil directed about $16 million from 1998 to 2005 to ideological and advocacy organizations that helped create uncertainty about the causes of global warming.

STRATEGY 5: FIGHT TRANSPARENCY

The Sources provide examples of a variety of ways in which industries fight information disclosure. Bero (2005) explains that when research didn't support Corporate Interests, the tobacco industry sometimes had it edited (through lawyers, for example), suppressed its dissemination, and sometimes even blocked its publication. Other tactics include choosing ignorance, intimidating those who threaten Corporate Interests, and fighting labeling requirements.

Choosing ignorance

The Sources provide a variety of examples of companies that possessed data suggesting toxicity that should have been reported to a regulatory agency or investigated further. Instead of sharing their findings, the companies ignored them; the information was filed away and not given further consideration. Robin (2010) discusses this pattern of behavior as part of the track record of PCBs, dioxins, Agent Orange, and rBGH. There are many other examples, such as the nonstick chemical C8, an "immortal" toxicant spotlighted in chapter I.7, and a class of chemicals known as aromatic amines, which are used by some manufacturers of dyes, rubber products, polyurethane foams, pesticides, pharmaceuticals, and semiconductors. Michaels (2008) writes that manufacturers knew that workers' exposure to aromatic amines was associated with higher incidences of bladder cancer:

> It seems to me that the companies knew almost everything all along. The German dye industry discovered that aromatic amines caused human bladder cancer in 1895. With the publication and dissemination of the 1921 report by the International Labour Organization, the uncontrolled exposure of dye workers to these carcinogens should have been eliminated. *Eliminated.* [emphasis in the original] Instead, the corporations' modus operandi was the same as it always is. Attack the science. Ignore the science. Demand of the science something neither it nor any institution possesses: absolute certainty.

Moreover, Michaels (2008) describes federal agencies as choosing ignorance on more than one occasion: "The less-information-the-better policy has been applied to many aspects of federal policy."

Intimidating opponents

Companies sometimes suppress information by intimidating whistleblowers, derailing the careers of individuals who threaten Corporate Interests, and even litigating. Companies haven't been above denigrating and undermining the scientists who have made discoveries that conflict with corporate goals

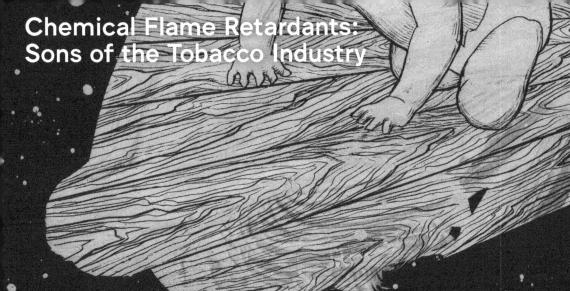

Chemical Flame Retardants: Sons of the Tobacco Industry

In addition to establishing deceptive scientific organizations around the world to confuse consumers about emerging evidence of harm, the tobacco industry collaborated with the chemical industry to create a new product, chemical flame retardants, to divert attention away from cigarette-initiated house fires and to alleviate pressure on Big Tobacco to create fire-safe cigarettes.

In May 2012, the *Chicago Tribune* published a seminal exposé, "Playing with Fire," about the manufactured demand for flame retardants. After reviewing thousands of government, scientific, and internal industry documents, the *Tribune* found the tobacco industry and chemical manufacturers to be part of a "decades-long campaign of deception" over the value of these products. These influential industries distorted science in ways that amplified the value of chemical flame retardants in preventing house fires (Hawthorne 2012).

Big Tobacco established a diversified Web of Influence to help its cause, including an association of top fire officials. Founded in 1989, the National Association of State Fire Marshals campaigned for Big Tobacco's cause for over a decade (Callahan and Roe 2012a). As a result, according to the NRDC (2014), "foam inside our sofas, recliners, and love seats [have been] saturated with pounds of toxic flame retardants." They're also found in our floor coverings and electronics, among other products.

Over decades, however, research linked chemical flame retardants to cancer, neurological deficits, developmental problems, and impaired fertility. As a double whammy, according to the *Tribune* series, these chemical flame retardants are "ineffective." Scientists have learned that flame retardants in household furniture do not offer meaningful protection against fire (Hawthorne 2014). In addition, we now know that flame retardants can escape from household products and settle in household dust. That's why young children, who often put things in their mouths from the floor where they play, generally have much higher levels of these chemicals in their bodies than their parents (Callahan and Roe 2012b). So Big Tobacco protected the popularity of toxic cigarettes by promoting the use of toxic chemical flame retardants.

As evidence of harm mounted, California updated its TB-117 flammability standard—which was largely responsible for why products sold outside California also contained these chemicals—to incorporate recent science. (Part II of this book discusses this further.) However, in the August 2014 article "Chemical Industry Fights for Flame Retardants," the *Chicago Tribune* reported that one of the largest manufacturers of flame retardants is suing California to block this updated flammability standard (Hawthorne 2014).

(Michaels 2008). Even independent researchers can experience abrupt withdrawal of funding or threats to their jobs or lives.

Such intimidation tactics have been widely documented for a variety of industries. In the food and agriculture sector, careers have been derailed, research data have gone missing, and threats to individuals' well-being have been made (Robin 2010). Campbell and Campbell (2006) write, "In the world of nutrition and health, scientists are not free to pursue their research wherever it leads. Coming to the 'wrong' conclusions, even through first-rate science, can damage your career. Trying to disseminate these 'wrong' conclusions to the public, for the sake of public health, can destroy your career." Even Oprah Winfrey, the media mogul, was sued for commenting on her show that she didn't want to eat another hamburger after learning about the cruel and unhealthy practices of some beef producers. (Ultimately, a jury ruled in her favor.)

Individuals who have raised questions about the safety of wireless technology (Davis 2008) or the wisdom of continued reliance on petroleum for energy have also been targeted for intimidation and censorship. Climatologists have even been threatened for documenting the need to control and reduce greenhouse gas emissions (Michaels 2008).

Fighting labeling requirements

Various reports discuss the food industry's opposition to food labeling. Brownell and Warner mention the beef industry's opposition to the labeling of fat content (Brownell and Warner 2009). Robin (2010) discusses the food industry's opposition to labeling products free of rBGH and genetically modified organisms (GMOs).

JustLabelIt.org (2014), an organization fighting for consumers' right to know what's in their food, reports that 90 percent of Americans want to know which foods contain GMOs. In 2014, Vermont became the first state to require food manufacturers to label foods made with GMOs. This law, known as Act 120, is scheduled to take effect in July 2016.

More than 60 countries already require labeling of genetically engineered foods (Kaldveer 2014). In the US, Connecticut and Maine have also passed mandatory labeling laws (Wheeler and Marcos 2015), while over 30 states are considering it.

Major players in the food industry have spent over $100 million fighting GMO labeling campaigns, according to the *Wall Street Journal* (Bunge and Gasparro 2014). In the meantime, four major industry food groups are suing the state of Vermont (No. 5:14-cv-117) for passing Act 120, claiming that the law is unconstitutional (Bunge and Gasparro 2014).

STRATEGY 6: DELAY LEVELING THE PLAYING FIELD TO MAXIMIZE SALES

My parents started a new life in a country where they didn't speak English fluently, had no support network, and had almost no money. They took risks and made great sacrifices as young parents in the hope that my brother and I could benefit from better opportunities for a brighter future. Appreciating this, I hoped that my life would be successful. But how does one define success? I've pondered this throughout my life.

Through various life experiences, I decided that success is complicated and difficult to define and that traditional appearances of success weren't most important to me. I decided that success couldn't be defined by clear metrics, like grades and money. Was I less successful because I earned a B on that exam that was graded on a curve after rejecting a chance to see an advance copy of the test? Was I less successful for playing honestly and not winning a close tennis match against a cheater?

One experience stands out for me. In a negotiations exercise in a business school class, we were divided into two groups or "parties." Each party was given information to embody (for example, each party represented a different company with unique perspective and information) and negotiation objectives. A person from each party then paired off to negotiate against each other. Towards the end of class, we posted our results on the blackboard and discussed keys to creating the best outcome.

I was surprised to learn that I was a pretty good negotiator. Only one person had negotiated a better outcome. I noticed that the key to his outperformance was his lack of concern for losing trust and likeability, which weakens his future negotiating power. Each party's unique set of information, however, also plays a role in the outcome.

In class, we learned about game theory and the idea of a "repeated game," in which reputation, trust, and likability matter when two parties need to repeatedly agree to terms of doing business with each other. Since then, I notice this dynamic often and find myself wondering about the value of sacrificing long-term value (such as health) to maximize short-term (such as financial) results. Success seems to depend on the game's duration: How many rounds do the involved parties engage? Also very important: Who has better *information*.

Years later, as I learned about Manipulative Business Strategies, I often thought about the outperformer in my negotiations class. The industries discussed in the Sources shared this same fixation on maximizing short-term outcomes, but they also worked to extend the duration of the game and keep the rules of the playing field unchanged for as long as possible. Their game plan drew on minimal regulation and managing information—or confusion—about threats of harm.

For example, after three scientists produced evidence that chlorofluorocarbons (CFCs, commonly known by the DuPont trade name Freon) were damaging the ozone layer, manufacturers attacked the science to create uncertainty. One goal of the uncertainty campaign, led by the public relations firm Hill and Knowlton, which had helped the tobacco industry, was to delay clear-cut regulatory action. Later, Hill and Knowlton would boast that its work on behalf of CFC manufacturers helped DuPont gain "two or three years before the government took action to ban fluorocarbons" (Michaels 2008). The science, however, was so strong that the three scientists won a Nobel Prize in Chemistry in 1995 for their work on the matter (Michaels 2008; NobelPrize.org 1995).

As I learned about dozens of examples in which this type of Manipulative Business Strategy was used successfully, I was both indignant and in awe of its effectiveness and sophisticated implementation. Many of the industries covered in this chapter were born or blossomed during the World Wars. They created products that supported war efforts in various ways: explosives, fertil-izers, pesticides, poison gas, plastics, and so forth. During peacetime, they evolved. Some are now dominant players in biotechnology and seed and food production. From a business perspective, their accomplishments are admirable. Below is a snapshot view of how powerful some of these noted industries are today:

— As of 2012, yearly revenues from global tobacco sales were estimated to be nearly $500 billion, generating combined profits for the six largest firms of $35.1 billion—more than $1,100 per second (Bowers 2012).

— ExxonMobil generated $420.8 billion in 2013. It was ranked number 1 on the 2012 Fortune 500 list (ExxonMobil 2014; Fortune 2012).

— A 2011 analysis projected that by 2018, global revenue from flame-retardant sales would hit $5.8 billion (Lee 2014). In 2014, it was estimated that the market for flame retardants would grow to $10.34 billion by 2019 (Markets and Markets 2014).

— The Doe Run Company, a premier metals mining company and a global lead producer, has annual revenue ranging from $600 million to $1 billion, depending on the price of lead (Hibbard 2012).

— World pesticide expenditures exceeded $35.8 billion in 2006 and $39.4 billion in 2007 (Grube et al. 2011). After years of decline, insecticide sales are now surging as American farmers are planting more corn, and previous genetic modifications, designed to safeguard crops from pests, have begun to lose their effectiveness (Berry 2013).

— Monsanto generated $14.9 billion in net sales in 2013 (Monsanto 2013).

— Global sales of dairy products are expected to reach $494 billion in 2015, and the US is predicted to account for 25 percent of this figure (Association for Packaging and Processing Technologies 2013).

— According to estimates by Insight Research Corp (IRC 2014; Telecompaper 2014), global revenues for telecommunications services will grow from $2.1 trillion to $2.4 trillion from 2014 through 2019.

While Manipulative Business Strategies do not account for the financial success of all industry leaders, they have given some companies an edge. The remarkable data points above indicate how savvy some industries have been in implementing their overall business strategies.

An ingredient to the success of these Manipulative Business Strategies has been, and continues to be, a general lack of awareness and information among consumers, government, and even those involved in litigation (such as judges and juries). With such clever Manipulative Business Strategies that are executed so well, consumers and responsible citizens of this planet need strategies too. We're on a lopsided playing field that most of us weren't aware even existed.

WHAT IS SUCCESS?

As a young immigrant, I held America in a special light, seeing it as the ultimate home of justice, humanitarianism, compassion, opportunity, and, of course, success.

In its nearly 250 years of existence, America has achieved phenomenal distinction. Its position as a superpower has been unrivaled. According to a ranking by the World Bank (2014), the US gross domestic product (GDP) led the world at $16.8 trillion dollars, which is 82 percent more than that of the second-ranked country, China, whose GDP was $9.2 trillion.

Within such a financially successful country, I expected Americans to have access to the best health care and to live longer. Therefore, it made sense to me that Americans spend more on health care than those from any other nation, "both absolutely and as a percentage of gross national product" (Crimmins, Preston, and Cohen 2011). In July 2014, *The Atlantic* reported that the US was expected to spend 18 percent of GDP on health care that year—6 percentage points more than the second-highest spender, the Netherlands (Fuchs 2014).

Yet, life expectancy, which is often used to measure population health, in the US is surprisingly low. According to a world ranking by the Central Intelligence Agency, the US is 42nd among the 223 countries ranked, with an average life expectancy of 79.56 years (CIA 2013).

Founded in 1961, the Organisation for Economic Cooperation and Development (OECD) was originally considered a club for rich countries that wanted to collaborate on improving the economic and social well-being of citizens around the world. It's now diversified to include 34 member countries. According to its website, "OECD member countries account for 63 percent of world GDP, three-quarters of world trade, 95 percent of world official development assistance, over half of the world's energy consumption, and 18 percent of the world's population" (OECD 2014).

Among the 34 OECD members, the US falls in the bottom quartile—in 27th place—for life expectancy, according to 2011 data. Compared with men and women from OECD countries with the longest life expectancies (Switzerland and Japan are first and second), American men and women have life expectancies that are 4.2 years and 4.8 years shorter, respectively (OECD 2013).

To recap: America has the highest GDP in the world and spends the most on health care, yet life expectancy is relatively low. Wealth doesn't necessarily buy health.

The reasons for this thought-provoking discrepancy are complicated and not entirely understood, but perhaps Manipulative Business Strategies play a role. In my research, I had to encounter repeated accounts of these strategies before I could believe that companies engaged in them, because the companies involved were so financially successful—and also American (though the strategies aren't limited to American companies). I assumed that America's companies held the same values as those of America's citizens. I learned that I was wrong. They've been so focused on excelling at their business objectives that some have intentionally confused us about health.

As large businesses inevitably fight regulation, transparency, and awareness (while predicting financial and job losses if their industries are more heavily regulated), consider the consequences of not changing: the pediatric and general health trends spotlighted in figures #01 and #02, respectively. We shouldn't have so many sick and uncomfortable people. Also, change always offers new opportunities. The EEA's 2013 report cites a few sources that present evidence that precautionary measures don't stifle innovation but encourage it.

As I continue to ponder how to define success for my children and myself, I often think of my mother. She frequently tells me that my husband and I work too much and are too busy. She reminds me, "You don't have anything without good health!"

CONSUMER STRATEGIES

This was the hardest chapter for me to write because I didn't want to disparage America, capitalism, or minimal government intervention. I am a proud American social entrepreneur.

However, it's important for individuals to become aware of the Manipulative Business Strategies that were, and still are, used by a wide variety of companies. With more awareness, the strategies become less effective.

The power of America resides in our freedom. The more informed we citizens are, the more powerful are our many freedoms. People deserve to know what's in their food, water, air, and household products as well as the potential risks to health and the environment. Individuals have to do their part to learn more too, because we are ultimately the ones responsible for what we put into and onto our bodies. Through our purchases and other behaviors, we often choose between health (long-term benefits) and convenience (short-term benefits), whether we are conscious of it or not.

With more information, everyone involved—companies, government, and individuals—can do more to support the right of each person to make *informed, conscious choices* and exercise self-regulation as he or she wishes. While collective action is powerful, individual concern and support are vital.

The strength of America depends on the participation and choices of its citizens. Undeniably, TSCA needs to be updated. We consumers can tell elected officials that we want improved laws, let regulatory agencies know that we're aware and concerned, and make it clear to manufacturers and retailers that we want safer products. Our system also needs higher standards: more toxicity testing, moral responsibility, accountability, unbiased checks and balances, and transparency. There should be less emphasis on proof of harm and more emphasis on proof of safety.

Fortunately, in America, individuals can create change. And, a growing portion of companies is conducting business in ways that are conscious of our Homes.

As my husband once said, "The beauty of capitalism in America is the power of the demand side to influence the supply side. Consumers have the ultimate control."

KEY POINTS

01. Sometimes businesses intentionally try to confuse the public and policymakers about the safety of their products. If you are confused about what to eat, what to buy, and other decisions that affect your health, it may be a result of an intentional effort.

02. Consumers should know about Manipulative Business Strategies so that they are on a level playing field and can protect themselves with consumer strategies. The more we are aware of industry's manipulative strategies, the less effective they become. Parts II and III of this book are full of tools you can use to form your individual strategy and evolve it as you become ready for more change.

03. The beauty of America is that informed and involved citizens have tremendous power.

04. As Mahatma Gandhi so wisely said: "If we could change ourselves, the tendencies in the world would also change. As a man changes his own nature, so does the attitude of the world change towards him.... We need not wait to see what others do."

Chapter I.13
Track Records of Substitutes

One day while I was at my office in early 2008, I received a thoughtful email from my nanny. She was proud and excited to share her research on BPA-free plastic food containers, which she thought was a safe option for my daughter, especially after speaking to her stepmother, who was a biologist.

As I've written already, public concern was growing over BPA found in plastic baby products. As a result, BPA-free products quickly populated stores. BPA-free was assumed, and marketed, to be safer.

Yet how would we know? I was instinctively suspicious of BPA-free plastics. I wondered: What was the purpose of BPA? How is that purpose being met in BPA-free products? Are the replacement chemicals better understood than BPA?

It turns out my instincts were on to something: Some BPA-free products are not safer.

This got me curious about the safety of other substitutes. I encountered several examples of one harmful chemical being replaced by another harmful chemical.

This section spotlights substitutes for BPA, chemicals used in mattress adhesives and toys, and flame retardants. This chapter's intention is to highlight that substitute chemicals are not always safer. And determining their safety or harm takes years; sometimes it can take the equivalent of a childhood or more.

OUR TRACK RECORD WITH A BPA SUBSTITUTE

Feared by some for its estrogenic activity, BPA in certain products has been banned by some states and countries, and voluntarily phased out by some manufacturers due to consumer and retailer demand. However, the safety of substitute chemicals is unknown and studying them is challenged by manufacturers legal right to protect their proprietary formulas.

Regardless, scientists are doing their best with their limited information. They're finding that some BPA-free plastics demonstrate estrogenic activity that are *at least* as high as—and sometimes higher than—the estrogenic activity from BPA-containing plastics! In some cases, products that had no estrogenic activity when they came off the shelf changed to have some after normal wear and tear from boiling, microwaving, dishwashing, and exposure to sunlight (Hamilton 2012).

Bisphenol S (BPS) has been a popular substitute for BPA in both plastics and cash register receipts. Structurally similar to BPA (the sole difference is that BPS uses sulfur instead of a carbon to link two phenol rings [Pestano 2012]), BPS poses similar concerns for health (*Consumer Reports* 2014b).

Whether this substitution produces a safer compound is yet to be determined, but preliminary studies raise concern. In early 2013, *Environmental Health News* reported results of a study by scientists at the University of Texas (Bienkowski 2013; Viñas and Watson 2013). At the low levels to which people are realistically exposed, BPS was found to disrupt estrogen (Bienkowski 2013). In fact, an August 2014 article in *Scientific American* points out that the Viñas and Watson study found that "even picomolar concentrations (less than one part per trillion) of BPS can disrupt a cell's normal functioning, which could potentially lead to metabolic disorders such as diabetes and obesity, asthma, birth defects, or even cancer" (Bilbrey 2014).

In 2014, the Endocrine Society published results of a study on the effects of an "environmentally relevant dose" of BPS on the hearts of 50 rats. The exposed female (but not male) rats experienced heart rhythm abnormalities, such as extra heartbeats, as well as a racing heartbeat, also known as ventricular tachycardia (Endocrine Society 2014b).

Another study, led by Kurunthachalam Kannan PhD, a research scientist at the New York State Department of Health, identified BPS in 16 varieties of paper from the US, China, Japan, and Korea (American

Chemical Society 2012; Pestano 2012; Liao, Liu, and Kannan 2012). In a news release on its website, the American Chemical Society summarized results of this study: "The researchers estimate that people may be absorbing BPS through their skin in larger doses than they absorbed BPA when it was more widely used—19 times more BPS than BPA" (American Chemical Society 2012). As with BPA, nearly everyone worldwide is exposed to BPS: Traces of it were found in 81 percent of urine samples from eight different countries (Bienkowski 2013).

OUR TRACK RECORD WITH MATTRESS ADHESIVES

Adhesives that join components of mattresses are usually made with a petroleum-based solvent. Historically, TCA (or 1,1,1-trichloroethane), a chlorinated solvent, was used in mattress adhesives until it was banned in 1996 after scientists learned that it was harming the ozone layer (IRTA 2000). Which chemical replaced TCA? Methylene chloride, a probable human carcinogen that may also affect the central nervous system (EPA 2013a).

OUR TRACK RECORD WITH LEAD IN TOYS

Like most people, I assumed that lead was no longer used in most products sold in the US, especially in children's products. After all, we now know that it's a potent neurotoxin and that no detectable amount of lead is safe for children (WHO 2010). As chapter I.11 made clear, this assumption doesn't reflect reality.

A surprising number of recalls have been enacted for toys and children's jewelry due to unacceptable levels of lead. For example, in 2007, the Consumer Product Safety Commission (CPSC) recalled 61 toys— over 25 million product units—due to their unacceptable lead levels (CPSC 2007).

Just as phthalates and cadmium can migrate from a vinyl shower curtain (discussed in chapter I.7), lead can migrate from children's products and become part of the dust that forms on the surface of lead-containing items as they gradually deteriorate. Heat, sun, and frequent handling can encourage this process. Paint with lead can also flake off and be ingested (*National Geographic* 2008). Lead can also

be ingested if children mouth the product or their contaminated hands (CDC 2013c; *National Geographic* 2008).

In an effort to reduce lead in household products, manufacturers have increasingly used cadmium as a substitute in paint, toys, and children's jewelry. However, cadmium is also a neurotoxin as well as a carcinogen that children can be exposed to when they handle, mouth, or swallow contaminated products (Mascarelli 2010). As with lead, analyses for cadmium have found high levels in children's products, and there have been a significant number of recalls because of it (Mascarelli 2010; Mead 2010).

OUR TRACK RECORD WITH FLAME RETARDANTS

As chapter I.12 introduced and parts II and III explain in more detail, we have an eventful history with chemical flame retardants: banning, phasing out, reintroducing toxic ones, and introducing modified versions of historical ones that have proved to be toxic. Some of the most commonly used flame retardants are not only toxic and persistent, but also inescapable: They pervade our environment and the food chain, enter our bodies, and remain within. The most notorious flame retardants include PBBs, PCBs, PBDEs, and Tris. In summary, our track record with flame retardants shows that we just replace one toxic flame retardant with another.

PBBs

Status: Discontinued in 1976
Why: PBBs can cause diseases of the nervous, immune, liver, kidney and thyroid systems (ATSDR 2004). They are probably human carcinogens (EPA 2014h).
Replaced by: PCBs

PCBs

Status: Banned in 1979
Why: Discovered to cause cancer and to accumulate in people, wildlife, and the environment (EPA 2014j). They can cause liver damage, cancer, and adverse effects on the immune, nervous, reproductive, and endocrine systems.
Replaced by: PBDEs

PBDEs

Status: Phased out in mid-2000s
Why: Studies have linked them to cancer,

liver toxicity (EWG 2003a), reduced fertility (Roan 2010; Harley et al. 2010; Louis et al. 2013), impairment to the brain and nervous system (including permanent damage if exposure occurs during critical stages of development), and fetal malformations (EWG 2003a).

Replaced by: Tris flame retardants

Tris flame retardants

Status: Still in use

Why it's a bad idea: Tris are structurally similar to banned chemicals like PCBs and DDT (Rahman et al. 2001) so they are linked to similar health threats: reduced IQ, learning disabilities, reduced fertility, thyroid disruption, and cancer (Gross 2013). The state of California listed TDCPP, one type of Tris flame retardant, as a carcinogen under Proposition 65 in October of 2011 based on laboratory studies that found increase incidence of kidney, liver, and testicular tumors as well as evidence of mutagenicity. It mutates DNA, disrupts hormones, and harms the nervous system (Schreder 2012).

KEY POINTS

01. We have a track record of sometimes substituting one harmful chemical for another. This is seen in the lengthy history of flame retardants, in our replacement of lead with cadmium in toys, in our substitution of BPS for BPA in plastics, and in our use of methylene chloride instead of TCA in mattress adhesives. Undoubtedly, other examples exist.

02. Replacement chemicals are sometimes structurally very similar to chemicals that are regulated due to their toxicity. Therefore, health effects of replacement chemicals may be similar to those of the regulated ones.

03. As toxic chemicals are regulated out of certain products, their makers find new opportunities to sell them. For example, Tris flame retardants were removed from children's pajamas in the late 1970s because these chemicals were proved to be toxic. They are still widely used today, however, in many other household products, including other items for children.

Chapter I.14
Opportunity Cost

In economics, "opportunity cost" is the benefit lost from having not made an alternative choice. I often thought of this concept while doing research for this book. I've wondered about the opportunity cost of not following a precautionary approach toward toxic or potentially toxic chemicals. While proof without a doubt is pursued over decades in laboratories and in the courts, with millions of dollars spent, how many healthy years are lost among too many innocent people?

In the cases of tobacco and asbestos, the opportunity cost of waiting to establish proof of harm was the many lives that were lost daily. Smoking kills an average of 1,300 Americans each day, including deaths from secondhand smoke (CDC 2014e). Asbestos causes 10,000 Americans to lose their lives each year (Reinstein 2010). Would precautionary measures and more awareness have saved some of these lives?

In general, the opportunity costs of our reactionary approach toward toxic or potentially toxic chemicals include many adverse health effects discussed in prior chapters: reproductive challenges, birth defects, rising incidence of a long list of chronic diseases and disorders, and the accumulating chemical burden in our environment—a legacy for future generations.

In this section, I examine a different kind of toxicant: the electromagnetic fields created from wireless and wired technologies. While these occur naturally, I consider them a toxicant because human activities have created, and continue to create, unnatural and unprecedented exposure levels for our bodies. As the sources of electromagnetic fields continue to expand, I worry about the opportunity cost of not following a precautionary approach toward them.

ANOTHER INVISIBLE REALITY: ELECTROMAGNETIC FIELDS

Electromagnetic fields (EMFs) and electromagnetic radiation (EMR) are the terms broadly used to refer to electric and magnetic fields created by natural and man-made sources. Electromagnetic fields are created by electric charges, and magnetic fields are made when current flows through wires and electrical devices.

Today, humans are exposed to two types of man-made EMFs. One is extremely low-frequency electromagnetic fields (ELF), which are emitted from electrical and electronic appliances, as well as power lines. The other is radiofrequency radiation (RF), which comes from wireless devices like cell phones and cordless phones, cellular antennas and towers, and broadcast transmission towers.

The WHO recognizes EMFs of all frequencies as "one of the most common and fastest-growing environmental influences, about which anxiety and speculation are spreading. All populations are now exposed to varying degrees of EMF, and the levels will continue to increase as technology advances" (WHO 2014c).

Increasingly, people from around the world are concerned about the unknown health effects of EMFs. The scientific evidence has been pursued for decades (WHO 2014e). While some experts claim that we already have proof that current exposures cause adverse health effects, debate continues and the subject remains controversial (EWG 2013a).

The health concerns are similar to those outlined for toxicants

The reported concerns about health threats from EMFs are similar to those associated with toxicants: The younger the life, the greater the potential damage, because children have unique vulnerabilities; adult vulnerabilities vary; and effects from chronic exposure to EMFs are unknown.

The BioInitiative Working group states: "Human beings are bioelectrical systems. Our hearts and brains are regulated by internal bioelectrical signals. Environmental exposures to artificial EMFs can interact with fundamental biological processes in the human body" (BioInitiative Working Group

2014a). More specifically, questions have been raised about links between EMFs and cancer, thermal versus nonthermal effects, an increase in free radicals in the body, and a weakening of the blood–brain barrier.

Whether risk assessments accurately assess for certain conditions that develop slowly over decades, such as cancer, is yet to be determined. The WHO recognizes that, given the latency period of something like brain cancer, mobile phones are so recent that there isn't enough data to judge their health effects. On its website, the organization states:

> While an increased risk of brain tumors from the use of mobile phones is not established, the increasing use of mobile phones and the lack of data for mobile phone use over time periods longer than 15 years warrant further research of mobile phone use and brain cancer risk. In particular, with the recent popularity of mobile phone use among younger people, and therefore a potentially longer lifetime of exposure, WHO has promoted further research on this group and is currently assessing the health impact of RF fields on all studied endpoints. (WHO 2013)

How are authorities responding to the controversial science?

Some authorities—such as the CDC (CDC 2014d), Federal Communications Commission (FCC 2012), and National Cancer Institute (NCI 2013)—are waiting for more data. Others—including schools and governments—have taken precautionary measures.

The American Academy of Pediatrics urged the FCC, in an August 2013 letter, to adopt radiation standards that safeguard children's health and wellness. The letter states:

> Children are not little adults and are disproportionately impacted by all environmental exposures, including cell phone radiation. Current FCC standards do not account for the unique vulnerability and use patterns specific to pregnant women and children. It is essential that any new standard for cell phones or other wireless devices be based on protect-
> ing the youngest and most vulnerable populations to ensure they are safeguarded throughout their lifetimes. (McInergy to FCC and FDA 2013)

Organizations that advocate less WiFi in schools, such as WiFi in Schools Australia, list more than a dozen countries—including Israel, France, England, Austria, and Canada—that require schools or public areas to restrict exposures to children and advise precautions in the use of wireless technologies. Increasingly, schools are banning wireless technologies in classrooms for the youngest grades.

In May 2011, the International Agency for Research on Cancer (IARC), an arm of the World Health Organization, reclassified microwave radiation from wireless communication devices and mobile phones as a Class 2B "possible carcinogen" (IARC 2011; NCI 2013). This is the classification also given to lead, DDT, and car exhaust (IARC 2014). The American Cancer Society (2014) explains that the IARC classification indicates that there could be some risk associated with cancer, but there is not enough evidence to establish a causal link and the issue needs to be studied further.

Certain states and foreign governments recognize electromagnetic sensitivity (EMS) as an adverse health impact from EMF exposure. For example, Connecticut acknowledges EMS as a "painful chronic illness"; Sweden recognizes it as a disability, and Canada recognizes it as a handicap (Environmental Health Association of Quebec 2014). Sweden and Denmark report a higher prevalence of electromagnetic hypersensitivity than do other countries. Symptoms vary by individual but can be "disabling" for some (WHO 2005).

In the meantime, in 1996, the WHO established the International EMF Project to pursue further scientific understanding of biological effects from exposure to EMFs. More information can be found on its website (www.who.ch/peh-emf).

Have Manipulative Business Strategies been used by the telecommunications industry?

Devra Davis PhD MPH is an accomplished scientist and academic. She has counseled leading officials of the US, United Nations,

European Environment Agency, WHO, World Bank, and others. She also served as a member of the Board of Scientific Counselors of the US National Toxicology Program (Environmental Health Trust 2014).

In her book *Disconnect: The Truth About Cell Phone Radiation, What the Industry Is Doing to Hide It, and How to Protect Your Family* (2010), Davis describes strategies she says are being used by the telecommunications industry to obfuscate emerging proof of harm and to intimidate researchers and others who communicate the emerging proof—even derailing promising careers. I was struck by the similarity to the patterns of behavior examined in chapter I.12. There's also been the common reaction that "more research is needed," which allows companies more time to grow as aggressively as possible before proof of harm is established. Over time, the truth slowly prevails, but at what cost?

While proof of harm is established, EMFs proliferate

After reading about concerns regarding our EMF exposures, I wondered again about success, as I first discussed in chapter I.12: From 2005 to 2013, the number of US smartphone subscribers increased from 3.5 million to 156 million (Breslow 2014; ComScore 2014). In 2013, global mobile data traffic grew 81 percent (Cisco 2014). As of 2013, there were an estimated five million cell phone towers worldwide (Tweed 2013; Saviva Research 2013), 190,000 of them in the US (Statistic Brain 2013). Davis (2010) reported that 50 percent of 8-year-olds and 75 percent of 12-year-olds in America have a cell phone.

From several metrics, the worldwide penetration of smartphones and other technologies into our lives is a huge success. However, the health effects of chronic exposures to EMFs is yet to be determined. Will this successful penetration result in net benefits for us?

While we wait and see how safe these unprecedented EMF exposures are, I incorporate precautionary measures to reduce my family's exposure whenever is practical, especially for my children. However, the erections of cell phone towers, proliferation of WiFi routers, and the explosive growth of "smart" devices and wireless technologies create inescapable EMF exposures that even the most conscientious person can't avoid.

I recognize that EMFs are another way that we are all interconnected as cell phone towers and other people's WiFi routers and cell phones surround us. More awareness and regulation are needed to protect us, and especially our children.

Tips for a precautionary approach to EMFs are given in chapter III.6.

KEY POINTS

01. While the invention and accessibility of wireless technologies and other devices that create EMFs have provided groundbreaking benefits, the adverse health effects are unknown and will take decades to understand better.

02. Currently, the existing body of science stirs controversy, with some authorities choosing precautionary measures and others waiting for more information.

03. Many of the unique biological vulnerabilities that were discussed in chapter I.3 and the Unintentional Potential Effects that were discussed in chapter I.8 may apply to the potential health threats of EMFs.

04. We are all interconnected in this.

Chapter I.15
It's Never Too Late!

Since my first child was born, I've met dozens of babysitters. These relatively young, educated women look healthy, strong, and vibrant. I've been surprised by their sincere interest in this book's topic, since I myself wasn't interested until I became concerned for my children.

I've been further surprised after hearing about changes they made after learning more. For example, I frequently hear about skin and energy improvements from changes in diet. The words of one seemingly healthy, glowing young woman in her early 20s has stuck with me: "I just want to feel better… I want more energy."

I have a very clear memory of browsing a woman's magazine in seventh grade and being excited to read the blurbs about how the vitamins in carrots and antioxidants in berries were good for my body. I have always loved learning about what foods will serve my body well, and I have always genuinely enjoyed eating fruits, vegetables, and seafood. I grew up not enjoying meats, fried foods, and fast foods. I always enjoyed striving to be healthier.

I also grew up playing a lot of tennis. I played varsity tennis from seventh to twelfth grade and even played on a college team for a semester. In between, I walked any chance I got, did aerobics, and jogged. My weight was always on the low end of the normal range, and my other health stats— blood pressure and cholesterol—were very "healthy," as my physicians reported.

I thought I was doing all the right things: I ate well, exercised, and maintained a healthy weight. So why did I always feel bad?

Until my mid to late 20s, my energy was low and would suddenly plummet. Feeling energized and having stable energy was rare for me. I also didn't have the stamina that might be expected for someone "so healthy." My biological systems felt out of control— blood sugar, thyroid, and menstrual cycle.

Today, in my early 40s, I feel better than I did in high school. What changed?

The key differences are that the quality of my diet improved and I significantly reduced my other sources of exposure to toxicants. The improvement—for myself, my babysitters, and my friends—resulted from experimentally avoiding one thing at a time.

GET SOME PERSPECTIVE, PLEASE!

Now that I have a good understanding of the role of toxicants in my family's health, I also have a broader perspective on well-being. Figure #08 summarizes it well: Toxicants are one among several variables that you can work on for more resilient health. Just as there are many interrelated causes of diseases and disorders, there are many factors leading to vibrant health and wellness.

The rest of this book is meant to empower you with tips on how to detox your Homes. But before we get there, the intention of this chapter is to emphasize that it's never too late to start feeling better. The emerging field of epigenetics is proving it.

THE HOPE IN THE UNKNOWN

Epigenetics is a burgeoning new field of science that is identifying the mechanisms by which environmental factors turn genes on and off. Just because you have a genetic predisposition for something, like breast cancer, doesn't mean that you'll inevitably develop it, and scientists are starting to understand why.

Through epigenetic research, we're realizing that it is not only our genes that govern our health. Environmental and lifestyle factors—factors that we can control—can determine whether genes will be expressed or remain silent (Duke Medicine 2005).

THE OPPORTUNITY IN EVERY CHOICE

When I cringe at my children's past toxic exposures, I remind myself of Maya Angelou's encouraging words: "I did then what I knew how to do. Now that I know better, I do better."

Our Bodies are Resilient

when we reduce their burdens and support their inherent capabilities.

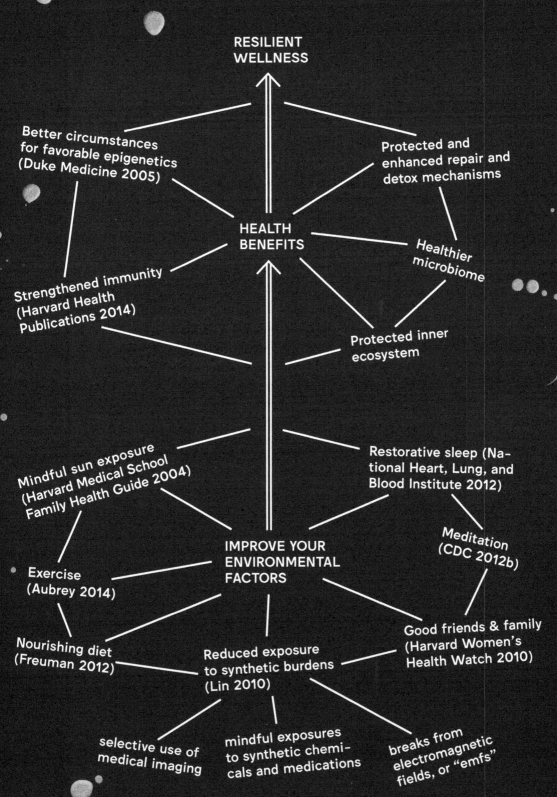

RESILIENT
WELLNESS

Better circumstances
for favorable epigenetics
(Duke Medicine 2005)

Protected and
enhanced repair and
detox mechanisms

HEALTH
BENEFITS

Healthier
microbiome

Strengthened immunity
(Harvard Health
Publications 2014)

Protected inner
ecosystem

Mindful sun exposure
(Harvard Medical School
Family Health Guide 2004)

Restorative sleep (Na-
tional Heart, Lung, and
Blood Institute 2012)

IMPROVE YOUR
ENVIRONMENTAL
FACTORS

Meditation
(CDC 2012b)

Exercise
(Aubrey 2014)

Good friends & family
(Harvard Women's
Health Watch 2010)

Nourishing diet
(Freuman 2012)

Reduced exposure
to synthetic burdens
(Lin 2010)

selective use of
medical imaging

mindful exposures
to synthetic chemi-
cals and medications

breaks from
electromagnetic
fields, or "emfs"

FIGURE #08

91

While environmental factors can promote disease, they can also nurture wellness (Duke Medicine 2005). Science is proving the opportunity in every choice. We have a lot more influence over our health than we previously understood. For example, studies on the interaction between genetics and nutrition have found that the nutrients in certain foods, such as cruciferous vegetables, can help protect against cancer (London et al. 2000; Sprouse 2014; Dashwood and Ho 2008; Zhang 2004). Diet can also help protect against toxicants (Merritt 2007). In 2007, researchers at Duke University found in animal studies that while early-life exposure to BPA could cause epigenetic damage, maternal dietary supplements—extra folate (largely found in green, leafy vegetables, like spinach) or extra genistein (found in legumes, like soy)—could counteract damaging BPA effects in offspring (Dolinoy, Huang, and Jirtle 2007; Jirtle 2012). The research is preliminary, and safe doses for humans are not yet known (Merritt 2007), since soy is also associated with estrogen-mimicking properties that can cause negative effects (O'Connor 2012). In another study, participants who drank a broccoli sprout beverage increased their excretion of the air pollutant benzene by 61 percent. This occurred from day one and was maintained throughout the 12-week study (Egner et al. 2014).

We each have a unique situation and unique sensitivities, so independent and critical thinking is important. In general, however, there's a lot that we can easily do to feel better and to position ourselves for more resilient health. It's never too late to reap the benefits from detoxing your choices! D-Tox, baby!

KEY POINTS

01. It's never too late to start improving your comfort, health, and energy!

02. Epigenetics is proving that environmental factors affect gene expression. Preliminary studies suggest that environmental factors can steer health toward wellness or disease.

03. If you're pregnant or hoping to become pregnant some day, then detoxing your choices is particularly meaningful because healthy choices can give your children—and maybe grandchildren—a healthier start.

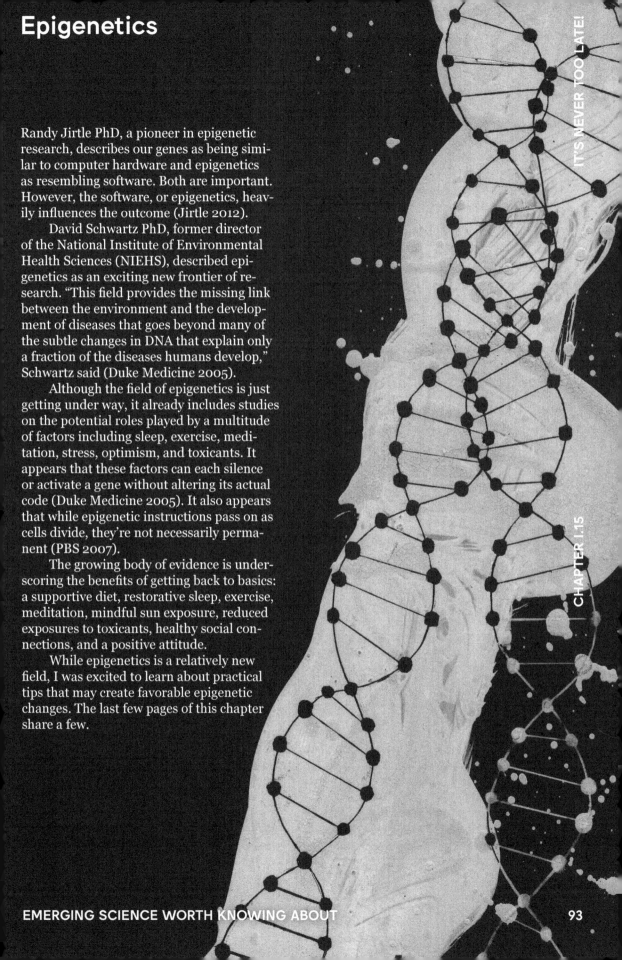

Epigenetics

Randy Jirtle PhD, a pioneer in epigenetic research, describes our genes as being similar to computer hardware and epigenetics as resembling software. Both are important. However, the software, or epigenetics, heavily influences the outcome (Jirtle 2012).

David Schwartz PhD, former director of the National Institute of Environmental Health Sciences (NIEHS), described epigenetics as an exciting new frontier of research. "This field provides the missing link between the environment and the development of diseases that goes beyond many of the subtle changes in DNA that explain only a fraction of the diseases humans develop," Schwartz said (Duke Medicine 2005).

Although the field of epigenetics is just getting under way, it already includes studies on the potential roles played by a multitude of factors including sleep, exercise, meditation, stress, optimism, and toxicants. It appears that these factors can each silence or activate a gene without altering its actual code (Duke Medicine 2005). It also appears that while epigenetic instructions pass on as cells divide, they're not necessarily permanent (PBS 2007).

The growing body of evidence is underscoring the benefits of getting back to basics: a supportive diet, restorative sleep, exercise, meditation, mindful sun exposure, reduced exposures to toxicants, healthy social connections, and a positive attitude.

While epigenetics is a relatively new field, I was excited to learn about practical tips that may create favorable epigenetic changes. The last few pages of this chapter share a few.

Fetal Origins

If you're pregnant, then your choices have special influence. And that influence may be even greater than you think: Fetal origins, another burgeoning field of science, is tracing adult-onset diseases to the prenatal period (Jirtle 2012).

As Annie Murphy Paul explains in her book *Origins: How the Nine Months Before Birth Shape the Rest of Our Lives*, a growing body of evidence is showing that in utero conditions—resulting from what your mother ingested, inhaled, and absorbed, as well as her emotional wellness—shape our lifelong vulnerability to disease, our appetite and metabolism, and our intelligence and temperament (Paul 2011).

THE BARKER HYPOTHESIS

One of the first milestones in the study of fetal origins of disease is associated with David J. Barker MD PhD. In 1989, after studying some 15,000 adults, Barker concluded that those born with low birth weight—often an indication of poor prenatal nutrition—were at greater risk for heart disease as adults (Barker et al. 1989). Barker theorized that with an inadequate food supply, "the fetus diverts nutrients to its most important organ, the brain, while skimping on other parts of its body—a debt that comes due decades later in the form of a weakened heart," according to an article by Paul, "The Womb. Your Mother. Yourself." (Paul 2010b). In 1995, the *British Medical Journal* dubbed this idea the "Barker Hypothesis."

Today, the Barker Foundation, which was headed by Barker until his passing in 2013, aims to improve the growth and development of babies and young children by promoting varied and balanced diets for girls and young women. The foundation's website (TheBarkerFoundation.org) lists the following as areas of further study for fetal origins: coronary heart disease, high blood pressure, stroke, type II diabetes and obesity, aging, osteoporosis, and breast and ovarian cancer.

STUDIES ON THE IMPACT OF SEVERE MALNUTRITION AND STRESS

Other studies have examined the development of schizophrenia in people who experienced extreme malnutrition and stress prenatally. Although the causes of schizophrenia are highly complex and not fully understood, a study based on 30 years of case records from Anhui Province in China indicate that prenatal factors might play a role. During China's Great Leap Forward in the mid-20th century, individuals living in that region experienced severe malnutrition due to famine. In comparison to children who were born at other times, children born of women who endured the famine were twice as likely to develop schizophrenia (Paul 2010a; St. Clair et al. 2005). Similarly, assessment of the health records of over 88,000 people born in Jerusalem between 1964 and 1976 found that the children of women who were in their second month of pregnancy in June 1967—the highly stressful time of the Six Day War—had a much higher likelihood of developing schizophrenia as young adults (Paul 2010a; Malaspina et al. 2008). According to Randy Jirtle PhD (2012), scientists who studied individuals born during or just after the Dutch famine of 1944–1945 found a doubling in the number of schizophrenia cases among those exposed to prenatal nutritional deficiency.

CHRONIC DISEASES MAY HAVE FETAL ORIGINS

In 1988, Theo Colborn PhD conducted groundbreaking research on the environmental pollution in and around the Great Lakes, which revealed that persistent synthetic chemicals were being transferred from mothers to offspring and causing harm in utero (Colborn, Dumanoski, and Myers 1997). She founded the Endocrine Disruption Exchange (TEDX), a nonprofit dedicated to sharing the latest science-based evidence on the impacts of EDCs on health (TEDX 2014a).

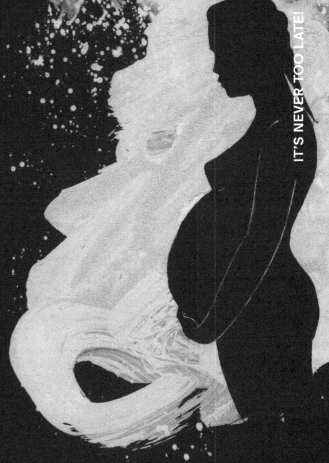

In researching the possible prenatal origins of cancer, TEDX reviewed more than 750 published articles—some 600 scientific studies and 150 review articles and commentaries spanning the years 1972 to 2007—focused on a wide range of environmental exposures and maternal factors such as illness and medication. The group found that increases in postnatal cancers were associated with maternal exposure to smoking, pesticides, radiation, industrial chemicals and fuels, metals, toxins in food and water, medication, alcohol, and recreational drugs (TEDX 2007). Collectively, the scientific community has found that exposure to EDCs during fetal life and puberty is linked to cancers (WHO and UNEP 2013; TEDX 2007).

In addition to cancer, the list of chronic diseases that are being associated with fetal exposure to EDCs is long. They include abnormal male gonadal development, infertility, ADHD, autism, intellectual impairment, diabetes, thyroid disorders (TEDX 2014b), cardiovascular disease, allergies, asthma, hypertension, diabetes, obesity, and mental illness (Paul 2010a), as well as conditions associated with old age like arthritis, osteoporosis, and cognitive decline (Paul 2011).

During the prenatal period, a mother's hormones direct the formation of her child's brain, heart, and other organs. Therefore, exposure to EDCs—even at minuscule levels—can cause permanent changes in the wiring and functioning of these organs, potentially positioning the body for health issues later in life. Accordingly, the WHO and UNEP 2013 report recommends, "endocrine disease prevention should begin with maternal and fetal health."

There is growing concern that maternal, fetal and childhood exposure to EDCs could play a larger role in the causation of many endocrine diseases and disorders [such as those in figure #02] than previously believed. (WHO and UNEP 2013)

EFFECTS CAN PERSIST THROUGH GENERATIONS

It turns out that pregnant women have unique influence not only on the foundation of their children's health, but also on their *future grandchildren*. Scientists have discovered that epigenetic changes can persist through generations (PBS 2007). For example, Michael K. Skinner PhD led a study on the impact of rats' fetal exposure to dioxins. The study revealed an increased incidence of multiple diseases in the first generation of exposed rats, and epigenetic changes persisted into the third generation (Manikkam et al. 2012; NIEHS 2012). The WHO and UNEP 2013 report also acknowledged that these epigenetic changes could persist into future generations of *people* and wildlife. So not only should a pregnant woman take special care of herself during this special time, but those around her should also treat her like a queen! The emerging proof that some epigenetic effects are transgenerational is another aspect of health that I hope society and lawmakers will recognize and address.

The Opportunity...

...in every bite

Nutritional epigenetics is a growing field of science that studies how nutrients affect gene expression. Researchers are finding nutrition to be "an attractive tool to prevent pediatric developmental diseases and cancer as well as to delay aging-associated processes," according to an article, "Epigenetics: A New Bridge between Nutrition and Health," published in Advances in Nutrition (Choi and Friso 2010).

Diet may protect against toxicants!
Extra folate (found in green leafy vegetables) may counteract the damaging effects of BPA in exposed offspring (Dolinoy, Huang, and Jirtle 2007; Jirtle 2012).

Omega-3 fatty acids
Found in fish, eggs, nuts, oils, some produce, and leafy greens, omega-3 fatty acids can offset the toxic effects of lead and mercury (EWG 2008).

Iron and calcium
Children with sufficient iron and calcium absorb less lead (EPA 2012b). Iron-deficient bodies are more likely to absorb cadmium, too (ATSDR 2012). Eggs, red meats, and beans are rich in iron. Green vegetables and beans offer calcium.

Iodine
Both the Institute of Medicine (Pearce 2008) and the EWG (2008) recommend higher levels of iodine during pregnancy and nursing because iodine can protect against perchlorate, which can disrupt thyroid functions and affect brain development during pregnancy and infancy.

Breast milk
Breast milk is the optimal nourishment for your child. According to the EWG (2008), breast milk helps protect babies from toxic chemicals.

...in every thought

Researchers at the Benson–Henry Institute for Mind Body Medicine at Massachusetts General Hospital, one of Harvard Medical School's teaching hospitals, have been studying how mind-body technologies can positively influence genes that are linked to stress and immunity (Bhasin et al. 2013). Through neuroimaging and genomics technology, they're proving that yoga and meditation can ward off disease. Other research has found that meditation can help prevent cardiovascular disease (Koike and Cardoso 2014).

Do yoga and meditate!

"Change Your Mind. Change the World."
— Center for Investigating Healthy Minds (2014), University of Wisconsin-Madison

Richard J. Davidson PhD, a world-renowned neuroscientist, is pioneering research that's showing how adaptable our brains are to our thoughts, behaviors and experiences. Recognized by *Time* magazine in 2006 as one of the 100 most influential people in the world, Davidson examines the biology of emotions and the brain's ability to change through experiences, mental training, and contemplative practices. His research has shown that qualities of the mind—kindness, compassion, altruism, forgiveness, mindfulness and well-being—can have a "robust and measurable effect on brain function and structure" (Affective and Clinical Neuroscience Laboratory 2014). For example, meditation can strengthen brain circuitry that is associated with happiness and positive behavior (Gilgoff 2010).

...in your attitude

Cultivate emotional vitality!

Laura Kubzansky PhD MPH, a professor of social and behavior sciences at the Harvard School of Public Health (HSPH), has been researching how emotions influence the development of diseases, including cardiovascular disease, lung function decline, and cancer (HSPH 2014). From a study that followed more than 6,000 men and women over 20 years, she found that enthusiasm, hope, engagement in life, and the ability to face stress with emotional balance appear to reduce the risk of coronary heart disease (Rimer 2011).

Another article published by the HSPH, "The biology of emotion—and what it may teach us about helping people to live longer," explains that a "vast scientific literature has detailed how negative emotions harm the body. Serious, sustained stress or fear can alter biological systems in a way that, over time, adds up to 'wear and tear' and, eventually, illnesses such as heart disease, stroke, and diabetes. Chronic anger and anxiety can disrupt cardiac function by changing the heart's electrical stability, hastening atherosclerosis, and increasing systematic inflammation" (Rimer 2011).

Be optimistic!
Researchers say that optimistic children may have fewer illnesses in adulthood. For example, Laura Kubzanky found that "optimism cuts the risk of coronary heart disease by half" (Rimer 2011).

Hug and connect!
Hugs and physical affection are also healthful. For example, when a mother rat withholds nurturing licks from its pup, that elicits a brain change that impairs the pup's response to stress as an adult (Duke Medicine 2005).
Studies show that people who are more "socially integrated" live longer and are healthier by a number of metrics (Cohen 2001).

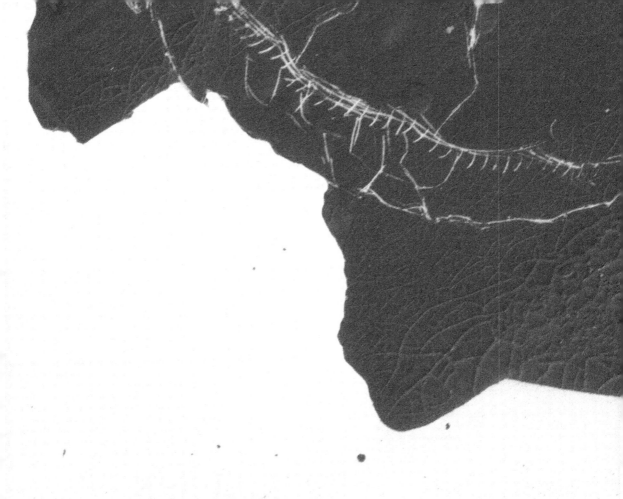

Part II

Household Repeat Offenders

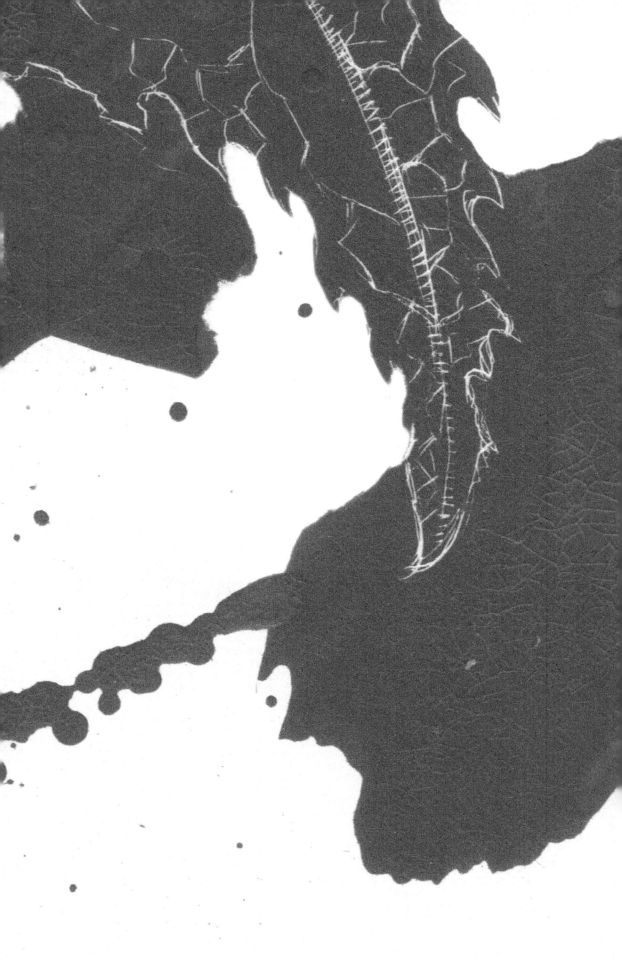

Part II Introduction

In the ancient language of Sanskrit, the term *avidya* refers to our inaccurate understanding or perception of reality or truth. T.K.V. Desikachar, an influential yogi and son of the great yoga master Sri Tirumalai Krishnamacharya, explains in his popular book *The Heart of Yoga: Developing a Personal Practice*:

> Avidya can be understood as the accumulated result of our many unconscious responses, the actions and ways of perceiving that we have been mechanically carrying out for years. As a result of those unconscious responses, the mind becomes more and more dependent on habits until we accept the actions of yesterday as the norms of today.... These habits cover the mind with avidya, as if obscuring the clarity of consciousness with a filmy layer.

I often thought of this term as I researched and completed part I. The information in part I helped clear up some of my avidya as it relates to consumer products, health, and our environment. I realized that my lifelong habits and preferences were formed as unconscious reactions to my cumulative exposures to advertising and marketing claims as well as from common practices of those around me. After becoming more informed by my research for this book, I have significantly reduced my exposure to many *conventional* things that were once part of my daily life, such as fragranced lotions and hair products, perfume, scented candles, aerosol and powdered products, and certain prepackaged foods.

Part II, intended to be referenced over time, provides informational building blocks through what I call "Household Repeat Offenders." The Household Repeat Offenders create an educational framework from which we can begin to make choices from a more informed understanding of the products we invite into our Homes. Even just skimming the details in part II will impress upon you the complex chemistry that creates our household products and built environments as well as the complex Unintentional Potential Effects, explained in chapter I.8, to which toxicants in products may contribute.

CONFUSION PROTECTS THE STATUS QUO

In evaluating which products may pose harm, my research taught me that the devil is in the details. However, even if you have the dedication to figure them out, you'll encounter a huge hurdle: lack of disclosure by manufacturers on what is in our products and what potential health risks they may pose. Moreover, some companies intentionally confuse consumers. Not only will companies and industries obscure emerging proof of harm, as chapter I.12 describes, but they will use labeling to confuse consumers.

In the spring of 2014, I was on a webinar hosted by the Sustainable Furnishings Council. The topic was greenwashing and how manufacturers of products could label responsibly. I learned that manufacturers use more than 430 labels—including "eco-friendly," "nontoxic," and "green." Some of these labels don't meet any standards, and others can't be verified. Sometimes they're simply not true.

WHAT'S A CONSUMER TO DO?

Becoming familiar with Household Repeat Offenders should help you navigate the confusion. The concept of Household Repeat Offenders was inspired by the understanding that ingredients create food. For example, just as most breads, cakes, cupcakes, and cookies result from a combination of flour, eggs, and sugar, many household products (like upholstered furniture and mattresses) are produced from pressed wood, adhesives, polyurethane foam, synthetic dyes, and conventional textiles.

Once you decide to avoid one type of component (or more) for health reasons, that avoidance acts as a filter, leaving you

Household Repeat Offenders (Part II)

II.1: TOXICANTS
No consumer-friendly indications on product labels

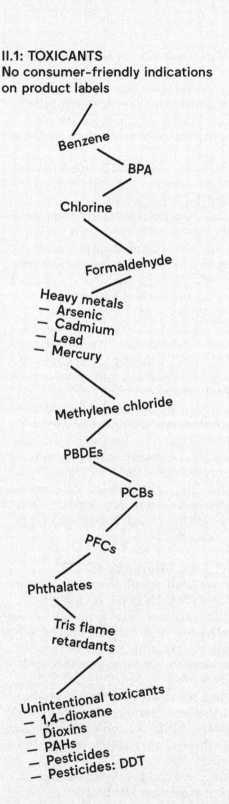

Benzene

BPA

Chlorine

Formaldehyde

Heavy metals
— Arsenic
— Cadmium
— Lead
— Mercury

Methylene chloride

PBDEs

PCBs

PFCs

Phthalates

Tris flame retardants

Unintentional toxicants
— 1,4-dioxane
— Dioxins
— PAHs
— Pesticides
— Pesticides: DDT

II.2: INGREDIENTS
Indications on product labels

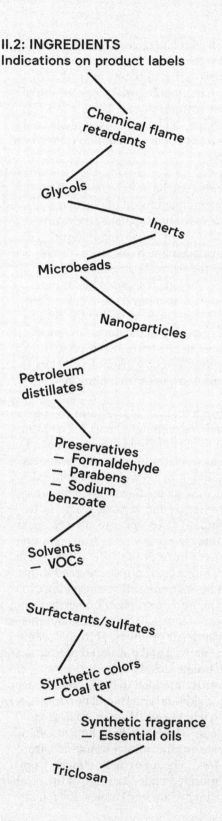

Chemical flame retardants

Glycols

Inerts

Microbeads

Nanoparticles

Petroleum distillates

Preservatives
— Formaldehyde
— Parabens
— Sodium benzoate

Solvents
— VOCs

Surfactants/sulfates

Synthetic colors
— Coal tar

Synthetic fragrance
— Essential oils

Triclosan

Tips (Part III)

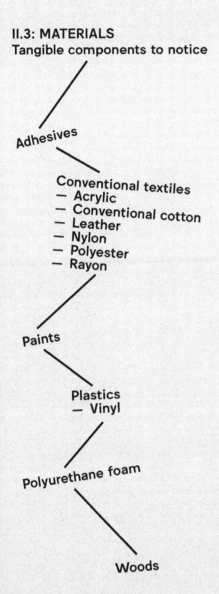

II.3: MATERIALS
Tangible components to notice

Adhesives

Conventional textiles
— Acrylic
— Conventional cotton
— Leather
— Nylon
— Polyester
— Rayon

Paints

Plastics
— Vinyl

Polyurethane foam

Woods

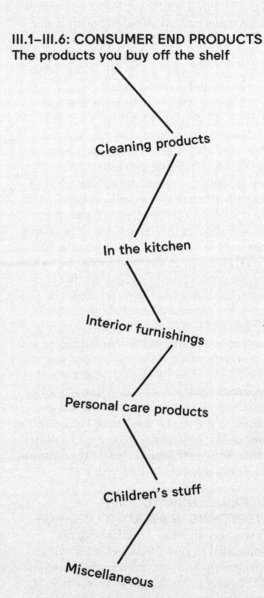

III.1–III.6: CONSUMER END PRODUCTS
The products you buy off the shelf

Cleaning products

In the kitchen

Interior furnishings

Personal care products

Children's stuff

Miscellaneous

with fewer (generally healthier) options. For example, in our diets, there are many kinds of sugar, including high-fructose corn syrup, brown rice syrup, cane syrup, agave, and maple syrup. When you decide to avoid one type of sugar, then that automatically eliminates many options. Similarly, with household products, once you decide to avoid certain ingredients and materials that pose risks, you will strategically filter out riskier purchases and possessions.

There are three main categories of Household Repeat Offenders: Toxicants of Concern, Ingredients of Concern, and Materials of Concern. These categories can be considered during different stages of manufacturing. For example, toxicants are generally chosen at the earliest stages when chemical formulas are created, ingredients are a product of the chemical formulas, and materials are a product of the ingredients. Part III focuses on the "end products," which are the products consumers buy, that contain these Household Repeat Offenders.

Overall, these Household Repeat Offenders will help you critically assess your purchases and edit your surroundings so you can declutter from a more informed perspective. This framework should inspire insightful questions as you navigate greenwashing and other marketing strategies; it will also empower you so you don't need to depend on lists, books, or websites to create a healthier home. Your confidence in your own common sense and instincts will strengthen too.

WARNING: HOW YOU SEE EVERYTHING IS ABOUT TO CHANGE
As you become more familiar with the Household Repeat Offenders, your avidya will clear up and you will become conscious of infinitely more things. Your fascination, curiosity, and awe of both human achievements and nature's brilliancy may grow too, as they did for me.

Chapter II.1
Toxicants of Concern

Chapter II.1, "Household Toxicants of Concern," includes some of the most common and pervasive household toxicants that I encountered. Their presence is not necessarily obvious from information disclosed on product labels; however, they can be detected in products from the ingredients and materials highlighted in chapters II.2 and II.3. You'll find these Household Repeat Offenders throughout part III as well.

THE INTENTIONS OF CHAPTER II.1

— Provide examples of the toxicants discussed in part I. These ingredients may be difficult to identify in the items in your home because they aren't necessarily noted on product labels.

— Highlight benefits of reducing our exposures to these types of toxicants. As you get to know them, remember the Unintentional Potential Effects.

— Spotlight products that may contain these toxicants to inform your instincts.

— Provide further explanation for why the D-Tox plan in part IV and the Simple Strategies in part III are worth incorporating.

Name of the subject Toxicant of Concern

OVERVIEW

This section provides a brief description of the subject toxicant. Even though certain toxicants are, and will continue to be, phased out of certain products, it's important to consider the track record of safety for replacement chemicals and their potential adverse health effects. Sometimes, as part I explained, substitute chemicals are similar in structure and toxicity to the toxic chemicals they replaced.

POSSIBLE HEALTH EFFECTS

While evidence is limited (but emerging), I share the potential adverse health effects I've discovered in my research.

POSSIBLE SOURCES OF EXPOSURE

Here I provide examples of products that may contain the subject toxicant. Being told that something is common isn't the same as realizing in which specific household products the Toxicant of Concern may reside.

This list is not comprehensive and the Toxicant of Concern may not necessarily be in the listed items. You can learn more by checking with individual manufacturers.

A CLOSER LOOK AT SOME TOXICANTS OF CONCERN

Specifically of certain heavy metals and Unintentional Toxicants.

TIPS

Information to help you reduce your exposures to the profiled toxicant.

EXPLANATION OF THE FORMAT

Benzene

OVERVIEW

Benzene is a clear, colorless, flammable liquid with a gasoline-like odor. Produced from coal and petroleum, benzene is commonly used by the chemical and pharmaceutical industries.

Benzene is a common air pollutant that is released from oil refineries, coal and oil combustion, gasoline vapors at gas stations, vehicle emissions, cigarette smoke, wood-burning fires, some adhesives, and other sources. Indoor concentrations of benzene are significant contributors to children's exposures, particularly in homes where people smoke.

POSSIBLE HEALTH EFFECTS

Benzene is a known carcinogen linked to several types of cancer, including leukemia, breast, lymphatic, and hematopoietic (Physicians for Social Responsibility 2015). According to the Worldwatch Institute, benzene can damage chromosomes (McGinn 2000).

POSSIBLE SOURCES OF EXPOSURE

We are exposed to benzene by breathing contaminated air and ingesting contaminated water. The main indoor sources of benzene are automobile exhaust in attached garages, environmental tobacco smoke, off-gassing fuels, and paint supplies. Benzene can also migrate through soil and foundations to enter basements or living spaces.

Contaminated Water
When contaminated groundwater is used indoors for dishwashing, laundry, or showering, benzene can contaminate indoor air. (EPA 2009a).

Exhaust
Motor vehicles.

Smoke
Cigarette smoke, and wood-burning fires.

Solvents
Degreasing products, developing agents, dyes, films, furniture waxes, gasoline, glues, lubricants, nylons, paints, and various other shop and industrial compounds.

BPA

OVERVIEW

BPA (bisphenol-A) was invented in 1891 as scientists were working to invent synthetic estrogen. It was not until the 1940s, however, that BPA became popular among manufacturers due to its ability to harden polycarbonate plastics. Since the 1960s, BPA has also been used to prevent metal cans from corroding or reacting with food (NY DOH 2011). By 2014, as a result of consumer concerns, BPA had been replaced in many products; however, the substitute chemicals are not necessarily safer and may be similar to BPA in chemical structure and toxicity (Bilbrey 2014).

Biomonitoring studies estimate that BPA is present in the bodies of most people (CDC 2013b), including in umbilical cord blood and breast milk (Gerona et al. 2013; Mendonca et al. 2014).

POSSIBLE HEALTH EFFECTS

Even with more than 800 studies on the potential health effects of BPA, more research is needed to understand the complex and wide-ranging impact of this ubiquitous chemical. BPA may contribute to altered sociosexual behavior (Porrini et al. 2005); asthma (Donohue et al. 2013); developmental disorders, such as attention deficit hyperactivity disorder (ADHD) and autism (Harley et al. 2013; Kaur et al. 2014); breast, uterine, and prostate cancer (Bienkowski 2014; Hiroi et al. 2004; Bienkowski and *Environmental Health News* 2014); reproductive system issues and changes for men and women (TEDX 2009; Weil 2012; Newbold, Jefferson, and Banks 2007; Henry 2013); diabetes (Alonso-Magdalena et al. 2010); heart disease (Melzer et al. 2012); increased aggressiveness (Perera et al. 2012); increased susceptibility to drugs of addiction (Jones and Miller 2008); inflammatory and autoimmune diseases (WHO and UNEP 2013); and obesity (Trasande, Attina, and Blustein 2012).

Of particular concern is the impact on fetuses, babies, and young children (NIEHS 2015). The EPA (2015a) reported that "because BPA is a reproductive, developmental, and systemic toxicant in animal studies and is weakly estrogenic, there are questions about its potential impact particularly on children's health and the environment." In 2008, the National Toxicology Program reported "some concern for effects on the brain, behavior, and prostate gland in fetuses, infants, and children at current human exposures to bisphenol A" (NTP 2008).

POSSIBLE SOURCES OF EXPOSURE

Epoxy Resins
Some adhesives, canned foods and beverages, composites, dairy equipment, dental materials, electrical laminates for printed circuit boards, metal parts of cars, office equipment, paints, pipes, protective coatings. The FDA banned BPA in infant formula in 2013 "because this use has been abandoned. FDA's action is based solely on a determination of abandonment and is not related to the safety of BPA" (FDA 2014a).

Food
Since BPA can leach from food and drink containers and is prevalent throughout our environment, diet is a major source of exposure. BPA leaches relatively easily into our foods and drinks and onto our hands as it is released from BPA-containing plastic and metal containers. Leaching occurs when BPA is broken down by detergents; heat from dishwashers, hot water, and microwaves; and normal wear and tear (WHO and UNEP 2013). Young children may have additional exposure due to putting things in their mouths more often than adults do (CDC 2013a).

Paper
BPA coats some types of paper (e.g., receipts from ATMs and cash registers, and carbonless and recycled paper).

Polycarbonate Plastic (#7):
Some automobiles, baby bottles, dental materials, digital media (e.g., CDs, DVDs), electrical and electronic equipment, eyeglasses, drink and food containers, medical devices, sports safety equipment, tableware, and water pipes.

PVC Vinyl (#3)
Some art and school supplies, cable and electrical wires, lunch bags, medical devices, rainwear, shower curtains, and toys.

Chlorine

OVERVIEW

Highly reactive, chlorine gas was the first chemical warfare agent used on a large scale during World War I. Today it is among the 10 highest-volume chemicals manufactured in the US. The EPA considers chlorine a pesticide (a disinfectant or an antimicrobial pesticide, to be exact) because of its ability to kill bacteria and viruses. Since it kills fungi and molds, the EPA also considers it a fungicide (EPA 2014b).

Chlorine has a variety of uses. It is widely found in solvents, pesticides, synthetic rubbers, re-frigerants, and cleaning products. It's commonly used as a bleaching agent in paper and cloth production. And household bleach is just chlorine diluted by water. Due to its antimicrobial and antifungal properties, it is commonly used to kill bacteria in drinking and swimming pool water, in sanitizing industrial waste and sewage, in foot baths, and, according to the EPA, even in the processing of food items including meat, fish, vegetables, fruits, and dairy. The EPA also notes that it's used in special batteries containing lithium or zinc (EPA 1994).

POSSIBLE HEALTH EFFECTS

When chlorine reacts with other compounds, potentially harmful Unintentional By-products may form. For instance, chlorine can form trihalomethanes when combined with naturally occurring matter (EPA 2013h). Trihalomethanes have strong links to bladder cancer, and are also suspected of being associated with colon and rectal cancer (Villanueva et al. 2004; EWG 2013).

POSSIBLE SOURCES OF EXPOSURE

The inhalation of chlorine gas is the most common exposure route, since chlorine becomes a gas at room temperature.

Cleaning Products
People using chlorine-containing household products, such as laundry bleach and swimming pool chemicals, are usually not exposed to chlorine gas. However, someone could be exposed to harmful levels if these household products are mixed with acid-containing household products, such as toilet bowl cleaners, or ammonia-containing household products like glass, metal, and oven cleaners.

Others
Drinking water, food, PVC vinyl (#3), and swimming pools.

Formaldehyde

OVERVIEW

Formaldehyde is a common volatile organic compound (VOC), meaning it exists as a gas at room temperature. Colorless and pungent-smelling, it is a chemical that is widely used by industries to manufacture building materials and various components of household products. Formaldehyde is also an Unintentional By-product that is created by combustion and other natural processes. Therefore, formaldehyde can be present in both indoor and outdoor environments.

Indoor formaldehyde levels depend primarily on the source, temperature, humidity, and air exchange rate (the rate at which outdoor air enters the indoor area). Therefore, indoor formaldehyde levels may change with the seasons and throughout the day: Levels may increase when temperatures and humidity are high, and may be lower on cooler, less-humid days. Being aware of these factors is important when one measures levels of formaldehyde (CPSC 2013). Some sources— such as pressed wood products containing urea-formaldehyde glues, urea-formaldehyde foam insulation, durable-press fabrics, and draperies—release more formaldehyde when new. As time passes, the formaldehyde released from these products and materials decreases.

POSSIBLE HEALTH EFFECTS

Formaldehyde has a vast array of potential negative health effects, including immune system toxicity, respiratory irritation, and cancer in humans (*National Geographic* 2008). Formaldehyde is recognized as a human carcinogen by the IARC (IARC 2004), and a neurotoxicant and developmental toxicant (EWG 2015k).

POSSIBLE SOURCES OF EXPOSURE

Adhesives
Phenol-formaldehyde and urea-formaldehyde.

Building Materials
Coatings, furniture (cabinets, dressers, shelves), insulation materials (fiberglass insulation and urea-formaldehyde foam insulation), paints, and subflooring.

Combustion Products
Auto exhaust, emissions from appliances (like gas stoves or space heaters) that burn fuels such as kerosene or natural gas, tobacco smoke, and wood smoke.

Composite Woods
Decorative wall coverings, hardwood and plywood paneling, medium-density fiberboards (MDF), particleboards, and pressed woods.

Home Furnishings
Durable- or permanent-press fabrics used in drapes and other home textiles.

Indoor Air
It is a major source of exposure for children (EPA 2007a).

Personal Care Products
Cosmetics, and hair straighteners. (Formaldehyde was once mixed into many personal care products as an antiseptic, but this use has declined.)

Others
May be in coatings for paper products, such as some wet-strength items, and as a disinfectant and preservative.

Heavy Metals

OVERVIEW

Heavy metals occur naturally, but human activity has boosted their concentrations. Some are toxic even at low concentrations, and some can cross the placenta and damage the fetal brain. Infants and young children are particularly vulnerable. Their exposure to some metals has been associated with learning difficulties, memory impairment, damage to the nervous system, and behavioral problems like aggressiveness and hyperactivity. Irreversible brain damage can occur from exposure to higher doses. Contaminated food can be a major source of exposure, and even more so for children than adults, "since they consume more food for their body weight than adults" (Imo et al. 2014).

The next few pages spotlight heavy metals that I found most frequently in my research of household products: mercury, lead, arsenic, and cadmium.

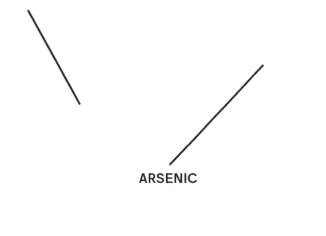

ARSENIC

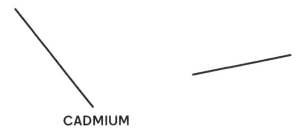

CADMIUM

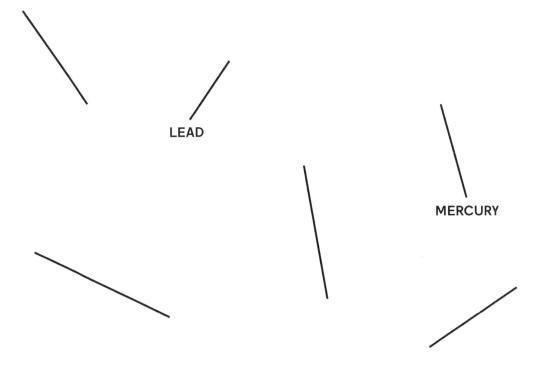

LEAD

MERCURY

Heavy Metals: Arsenic

ARSENIC OVERVIEW

Arsenic is a naturally occurring metal, but people have higher levels of exposure than nature intended because of human activities.

According to the EPA, food is a major source of exposure to arsenic for most individuals (EPA 2013b). There has not been US regulation of arsenic in food, but the FDA has been investigating this further since diet may introduce significant exposures to arsenic. Arsenic is also found in drinking water.

POSSIBLE HEALTH EFFECTS

Arsenic is a carcinogen and has been linked to a number of adverse health effects, including skin lesions, developmental effects, cardiovascular disease, neurotoxicity and diabetes (WHO 2012).

POSSIBLE SOURCES OF EXPOSURE

Diet

Fish, rice, rice products, and water are common sources of exposure (Meharg, Deacon, et al. 2008; Meharg, Sun, et al. 2008; Williams et al. 2005). Rice is incorporated into many foods (sometimes in the form of organic brown rice syrup); and they (such as cereals, crackers, and rice drinks) can be significant dietary sources of arsenic (Sun et al. 2009; Meharg, Deacon, et al. 2008).

Young children are especially vulnerable to dietary arsenic exposure because of their greater food consumption relative to their body weight (Alexander et al. 2009). Infants fed rice cereal at least once daily may exceed the daily arsenic exposure limit of 0.17 μg/kg body weight (Meharg, Sun, et al. 2008).

Other

Tobacco.

Heavy Metals: Cadmium

CADMIUM OVERVIEW

A naturally occurring metal, cadmium is used in batteries, pigments, coatings, platings, stabilizers for plastics, and other applications. It's also been used as a substitute for lead in consumer products.

Cadmium is so pervasive that diet is the main source of exposure for nonsmokers in the US (ATSDR 2015b).

POSSIBLE HEALTH EFFECTS

Chronic exposure to low levels of cadmium can lead to kidney damage. It can also weaken bones.

Prenatal exposure may impair learning and behavior. According to HealthyStuff.org (2015), "cadmium exposure is associated in animal studies with developmental effects, including possible decreases in birth weight, delayed sensory-motor development, hormonal effects, and altered behavior."

Cadmium is also recognized as a human carcinogen by the US Department of Health and Human Services and the IARC. The EPA has stated that cadmium is a probable human carcinogen (ATSDR 2015b).

POSSIBLE SOURCES OF EXPOSURE

Diet
Cadmium is found in leafy vegetables such as lettuce and spinach, as well as in grains, peanuts, potatoes, soybeans, and sunflower seeds.

Smoking
Tobacco leaves accumulate cadmium. Smokers have been found to have roughly twice as much cadmium in their bodies as nonsmokers (ATSDR 2015b).

Toys
Clothing accessories, jewelry, and some toys that are treated with paint and surface coatings.

Heavy Metals: Lead

LEAD OVERVIEW

Commonly found in rocks and soils worldwide, lead is a toxic metal that was widely used in consumer products. Lead cannot be detected through the use of sight, smell, or taste.

Although the US banned lead from paint and gasoline in the 1970s, it still pervades our environment and is still found in a wide variety of consumer products, including children's items. Even children who seem healthy can have high levels of lead in their bodies (HUD 2003).

POSSIBLE HEALTH EFFECTS

According to Melissa Hendricks (2000), former senior science writer for *Johns Hopkins Magazine*, "Breathing or swallowing lead particles or dust can cause serious neurological impairments … resulting in delayed physical and mental development, lower IQ, and reduced attention span. At high levels, lead can cause convulsions, coma, and death." The EPA considers lead a probable human carcinogen (EPA 2013d).

Lead can affect all organs, particularly the brain and nervous system and the cardiovascular, gastrointestinal, renal, endocrine, immune, and hematological systems. For the developing brain, low levels of lead exposure can cause permanent loss of intelligence, shortened attention span, and behavioral disorders. During critical periods of development, lead exposure can cause other permanent damage as well (WHO 2010a).

Risk is highest for fetuses and for children up to six years old (California Department of Public Health 2015). For them, there is no safe level of exposure (CDC 2013c).

POSSIBLE SOURCES OF EXPOSURE

Air
Lead can be emitted into the air from industrial sources and leaded aviation fuel.

Drinking Water
This can be contaminated from plumbing that has lead or lead solder. (If you think your plumbing has lead in it, let your water run a few minutes before using, and use only cold water for cooking and drinking.)

Dust and Soil
Dust and outdoor soil may contain lead from exterior paint or other sources, such as leaded gasoline used in the past. Indoor dust can contain lead from soil tracked into the home on the bottom of shoes.

Folk Remedies
Azarcon and greta (used to ease upset stomachs) and other traditional medicines may contain lead.

Hobbies
Creating pottery or stained glass, or refinishing furniture, may expose you to lead.

In the Kitchen
Lead may be used in crystal or in glazes for porcelain or pottery. Food may also be contaminated with lead from both the natural environment and through food packaging, food processing, and other storage materials.

Lead Paint
In homes built before 1978, paint remains a key source of lead for many children. Approximately 38 million homes in the US still have lead-based paint. In most cases, if this paint is in good condition, it is not a hazard.

Occupational Exposure
Jobs in construction and those involving batteries, heavy metals, paints, and pottery carry risk of exposure to lead.

PVC
This can be found in children's rain coats, electrical cords (being phased out), flooring, older window blinds, shower curtains, toys, wallpapers, and more.

Renovations
These can disturb lead from paint, distributing it into the environment.

Toys and Furniture
Some imported and old painted items pose a risk.

Heavy Metals: Mercury

MERCURY OVERVIEW

Mercury is a naturally occurring heavy metal. There are three types: elemental, inorganic, and organic.

Naturally found in rock and soil, mercury is also created from industrial processes, including the burning of fossil fuels and solid wastes. Disposal of mercury-containing products also increases its environmental presence. As a result of its prevalence in our environment, mercury is found throughout our diet.

POSSIBLE HEALTH EFFECTS

Mercury, a neurotoxin, is considered toxic in any form (EPA 2013f). The American Academy of Pediatrics has recommended minimizing exposure to any form of mercury to optimize children's health and nervous system development (Goldman, Shannon, and the Committee on Environmental Health 2001). According to NIEHS and EPA (2013), prenatal exposure to mercury and other heavy metals may also contribute to congenital malformations and miscarriage.

POSSIBLE SOURCES OF EXPOSURE

Diet

Food is the main exposure source. Mercury is found in fish (especially predators) and processed foods. Some studies have found mercury in high-fructose corn syrup (HFCS), which is in many processed foods (Dufault et al. 2009; Wallinga et al. 2009). Common foods that contain HFCS include baked goods, beverages (fruit juices and soft drinks), breads, breakfast bars, cereals, crackers, fruit yogurts, ketchups, lunch meats, salad dressings, soups, and many foods marketed to children, like candy and macaroni and cheese.

Medical Pharmaceutical Products

Antibiotics, contact lens' solutions, ear and eye drops/eye ointments, hemorrhoid relief ointments, nasal sprays, and thermometers.

Personal Care Products

Lotions, mascaras, skin creams, and soaps.

Others

Certain appliances, automotive parts, electronics, imported necklaces with glass pendants, lamps, and light bulbs.

Methylene Chloride

OVERVIEW

Methylene chloride, also known as dichloromethane, is a colorless liquid that emits a mild and sweet odor. It evaporates easily but does not readily burn. Methylene chloride is widely used as an industrial solvent as well as in the manufacturing of many consumer products. In addition to aerosol products and paint thinners, it is in many other items such as mattresses, building materials, and even decaffeinated coffee.

POSSIBLE HEALTH EFFECTS

The EPA has classified methylene chloride as a suspected human carcinogen; it is known to cause cancer in animals. In humans, it primarily affects the nervous system, possibly causing decreased visual, auditory, and motor function (EPA 2013g). Symptoms may include mental confusion, light-headedness, nausea, vomiting, and headache (OSHA 2003). The effects are reversible once exposure ceases (EPA 2013g). If exposure is chronic and high, then effects on the nervous system can be long-lasting and possibly permanent (NRDC 2014).

POSSIBLE SOURCES OF EXPOSURE

Consumers can inhale off-gassing vapors or absorb it through dermal contact, but amounts absorbed through the skin are usually small. The exception is when methylene chloride is trapped against the skin by apparel, which can lead to high absorption levels and even chemical burns. You may be exposed by breathing contaminated air, eating or drinking contaminated food or water, or using methylene chloride-containing consumer products (ATSDR 2015c).

Aerosol Products
Aerosol spray deodorants, spray paints, and spray shoe polishes.

Food
Decaffeinated coffees, hops (including beers), and spices.

Household Goods
Conventional mattresses, glues, lubricants, paint removers, paints, rust removers, shoe polish, solvents, spot removers, water repellents, wood floor and panel cleaners, and wood stains and varnishes.

Others
Artificial snow, automotive cleaners, glass frostings, pesticides, and photographic film processing.

PBDEs

OVERVIEW

PBDEs (polybrominated diphenyl ethers) were used as flame retardants in various consumer products for several decades until they were voluntarily phased out in the mid-2000s due to health concerns. PBDEs are structurally similar to both PCBs and PBBs and have the potential for similar behavior.

PBDEs belong to a broader class of flame retardants called brominated flame retardants (BFRs) and were among the most common BFRs used. While there are dozens of varieties of PBDEs, three draw the most attention: penta-, octa-, and deca- BDEs.

In 2004, penta and octa were phased out in the US. In 2009, the two largest producers and the largest importer of decaBDE in the US pledged to phase out decaBDE by 2013; the EU has banned all three. They remain a concern because they are still found in household products manufactured before the bans.

Despite the phaseout of pentaBDE and octaBDE in 2004, researchers from the CDC found that 97 percent of Americans have detectable levels in their body (Sjodin et al. 2008). Moreover, the EPA reported that levels may be increasing (EPA 2015d). A potential source of exposure may be imported products. DecaBDE may also break down in the environment into more toxic and bioaccumulative compounds.

POSSIBLE HEALTH EFFECTS

While research on the health effects of PBDEs on humans is limited (but emerging), animal studies have linked PBDEs to a variety of adverse health outcomes. According to the Agency for Toxic Substances & Disease Registry, even moderate amounts of PBDEs in animal studies affected the thyroid gland, liver, neurobehavioral development, and the immune system and may have contributed to cancer. Because of their developing nervous system and thyroid, fetuses and children may be more vulnerable to the effects of PBDE exposure (ATSDR 2004). Since "thyroid hormones regulate metabolism and are critical to normal development of the baby's brain and nervous system" (NIEHS and EPA 2013), disruption of thyroid hormones during pregnancy is of concern. While proof of harm to humans was not established, concern was serious enough that the two largest US manufacturers of PBDEs voluntarily phased it out (Washington Toxics Coalition 2009).

POSSIBLE SOURCES OF EXPOSURE

PBDEs don't bind to foam, plastic, or other materials that contain them. Instead, they leach into the environment and make their way into our bodies. The release of these chemicals may continue through normal wear and tear.

Diet
Breast milk, dairy, eggs, fish, and meat.

Electronics
Computers, TVs, and other devices.

Interior Furnishings
Bedding, carpets, clothing, foam furniture, lighting, textiles, and hundreds of other consumer products, as well as dust that accumulates on interior surfaces.

Vehicles
Interior upholstery and rugs in airplanes and automobiles.

Other
Wire insulation.

PCBs

OVERVIEW

While regulated by the Stockholm Convention on POPs and no longer commercially produced in the US, PCBs (polychlorinated biphenyls) are still manufactured and used in developing countries. Experts have estimated that of all PCBs ever produced, up to 70 percent are still in use or in the environment. These PCBs are often found in landfills where they can seep into groundwater (McGinn 2000). PCBs may be present in products and materials made before the 1979 ban.

Decades after being banned, PCBs continue to persist in the environment, to bioaccumulate in the food chain, and to have adverse health effects. While levels are decreasing in the US, diet remains a major source of exposure (ATSDR 2000).

POSSIBLE HEALTH EFFECTS

The EPA has categorized PCBs as a probable human carcinogen. PCBs can cause liver damage and have adverse effects on the immune, nervous, reproductive, and endocrine systems (EPA 2013c). PCBs may also cause liver and breast cancer as well as non-Hodgkin's lymphoma; attention deficits among boys; lower testosterone levels; and autoimmune thyroid disease (EPA 2013c; CDC 2015; Sagiv et al. 2012; Schell et al. 2014; WHO and UNEP 2013).

The EPA (2009b) reported that early PCB exposure was linked to low birth weight, neurobehavioral developmental delays, cognitive deficits, changes in production of thyroid hormones, and altered reproductive system development in males and females.

POSSIBLE SOURCES OF EXPOSURE

Diet
Since the environment is so contaminated with PCBs, diet is a major source of exposure (ATSDR 2000). Most commonly, PCBs are found in dairy products, fish, human breast milk, and meat.

Electrical Equipment
Busings, capacitors, electromagnets, reclosers, switches, transformers, and voltage regulators. Also old appliances or electrical devices that contain cable insulation; coolants in electrical installations; fluorescent light bulbs; PCB capacitors; and thermal insulation including cork, felt, fiberglass, and foam.

Others
Adhesives, caulking, finishes on floors treated in the 1960s, oil-based paints, plastics, oils used in hydraulic systems and motors, tapes, and carbonless copy paper.

PFCs

OVERVIEW

PFCs (perfluorochemicals) are a class of chemicals that are widely used in water, grease, and stain repellents (EWG 2015b). They were, and may still be (formulas change sometimes), found in Stainmaster, Gore-Tex, and Teflon fabric coatings and sprays.

There are hundreds of PFCs, most of which are not well understood. Included in this class are perfluorooctane sulfonic acid (PFOS) and perfluorooctanoic acid (PFOA or C8). Perfluorinated acids have been compared to PCBs and DDT but are more persistent than either: While PCBs and DDT break down over decades, some PFCs do not. In fact, they might be the most persistent man-made chemicals ever created. They don't biodegrade but accumulate in the environment and in humans. When Congress banned PCBs in 1976, less was known about PCBs than is currently known about perfluorinated acids (Lee 2003).

From biomonitoring studies conducted in 2003–2004, the CDC estimated that PFCs can be found in nearly all Americans (CDC 2013d).

In one test, PFCs were found in the blood of more than 98 percent of Americans (Calafat et al. 2007); in another, they were found in 100 percent of 293 infants tested (Apelberg et al. 2007), indicating that PFCs are present in the blood supply to the fetus. PFCs are often in children's blood at higher levels than in adults. They may also reduce the effectiveness of childhood vaccinations (Grandjean et al. 2012).

POSSIBLE HEALTH EFFECTS

C8, the principal component of a popular water and stain repellent, may cause a variety of cancers (liver, pancreatic, testicular, and breast), hypothyroidism, birth defects, and damage to the immune system (EWG 2003b). Once inside the body, C8 concentrations persist for a long time (CDC 2013e). In 2003, the EWG predicted that PFCs would "supplant DDT, PCBs, dioxin, and other chemicals as the most notorious, global chemical contaminants ever produced" (EWG 2003a).

The young (including fetuses) are especially susceptible to the adverse health effects of chemicals like PFOA and PFOS, which may impede development of the brain as well as the reproductive, immune, and endocrine systems (Cone and *Environmental Health News* 2012). 3M, manufacturer of Scotchgard, began the phaseout of PFOS in 2000, following pressure from the EPA over the chemical's developmental and reproductive toxicity. PFCs have been linked to low birth weight, high cholesterol levels, abnormal thyroid levels, liver inflammation, a weakened immune system, and developmental damage (EWG 2015b; NIEHS 2012).

POSSIBLE SOURCES OF EXPOSURE

Cleaning Products
Household cleaners.
Household Dust
In the Kitchen
Coatings on fast food packaging and food wrappers, delivery/takeout food containers, the inner lining of microwave popcorn bags, nonstick pans, packaged food containers, paper plates, and pet food bags.
Interior Furnishings
Carpets, certain fabrics, and furniture.
Personal Care Products
Cosmetics, and dental flosses.
Others
Clothing, electrical wires, eyeglasses, and rain gear.

Phthalates

OVERVIEW

There are approximately 25 types of phthalates used in consumer and industrial products (Freinkel 2011). They are valued for their oily properties (Smith and Lourie 2009). The most common ones are highlighted in the table on the next page.

The EPA estimates that over 470 million pounds of phthalates are produced in the US each year (EPA 2012c). Phthalates serve a variety of purposes, such as the softening of hard plastics, aiding lotions in penetrating and softening skin, allowing fragrances to last longer, giving products a silky feel, suspending colors and scents, and helping keep nail polish from chipping.

Various types of phthalates have been detected in almost everyone who has been tested (CDC 2013f). However, phthalates exit the body quickly, so reducing one's exposure is effective in reducing body burdens.

POSSIBLE HEALTH EFFECTS

Since there are more than two dozen types of phthalates, potential effects vary especially since they can disrupt hormones. A few potential effects are listed below:
— Can cause liver and kidney abnormalities and may contribute to cancer (ATSDR 2002).
— Incineration of phthalates produces dioxins, among the most potent carcinogens ever tested (McGinn 2000).
— Linked to birth defects in the male reproductive system; the immature male reproductive system seems particularly vulnerable to phthalates (EPA 2007b).
— May be associated with infertility (ATSDR 2002).
— May be linked to obesity, breast cancer, and precocious puberty in girls; endometriosis; and developmental abnormalities (Teitelbaum et al. 2012; Stahlhut et al. 2007; Reuben 2010; Pitre 2014; EPA 2007b).
— May be linked to allergies, asthma, and other similar disorders (Bornehag et al. 2004).
— Some produce less severe or no health effects (EPA 2012c).

POSSIBLE SOURCES OF EXPOSURE

People are exposed to multiple phthalates, starting prenatally. The EPA says diet is a main route of exposure (EPA 2007b). Like BPA, phthalates leach from plastic food packaging and from plastic items used in the food manufacturing process (like plastic tubing). Heat facilitates leaching, and phthalates are attracted to hot and fatty foods. Phthalates may migrate out of products onto hands or furniture and contaminate the dust throughout the home. We are exposed through ingestion, inhalation, skin absorption, and contact with some medical equipment.

Building Materials
Adhesives and glues, caulking, floor tiles, lubricants, and paint treatments.

Children's Products
High chairs, lunch boxes, pacifiers, personal care products, toys, and more.

Cleaning Products
Air fresheners, and detergents.

Fragrance
Additives to many of the products mentioned above, and candles.

In the Kitchen
Drink and food containers, food, and food packaging.

Medical Products
Blood bags, intravenous fluid bags, medical tubing, nutritional supplements, and pharmaceutical pills.

Personal Care Products
Cosmetics, eye shadows, hairsprays, insect repellents, liquid soaps, moisturizers, nail polishes, and perfumes.

Others
Binders, film, flexible plastics, interiors of most new cars, pesticides, raincoats, sex toys made of "jelly rubber," shower curtains, soft plastic fishing lures, sports equipment, textiles, tubing (such as water pipes), upholstery, and vinyl products.

COMMON PHTHALATES AND EXAMPLES OF THEIR USES
There are more than two dozen types, but the nine below are widely used.

Phthalate	Uses
BBP*	Adhesives, industrial solvents, sealants, and vinyl flooring.
DBP*	Adhesives, caulks, cosmetics, industrial solvents, and medications.
DCHP	Stabilizer in polymers and rubbers.
DEHP*	One of the most commonly used and produced phthalates in the US, DEHP is found in soft plastics, including plastics used in cleaning solutions, construction materials, cosmetics, food containers, food packaging, home products, medical supplies, toys, and tubing. It is the most common phthalate found indoors (WHO and UNEP 2013; Schettler 2006).
DEP	Ubiquitous in personal care products, it is found in colognes, cosmetics, lotions, perfumes, shampoos, and soaps, as well as industrial solvents and medications. In cosmetics, it adds lubrication to enable lotions to penetrate and soften the skin and helps fragrances last longer. It is also found in adhesives and caulks.
DIBP	Adhesives, caulks, cosmetics, and industrial solvents.
DINP*	DINP softens hard plastics and is found in vinyl toys. It is known to damage the liver and kidneys. When children mouth soft PVC toys, they can ingest DINP. The EU banned soft PVC teething toys in December 1999; and in 2002 Japan issued a ban on DINP in toys that might be mouthed by children under 6 years old (National Environmental Trust 2004). Years later, in 2009, the US CPSC took similar action.
DMP	Insect repellents, and plastics.
DOP	Soft plastics.

* The Consumer Product Safety Improvement Act (CPSIA) banned these from certain baby and children's products as of February 2009. However, avoiding exposure to threatening phthalates is complex. For example, three phthalates included in the CPSC's ban (DINP, DIDP, and DnOP) are illegal only for teethers and other items that children may put into their mouths. In addition, other threatening phthalates may be used; such as DnHP, which is known to cause cancer but has not been banned.

Tris Flame Retardants

OVERVIEW

Widely used in children's sleepwear in the 1970s, Tris flame retardants became even more popular in the 2000s as manufacturers sought a replacement for toxic PBDEs. They were banned or phased out from children's sleepwear after studies showed them to be harmful to human health.

Tris has not gone away. One type, TDCPP, continues to be widely used, at concentrations of up to 5 percent (by weight), in consumer products including nursery items, strollers, and nursing pillows. TDCPP is also used in foam-padded furniture such as couches, chairs, and sofa beds. Tris continues to be detected in household dust and in the bodies of biomonitoring subjects.

POSSIBLE HEALTH EFFECTS

Flame retardants have a structure similar to that of banned chemicals like PCBs and DDT, so they are linked to similar health impacts: reduced IQ, birth defects, reduced fertility, thyroid disruption, and cancer (Green Science Policy Institute 2015b). California listed TDCPP as a carcinogen under Proposition 65 in October 2011 based on studies that found that the chemical caused increases in kidney, liver, and testicular tumors and was linked to mutagenicity. TDCPP also mutates DNA, disrupts hormones, and harms the nervous system (Schreder 2012). Meeker and Stapleton (2010) suggested that TDCPP may impair male fertility.

Regarding increased cancer risk, many regulatory bodies in the US and around the world consider the maximum acceptable level of cancer risk to be one excess case per million people. In the case of TDCPP, the CPSC has estimated the number of excess cancer cases from exposure at 300 per million, which puts TDCPP's carcinogenic potential at 300 times the maximum acceptable level (Schreder 2012).

POSSIBLE SOURCES OF EXPOSURE

Baby Items
Car seats, high chairs, nursing pillows, strollers, toys, and other children's products.

Electronics
Computers and televisions.

Foam Cushioning
Airplane, car, furniture, and mattresses interior padding.

Interior Furnishings
Adhesives, non-apparel textiles, paints, rubbers, the undercoating of carpets, upholstery, and varnishes.

Plastics
PVC vinyl.

Unintentional Toxicants

OVERVIEW
Some Unintentional Toxicants, discussed in part I, are toxic, and can be even more toxic than their parent compounds. This section spotlights four: PAHs, dioxins, 1,4-dioxane, and pesticides.

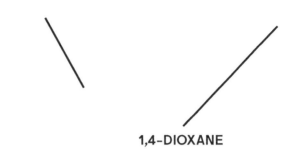

1,4-DIOXANE

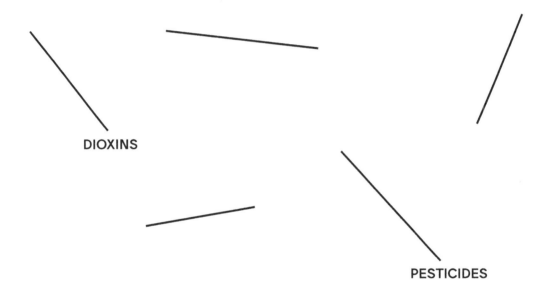

DIOXINS

PESTICIDES

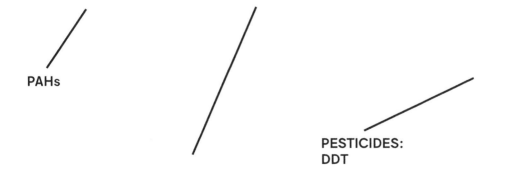

PAHs

PESTICIDES: DDT

Unintentional Toxicants: 1,4-Dioxane

1,4-DIOXANE OVERVIEW

1,4-dioxane is an unintentional by-product from manufacturing processes or from a mixture of ingredients. It is also intentionally used as a stabilizer and solvent in some personal care products.

Studies have found 1,4-dioxane in the following percentages of products tested:
— 22 percent of the 25,000 personal care products in the Skin Deep database, including many children's products (EWG 2007)
— 97 percent of hair relaxers (EWG 2007)
— 57 percent of baby soaps (EWG 2007)
— 15 percent of shampoos (these contained levels of dioxane exceeding the FDA's suggested maximum of 10 parts per million; *National Geographic* 2008)

POSSIBLE HEALTH EFFECTS

The Department of Health and Human Services considers 1,4-dioxane a reasonably anticipated human carcinogen (ATSDR 2015a), which the EWG (2007) says can penetrate the skin. The FDA monitors products for the chemical, but has yet to recommended an exposure limit. While the FDA encourages manufacturers to remove 1,4-dioxane, this is not required by federal law.

Under Proposition 65, 1,4-dioxane is classified in California as a carcinogen (CA EPA 2010). According to the US EPA, 1,4-dioxane has been linked to neurotoxicity, kidney damage, and respiratory issues (EPA 2013j).

The key concern is accumulated exposure. For example, during one bath, a baby could be exposed to 1,4-dioxane from baby shampoo, bath bubbles, and body wash, as well as other contaminated personal care products.

POSSIBLE SOURCES OF EXPOSURE

Since it is sometimes unintentionally present, you won't see 1,4-dioxane listed on product labels. However, it tends to be in those products that produce suds.
Children's Stuff
Body washes, bubble bath products, and shampoos.
Cleaning Products
Laundry detergent and liquid soaps.
Personal Care Products
Body washes, bubble bath products, and shampoos.

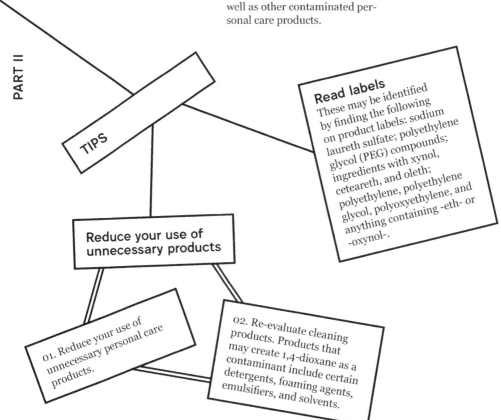

TIPS

Read labels
These may be identified by finding the following on product labels: sodium laureth sulfate; polyethylene glycol (PEG) compounds; ingredients with xynol, ceteareth, and oleth; polyethylene, polyethylene glycol, polyoxyethylene, and anything containing -eth- or -oxynol-.

Reduce your use of unnecessary products

01. Reduce your use of unnecessary personal care products.

02. Re-evaluate cleaning products. Products that may create 1,4-dioxane as a contaminant include certain detergents, foaming agents, emulsifiers, and solvents.

Unintentional Toxicants: Dioxins

DIOXINS OVERVIEW

Dioxin and dioxin-like compounds are a family of more than 150 substances formed as industrial by-products during waste incineration, chemical manufacturing, PVC production, paper bleaching, metal smelting, production of pesticides and chlorinated chemicals, and a variety of other processes.

According to the US Department of Health and Human Services' National Toxicology Program, the average American has measurable levels of dioxins in their bodies (NTP 2014). Once dioxins have entered the body, they endure a long time because of their chemical stability and their ability to be absorbed by fatty tissue, where they are stored. Their half-life in the body is estimated to be seven to eleven years. In the environment, dioxins tend to bioaccumulate and biomagnify throughout the food chain.

POSSIBLE HEALTH EFFECTS

Targeted by the Stockholm Convention (2015) of POPs, dioxins have been studied more than most chemicals. Dioxins are known to be toxic at a few parts per trillion, which is less than a single drop in a backyard pool (Martin 2010). In 1985, the EPA described dioxins as "among the most potent carcinogens tested in rodents" (EPA 1985).

Dioxins have the potential to cause a wide range of adverse health effects in humans. For example, it can damage the reproductive system, contributing to increased risk of pelvic inflammatory disease, endometriosis, reduced fertility, lowered sperm count, and birth defects (Hollender and Zissu 2010; Rier and Foster 2002; EPA 2014a; EPA 2015e). Dioxins also affect the nervous system, immune system, the adult and fetal endocrine system, and the developing nervous system (EWG 2015f; Birnbaum 1994; WHO 2014). In 1997, the IARC stated that dioxins are carcinogenic to humans (IARC 1997). *National Geographic's Green Guide* (2008) stated, "The average American's risk of contracting cancer from dioxin exposure may be greater than 1 in 1,000. That's 10 to 1,000 times higher than the government's current 'acceptable' standard for environmental carcinogens."

There is no acceptable level of dioxin exposure; the real dangers are in repeated contact (Hollender and Zissu 2010).

POSSIBLE SOURCES OF EXPOSURE

Diet
Animal fat is a major source of exposure through dietary intake.
Others
Cleaning products, like chlorine bleach and pool cleaners; personal care products, such as tampons; and products that contain bleached paper pulp. Air and water can also contribute to our body burden of dioxins.

Unintentional Toxicants: PAHs

PAHS OVERVIEW

PAHs (or polycyclic aromatic hydrocarbons) are carcinogenic by-products of combustion.

PAHs pervade our air and diet. In fact, food appears to be the major source of PAH intake in industrialized countries (Srogi 2007). Coal and biomass (living and dead vegetation) burned for cooking and heating can increase indoor concentrations of PAHs. Additionally, PAHs are found in coal tar from roofs and surface coatings (NTP 2014).

POSSIBLE HEALTH EFFECTS

PAHs are reasonably thought to be a human carcinogen, according to the National Toxicology Program (NTP 2014). PAHs have also been linked to lower birth weight in babies of exposed mothers, and to autoimmune thyroid disease (WHO 2010b; WHO and UNEP 2013).

POSSIBLE SOURCES OF EXPOSURE

By-products of Combustion
Burning fossil fuels and wood in automobiles, coal burners, diesel-fueled engines, refuse fires, and residential heating; also tobacco smoke.

Coal Tar
Used for roofing and surface coatings; may be tracked inside the home.

Food
Charred or grilled meats, contaminated cereals and vegetables, contaminated water, and smoked foods.

Unintentional Toxicants: Pesticides

PESTICIDES OVERVIEW

Pesticides are unique among other chemicals that are released into the environment because they were created to kill organisms—insects, plants, and fungi—that we consider pests (EWG 2010). Subclasses include herbicides, insecticides, fungicides, rodenticides, pediculicides, and biocides.

However, the popular use of persistent pesticides has led to the unintentional contamination of our food supply as well as house dust.

It is estimated that global production of pesticides equaled 200 million pounds in 1945 (McGinn 2000), and that by 2007, global use of pesticides was approximately 5.2 billion pounds. In 2007, the US accounted for more than one-fifth (1.1 billion pounds) of the total (EPA 2013a). According to the Worldwatch Institute, pesticides have become much more acutely toxic since 1945 as manufacturers sought to decrease low chronic toxicity without losing efficacy (McGinn 2000). Since 1984, an average of 18 new pesticides have entered the market each year (Cox 2002).

POSSIBLE HEALTH EFFECTS

According to the EPA (2011b), health effects of pesticides include irritation to eyes, nose, and throat; damage to the central nervous system and kidneys; and increased risk of cancer. According to Greenop et al. (2013), childhood brain tumors are also associated with pesticide exposure.

According to the NRDC, some pesticides (including insecticides, herbicides, fumigants, and fungicides) are potential hormone disruptors and may be associated with a long list of adverse health effects, such as those discussed in chapter I.8 (NRDC 2015a).

The risks that pesticides pose are especially great for children (EPA 2012a), including those who have experienced in utero exposure (NRDC 1997). There is strong evidence associating prenatal pesticide exposure with neurodevelopmental impairment (Jurewicz and Hanke 2008; Bouchard et al. 2011).

POSSIBLE SOURCES OF EXPOSURE

Diet
It is a major source of exposure, especially to banned, persistent pesticides like DDT.

Indoors
Consumer products, including triclosan, a registered pesticide, in antibacterial products and toothpastes, dirt and dust, and indoor pest control applications (including flea and tick products for pets).

Outdoors
Pest control and treated lawns. Pesticides can also be used around lakes and roadsides.

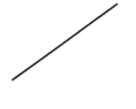
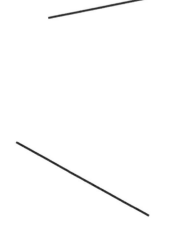
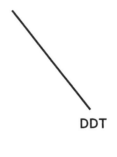
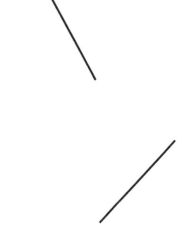

DDT

Unintentional Toxicants: Pesticides: DDT

DDT OVERVIEW

DDT is an important pesticide in the history of environmental toxicants. It was first synthesized in 1874, and in 1939 its insecticidal properties were discovered. DDT subsequently served effectively in fighting insect-borne diseases, such as malaria and typhus.

Given its effectiveness and relatively low cost, DDT's commercial appeal grew, and it began to be widely used to protect "crop and livestock production, institutions, homes, and gardens" from insects (EPA 2015b). In the US, DDT was used extensively on agricultural crops, particularly cotton, from 1945 to 1972. Households commonly applied DDT to porches, window screens, and baseboards. The dry cleaning industry also used solutions that contained DDT to mothproof woolens.

In 1962, Rachel Carson published the historic book *Silent Spring*, which attracted attention to the heavy use of this highly persistent chemical. It inspired government to take a closer look at DDT and eventually led to DDT's ban in the US. Since that time, scientific studies have continued, and substantial data now confirm Carson's research suggesting its harm to both wildlife and humans. While DDT was banned decades ago, we are still exposed to it through our diet.

DDT is now considered one of the most notorious pesticides and is regulated by the Stockholm Convention, though it remains a valuable public health tool in parts of the tropics. DDT's use around the world is associated with increased pesticide resistance by many insect species.

Since 1940, an estimated 4 billion pounds have been produced and used worldwide (EPA 2015c).

POSSIBLE HEALTH EFFECTS

DDT is recognized by the EPA (2011a) as a probable human carcinogen. It is known to affect the nervous system and may produce reproductive effects as well. In human studies, DDT has been associated with low sperm count, premature birth, and impaired breastfeeding (Steingraber 2010).

POSSIBLE SOURCES OF EXPOSURE

Contaminated Air and Water
Air and water near contaminated waste sites and landfills can contain higher levels of DDT.

Diet
It is a major source of exposure to DDT, which was banned in 1972. However, contamination is at very low levels. At the same time, the bioaccumulation of repeated exposures is cause for concern. Since other countries still use DDT as a pesticide, imported contaminated foods is a common source. Infants may be exposed through breast milk. The following foods tend to be contaminated: fatty meat, fish, leafy and root vegetables, and poultry.

Chapter II.2
Ingredients of Concern

In chapter II.2, I profile the most common ingredients in household products ("Ingredients of Concern") that may expose us to Toxicants of Concern or other threatening exposures. The difference between Toxicants of Concern and Ingredients of Concern is that Ingredients of Concern can often be detected from product labels.

They reappear throughout a range of household products, as part III details. One example is solvents, which are a major source of potentially harmful VOCs. Solvents are a common component of paints, glues, art and office supplies, cleaning products, nail polish, and nail polish remover. By being more aware of solvents, you will narrow your product considerations for healthier options.

THE INTENTIONS OF CHAPTER II.2

— Briefly communicate the complexity of product formulations.

— Highlight why it's important to read labels.

— Provide tips on reading product labels to assess the presence of harmful ingredients, which communicates why using fewer products helps all of our Homes.

— Quickly show why the Simple Strategies throughout part III are worth incorporating.

— Call attention to products that may contain these ingredients to help you "edit" your possessions and purchases.

Name of the subject Ingredient of Concern

OVERVIEW
This provides brief insight into the subject Ingredient of Concern.

POSSIBLE HEALTH EFFECTS
Same as in chapter II.1: This section highlights possible adverse health effects towards which the subject Ingredient of Concern may contribute.

POSSIBLE SOURCES OF EXPOSURE
Same as in chapter II.1: This is a list of products that may contain the subject ingredient. It quickly communicates how prevalent the Ingredient of Concern is and provides ideas on which of your products you can re-evaluate.

HOUSEHOLD REPEAT OFFENDERS

Toxicants
This lists toxicants that may be in the Ingredient of Concern and that are also profiled in chapter II.1.

Materials
This lists Materials of Concern, profiled in chapter II.3, that may contain the Ingredient of Concern.

REPEAT ISSUES
Discussed in other parts of the book.

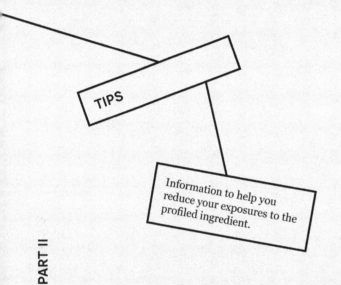

TIPS

Information to help you reduce your exposures to the profiled ingredient.

A CLOSER LOOK AT SOME INGREDIENTS OF CONCERN
Specifically of certain Preservatives, Solvents, Synthetic Colors, and Synthetic Fragrance.

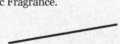

Chemical Flame Retardants

OVERVIEW

Chemical flame retardants are a group of chemicals intended to deter ignition. Manufacturers began to use chemical flame retardants in order to comply with a flammability requirement enacted in 1975 by the state of California, known as TB 117. TB 117 required cushioning material—usually polyurethane foam, which is highly flammable—from withstanding a flame for at least 12 seconds. For practical reasons, this became the de facto standard, so products sold even outside California generally have contained these chemical flame retardants. This resulted in furniture like sofas, recliners, and love seats being saturated with pounds of flame retardants (NRDC 2015b). In a test of 101 American sofas purchased between 1985 and 2010, 85 percent contained flame retardant chemicals in the foam (Stapleton et al. 2012).

In 2013 California revised its TB 117 standard. The replacement standard, TB 117-2013, allows manufacturers to meet a flammability standard without chemical flame retardants. Effective January 1, 2014, the flammability requirement for the cushioning of products was replaced by a "smolder test" for the covering material (e.g., fabric). Manufacturers had until January 1, 2015 to comply.

Experts seem pleased with the revised standard, TB 117-2013. However, TB 117-2013 does not ban the use of chemical flame retardants in cushioning or the covering material. Products that were created from materials and products made before the revised requirement may contain them. Furthermore, it's unclear whether chemical flame retardants will be used on fabric coverings, as manufacturers will have to meet flammability requirements by adding more smolder-resistant cover fabrics, or smolder-resistant barriers between the fabric and upholstery filling.

In the 2013 HBO documentary *Toxic Hot Seat*, Linda S. Birnbaum PhD, one of the nation's leading toxicologists, and Arlene Blum PhD, whose research was instrumental in banning Tris flame retardants from children's pajamas in the 1970s, explained that flame retardants are not effective and actually increase risk to humans and wildlife. During a fire they create toxic fumes (such as carbon monoxide) and soot. Most fire-related deaths and injuries are actually the result of inhaling these gases.

Even as certain flame retardants become regulated for their toxicity, remember that substitute formulas are not necessarily safer. According to researchers at the EPA (Birnbaum and Staskal 2004), there are more than 175 different types of flame retardants. Because they are sometimes chemically similar, they may cause similar health effects.

POSSIBLE HEALTH EFFECTS

Flame retardants have been linked to immune, endocrine, reproductive, developmental, and nervous system complications (Green Science Policy Institute 2015a). Brominated flame retardants may also increase the risk of cancer (Congleton 2013). Many are also linked to reduced IQ, learning disabilities, reduced fertility, thyroid disruption, and ecotoxicity (Gross 2013; Hawthorne, Nieland, and Eads 2012). Some currently used retardants have chemical structures similar to those of banned chemicals like PCBs and DDT and are believed to cause similar harm (Green Science Policy Institute 2015b).

POSSIBLE SOURCES OF EXPOSURE

Dust is a main source of exposure (Stapleton et al. 2011): It is estimated that 82 percent of human exposure to PBDEs occur from inhaling contaminated dust particles (Lorber 2008). PBDEs, Tris flame retardants (TCEP and TDCPP), and more have been detected in breast milk, drinking water, fish, food, house dust, indoor air, semen, surface water, and urine (Schreder 2012). Infants using products with TDCPP have been found to have exposure levels exceeding government guidelines. Tip Report 2 lists sources of exposure. Other possible sources are listed below.

Children's Stuff
Car seats, crib mattresses, high chairs, night gowns, nursing pillows, pajamas, play pens, and stuffed toys.

Electronics
Alarm clocks, computers, telephones, and televisions.

Interior Furnishings
Carpets, mattresses, and upholstered furniture.

HOUSEHOLD REPEAT OFFENDERS

Toxicants
— Formaldehyde
— PCBs
— PBDEs
— Tris flame retardants

Materials
— Conventional textiles
— Polyurethane foam

REPEAT ISSUES
— Carcinogenicity
— Chemical flame retardants contributing to body burdens; children's body burdens tend to have higher concentrations of flame retardants than adults do.
— Hormone disruption
— Petroleum-based ingredients
— Unintentional Potential Effects
— Unique vulnerabilities

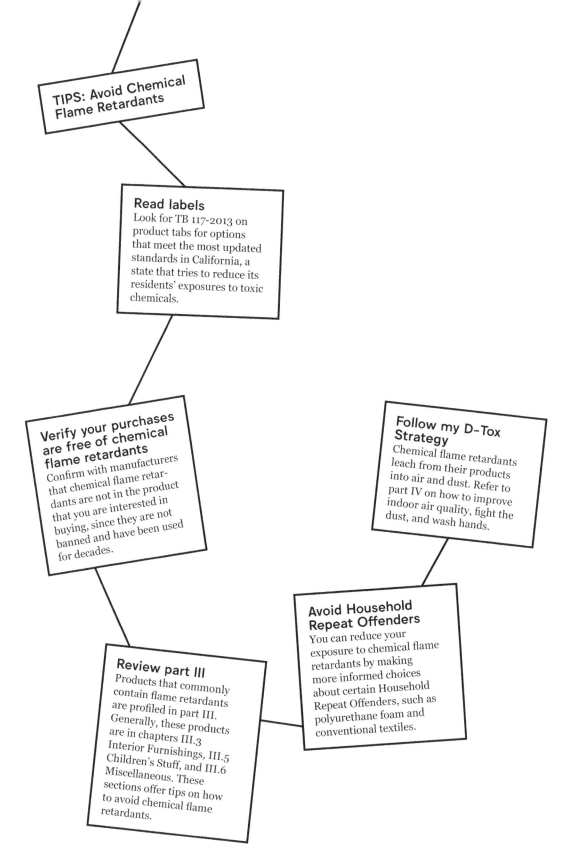

TIPS: Avoid Chemical Flame Retardants

Read labels
Look for TB 117-2013 on product tabs for options that meet the most updated standards in California, a state that tries to reduce its residents' exposures to toxic chemicals.

Verify your purchases are free of chemical flame retardants
Confirm with manufacturers that chemical flame retardants are not in the product that you are interested in buying, since they are not banned and have been used for decades.

Follow my D–Tox Strategy
Chemical flame retardants leach from their products into air and dust. Refer to part IV on how to improve indoor air quality, fight the dust, and wash hands.

Avoid Household Repeat Offenders
You can reduce your exposure to chemical flame retardants by making more informed choices about certain Household Repeat Offenders, such as polyurethane foam and conventional textiles.

Review part III
Products that commonly contain flame retardants are profiled in part III. Generally, these products are in chapters III.3 Interior Furnishings, III.5 Children's Stuff, and III.6 Miscellaneous. These sections offer tips on how to avoid chemical flame retardants.

Glycols

OVERVIEW

Glycols, a kind of alcohol, are ingredients that help clean and prevent the loss of moisture in the skin. Some compounds can actively attract moisture. Glycols also increase the effect of preservatives.

POSSIBLE HEALTH EFFECTS

The FDA stated that glycols may cause adverse reactions in some individuals. Health effects from some glycols include contact dermatitis, damage to the reproductive system, birth defects, kidney damage and liver abnormalities (*National Geographic* 2008).

POSSIBLE SOURCES OF EXPOSURE

Children's Stuff
Baby wipes, and other personal care products.

Personal Care Products
Anti-aging products, body washes, facial cleansers, foundations, hair dyes, liquid soaps, mascaras, moisturizers, shampoos, and sunscreens.

HOUSEHOLD REPEAT OFFENDERS

Toxicants
— Unintentional Toxicants, such as 1,4-dioxane

REPEAT ISSUES
— PEGs/Ceteareth/Polyethylene compounds. These glycols may be contaminated with 1,4-dioxane (probable carcinogen) and ethylene dioxide (known human carcinogen) (EHANS 2011). PEG is also made from the same chemical used in antifreeze, hydraulic fluids, plasticizers, and solvents. PEG facilitates penetration of skincare products deeper into the skin, thereby allowing increasing amounts of other chemicals and toxins to reach the bloodstream.
— Propylene glycol is related to PEG and is recognized as a neurotoxin by the NIOSH. It may cause kidney damage (EHANS 2011).
— Unintentional Potential Effects

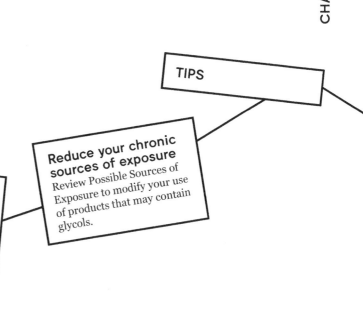

TIPS

Reduce your chronic sources of exposure
Review Possible Sources of Exposure to modify your use of products that may contain glycols.

Read labels
Glycols may be listed on labels as glycerin, hyaluronic acid (sodium hyaluronate), propylene glycol, ethylene glycol, diethylene glycol, polyethylene glycol (PEG), and butylene glycol.

Inerts

OVERVIEW

Some product ingredients can be generally categorized as active ingredients, the chemicals that actually do the work, and inert ingredients, those that are not directly involved in the marketed function of the product. This doesn't necessarily mean that inerts are harmless. They can be a source of toxicants.

Examples of inert ingredients are buffering agents, detergents, dispersal agents and carriers, dyes, fillers, fragrances, preservatives, propellants, solvents, wetting agents, and other elements that help to stabilize and dispense, as well as boost the potency, effectiveness and ease of various products (Hollender et al. 2006).

Product labels aren't required to disclose inert ingredients (except for the most toxic ones known), even though inert ingredients can be more toxic than active ones.

POSSIBLE HEALTH EFFECTS

Though their name suggests otherwise, inert ingredients can be quite active in the human body. The EPA allows some 1,400 chemicals to be called inert. Of these, 40 are known carcinogens or neurotoxins and 64 are potentially toxic. The health effects from most inerts have never been studied (Hollender et al. 2006).

POSSIBLE SOURCES OF EXPOSURE

Cleaning Products
Antibacterial products.
Personal Care Products
Many personal care products include inert ingredients, such as buffering agents, fragrances, preservatives, and dyes. They include cleansers, shampoos, hair sprays, and more.
Pesticides
Synthetic Fragrance

REPEAT ISSUES

— Carcinogenicity
— Neurotoxicity
— Petroleum-based ingredients
— Unintentional By-products
— Unintentional Potential Effects
— Unintentional Toxicants

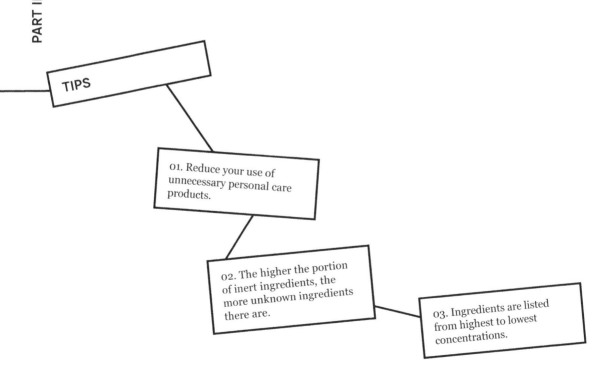

TIPS

01. Reduce your use of unnecessary personal care products.

02. The higher the portion of inert ingredients, the more unknown ingredients there are.

03. Ingredients are listed from highest to lowest concentrations.

Microbeads

OVERVIEW

Microbeads are extremely small pieces of plastic—anywhere from 0.5 to 500 micrometers in size—that are used in hundreds, if not thousands, of different personal care products. They add exfoliating properties, color, or texture.

However, they don't biodegrade, and our water treatment systems aren't equipped to manage them. So they accumulate in our marine environments, and continue to leach toxicants into their surroundings as they absorb other toxicants, including pesticides, phthalates, heavy metals, and POPs. Since they persist and are increasing in concentration, marine life have been absorbing and ingesting the microbeads, which, ultimately, we consume.

Fortunately, some states have restricted microbeads. In May 2015, California banned them in personal care products.

POSSIBLE HEALTH EFFECTS

Since the accumulation of microbeads in our environment and food web is relatively new, the health effects will take time to understand. However, dentists are reporting that microbeads in toothpaste can become trapped in the gums and crevices between the teeth. This can trap bacteria, which can lead to more serious consequences, like periodontal disease.

POSSIBLE SOURCES OF EXPOSURE

Personal Care Products
Exfoliating scrubs, face washes, moisturizers, shaving creams, shower gels, and toothpastes.

HOUSEHOLD REPEAT OFFENDERS

Toxicants
— Heavy metals
— Pesticides
— Phthalates

Materials
— Plastics

REPEAT ISSUES
— Bioaccumulation may occur
— Petroleum-based ingredients
— Trails of Contamination of our Homes persist through a potentially eternal Life Cycle.
— Unintentional Potential Effects

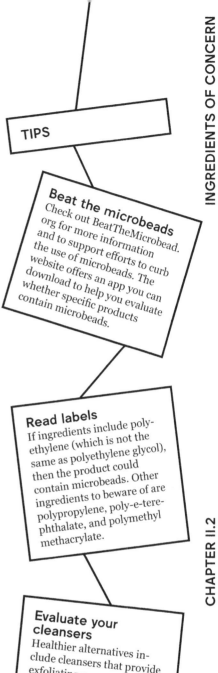

TIPS

Beat the microbeads
Check out BeatTheMicrobead. org for more information and to support efforts to curb the use of microbeads. The website offers an app you can download to help you evaluate whether specific products contain microbeads.

Read labels
If ingredients include polyethylene (which is not the same as polyethylene glycol), then the product could contain microbeads. Other ingredients to beware of are polypropylene, poly-e-terephthalate, and polymethyl methacrylate.

Evaluate your cleansers
Healthier alternatives include cleansers that provide exfoliating properties with ground nut shells or salt crystals; and natural materials that facilitate exfoliation, such as a loofah.

Evaluate your toothpaste
Make sure your toothpaste doesn't contain microbeads.

Nanoparticles

OVERVIEW

With the advent of nanotechnology, which manipulates materials at microscopic levels (generally 5 to 500 nanometers), nanoparticles have become popular in a wide range of consumer products. In sunscreens and cosmetics, titanium dioxide and zinc oxide nanoparticles are now common because they provide better sun protection than larger particles, as well as easier blendability and better translucency. In fabrics, nanoparticles may be added to create antimicrobial and resistant properties. In food, they may be used to enhance color and texture. They have been embraced by the industries of biotechnology and pharmaceuticals. The global market reached almost $25 billion in 2013.

While the health effects are not fully understood, early studies raise concern. Given their minute sizes, nanoparticles are easier to inhale. The EWG says that 800 to 80,000 nanoparticles "can line up across the breadth of a single human hair" (EWG 2011). Inhaling zinc, which is popular in sunscreens, may irritate lungs. Titanium dioxide nanoparticles, popular in many products, are possibly carcinogenic when inhaled (EWG 2015l). Once in the body, they may reach organs, cross the placenta, enter the brain, and damage cell DNA (Ostiguy et al. 2010). According to the NRDC, "animal studies suggest that some nanomaterials can cause inflammation, damage brain cells and cause pre-cancerous lesions" (NRDC 2011b).

POSSIBLE HEALTH EFFECTS

Since the widespread use of nanotechnology is relatively recent, there is not enough data to study the long term human health effects. However, one major concern is that nanoparticles' minuscule size makes it easier for them to be inhaled, travel to organs and cells in living organisms, and poten-

tially cross the placenta and blood-brain barrier. Preliminary studies find nanoparticles to have adverse effects on the behavior and metabolism of wild fish (Mattsson et al. 2015). Laboratory studies found that exposed mice experienced inflammation and damage to DNA and chromosomes; mice exposed prenatally were born with genital malformations and neurological damage (Trouiller et al. 2009; Takeda et al. 2009).

POSSIBLE SOURCES OF EXPOSURE

In the Kitchen
Food, like dairy, doughnuts, and sweets (like candy, frosting, and gum), and food packaging.
Personal Care Products
Cosmetics (e.g., concealers and foundations), creams, and sunscreens.
Others
Anti-graffiti coatings for walls, batteries, ceramic coatings for solar cells, clothing, crack-resistant paints, dietary supplements, electronics, plastics (as they break down), scratchproof eyeglasses, self-cleaning windows, sporting equipment, and stain-repellent fabrics.

REPEAT ISSUES

— Lack of disclosure. For example, while "cosmetics manufacturers are not required to disclose the presence of nanoparticles in products" (EWG 2015k), the EU requires that "nano" be stipulated when nano-size ingredients are used (Stafford 2009).
— The "opportunity cost" of exponential growth without understanding of long term consequences

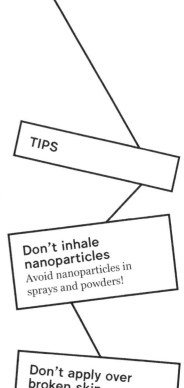

TIPS

Don't inhale nanoparticles
Avoid nanoparticles in sprays and powders!

Don't apply over broken skin
Incorporated into creams and lotions (e.g., sunscreen, foundations, and concealers), titanium dioxide and zinc oxide nanoparticles appear to pose low health risk. Avoid applying creams with nanoparticles over cuts, however.

Petroleum Distillates

OVERVIEW

Petroleum distillates are chemicals made from coal tar or crude oil that have been distilled in a refinery, processed, then purified further. There are many types with as many characteristics and uses. They may have a gasoline- or kerosene-like odor.

These products can contain trace amounts of benzene, toluene, xylene, and other chemicals that may have similar health effects.

Petroleum distillates are required to be disclosed on product labels so that in case of accidental consumption, doctors and emergency medical professionals can know how to respond. Used as anti-foaming agents and solvents, they are also added to personal care products to seal in moisture.

POSSIBLE HEALTH EFFECTS

The EWG considers petroleum distillates to be persistent or bioaccumulative and of moderate to high toxicity concern in humans, meaning these products are possible human carcinogens (EWG 2015h). They can contain trace amounts of benzene and other aromatic hydrocarbons, like toluene and xylene, which have similar negative effects.

POSSIBLE SOURCES OF EXPOSURE

Petroleum distillates are prohibited or restricted in the EU but are found in several US products.

Personal Care Products
Foot powders, glosses, hair styling products, lip balms, lipsticks, and mascaras.

HOUSEHOLD REPEAT OFFENDERS

Toxicants
— Benzene
— Coal tar
— Solvents

ADDITIONAL OFFENDERS
— Toluene
— Xylene

REPEAT ISSUES
— Petrochemical ingredients
— Trails of Contamination
— Unintentional By-products, such as 1,4-dioxane
— Unintentional Potential Effects

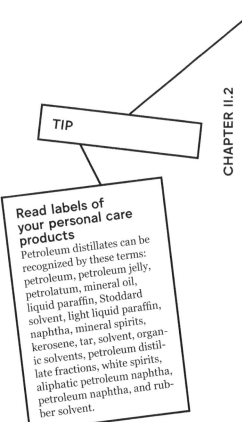

TIP

Read labels of your personal care products
Petroleum distillates can be recognized by these terms: petroleum, petroleum jelly, petrolatum, mineral oil, liquid paraffin, Stoddard solvent, light liquid paraffin, naphtha, mineral spirits, kerosene, tar, solvent, organic solvents, petroleum distillate fractions, white spirits, aliphatic petroleum naphtha, petroleum naphtha, and rubber solvent.

Preservatives

OVERVIEW

Preservatives are designed to help the consumer by extending a product's shelf life and preventing the growth of microbes that could cause infection. In recent years, however, there has been increasing concern that preservatives may harm us too.

The next few pages spotlight three common preservatives: parabens, formaldehyde, and sodium benzoate.

HOUSEHOLD REPEAT OFFENDERS

Toxicants

— Formaldehyde: Formaldehyde may be found in deodorants, hair products, lotions, mouthwash, nail products, shampoos, shaving creams, and soaps (EHANS 2011).

ADDITIONAL OFFENDERS

— Benzyl alcohol and isopropyl alcohol: There is evidence that they both are neurotoxic. Be extra mindful with children under three years old; benzyl alcohol may be found in baby wipes, hand sanitizers, lotions, and sunscreens (EHANS 2011).

— Boric acid and sodium borate: They are considered unsafe for babies or for damaged skin. They may be found in diaper rash creams and moisturizers, so look for them on product labels (EHANS 2011).

— Bronopol (2-Bromo-2-Nitropropane-2,3-Diol): It can harm the lungs, immune system, and skin, and may disrupt hormones. Bronopol can break down into formaldehyde and nitrosamines, suspected carcinogens, and may be found in baby wipes, body washes, conditioners, and liquid soaps (EHANS 2011).

— Butylated hydroxy anisole (BHA) and butylated hydroxy toluene (BHT): BHA is "reasonably anticipated to be a human carcinogen" by the US National Toxicology Program (NTP 2014). BHT may promote tumors and disrupt hormones and may be found in some eyeshadows, lipsticks, and other cosmetics. BHA is regulated in the EU because it can cause skin depigmentation (EHANS 2011).

— Thimerosal: A preservative that contains mercury. Used in some mascaras.

— Iodopropynyl butylcarbamate: A registered pesticide that is used not only as a wood preservative, but also in baby wipes, moisturizers, shampoos, sunscreens, and other cosmetic products (EHANS 2011).

REPEAT ISSUES

— Body burden: Ingredients from personal care products like methylparaben have been detected in most people (CDC 2010).

— Lack of transparency and disclosure: It is hard to know which harmful or threatening preservatives may be in your product from reading the label.

— Lack of unbiased safety reviews

— Petroleum-based ingredients

— Unintentional By-products, such as formaldehyde, may contaminate the product.

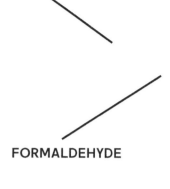

FORMALDEHYDE

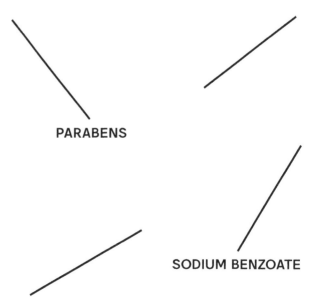

PARABENS

SODIUM BENZOATE

Preservatives: Formaldehyde

FORMALDEHYDE OVERVIEW

Formaldehyde is sometimes intentionally used in consumer products (e.g., as a preservative). It can also be unintentionally present as contamination from the manufacturing process, or as a breakdown product from other ingredients.

POSSIBLE HEALTH EFFECTS

Recognized as a human carcinogen by the IARC (IARC 2004), formaldehyde causes cancer of the throat, nose, and blood. Other adverse health effects include irritation of the eyes, nose, throat and skin and menstrual cycle disruption (Tox Town 2014a).

POSSIBLE SOURCES OF EXPOSURE

Children's Stuff
Bath soaps, and shampoos.
Cleaning Products
Carpet cleaners, dishwashing liquids, fabric softeners, and lacquers.
Food
Formaldehyde occurs naturally in our diet and is also added in some foods as a preservative, unintentional contaminant, or bacteriostatic agent in some foods, such as cheese.
Home Improvement Products
Foam insulation, paints, and wood products.
Interior Furnishings
Carpets, and permanent press coating on fabrics.
Personal Care Products
Bath soaps, body washes, colored cosmetics, hair dyes, hair gels, hair-smoothing products, nail and eyelash adhesives, and nail polishes.
Other
Medicines.

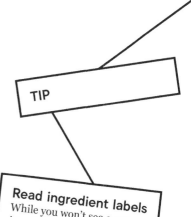

TIP

Read ingredient labels
While you won't see a warning of the possible presence of formaldehyde on product labels, look for common preservatives that may release formaldehyde, including DMDM hydantoin, quaternium-15, sodium hydroxymethylglycinate, 2-bromo-2-nitropropane-1,3-diol (bronopol), urea compounds, imidazolidinyl urea (Germall 115), and diazolidinyl urea (Germall II).

Preservatives: Parabens

PARABENS OVERVIEW

Parabens are used as preservatives and may disrupt hormones (EHANS 2011).

POSSIBLE HEALTH EFFECTS

According to the Campaign for Safe Cosmetics (2012), health concerns include cancer, endocrine disruption, reproductive toxicity, immunotoxicity, neurotoxicity, and skin irritation. In fact, Denmark banned propyl- and butyl- parabens for children up to three years of age in 2011. Parabens have been detected in the bodies of virtually all Americans who have been studied, according to the CDC (2010).

POSSIBLE SOURCES OF EXPOSURE

Food
Canned goods, jarred foods, and processed foods.

Personal Care Products
Conditioners, facial and shower cleansers and scrubs, shampoos, sunscreens; and leave-on skin products such as cosmetics and creams (rinse-off requires less preservatives). According to EWG's 2004 product assessment, 57 percent of all products contained paraben preservatives (Houlihan 2015).

Pharmaceuticals
Anesthetics, contraceptives, pills, and syrups (Andersen 2008).

TIP

Read ingredient labels
Commonly used parabens go by many names: butyl, ethyl, methyl, propyl, isopropyl, and isobutylpropyl parabens.

Preservatives:
Sodium Benzoate

SODIUM BENZOATE OVERVIEW

Sodium benzoate is commonly used as a preservative in personal care products and as a coloring in food and beverage products. A study of approximately 300 children in the UK suggested that sodium benzoate, when ingested with artificial colors, contributes to hyperactivity in children (McCann et al. 2007).

POSSIBLE HEALTH EFFECTS

A study by McCann et al. (2007) was the first to link artificial colors and food additives to hyperactivity in children. Sodium benzoate, a preservative, caused some children to become more hyperactive and more distractible.

POSSIBLE SOURCES OF EXPOSURE

Baby Products
Shampoos, sunscreens, and wipes.
Cleaning Products
Household cleaning wipes, laundry detergents, metal cleaners, and toilet bowl cleaners.
Diet
Fruit juices, salad dressings, soft drinks, and other foods.
Interior Furnishings
Carpet care, fabric treatments, and wood treatments.
Personal Care Products
Anti-aging products, applications for joint and muscle soreness, cleansers (body and facial), conditioners, cosmetics, facial treatments, hair bleach and hair color products, hair sprays, insect repellents, moisturizers, mouthwashes, nail polishes, shampoos, sunless tanning agents, and toothpastes.
Pharmaceuticals and Health Care Items
External analgesics (topical pain relief); feminine care products; lubricants and spermicides; medications for nausea, oral pain relief, and vomiting; nipple creams for breastfeeding moms; and treatments for earaches, foot ailments, varicose veins, and yeast infections (The Good Guide 2015).

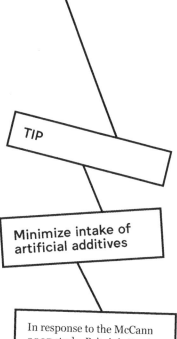

TIP

Minimize intake of artificial additives

In response to the McCann 2007 study, Britain's Food Standards Agency immediately warned parents to limit their children's intake of additives if they noticed a change in behavior. There was no official response by American organizations.

James Perrin MD, professor of pediatrics at Harvard, told *Time* magazine, "My guess is that if we do similarly systematic work with other additives, we'd learn they, too, have implications for behavior." With tens of thousands of new food and beverage products introduced each year, children face "tremendous numbers of new opportunities for things that may not be good for them," Dr. Perrin adds. (Wallis 2007)

Solvents

OVERVIEW

Solvents are major components in many products. While solvents can be in solid, liquid, or gas form, they are usually in liquid form.

Solvents can be made from natural sources, such as water and turpentine, but most are petroleum-based. Although water is the universal solvent, chemicals are generally added to enhance performance. Below are some functions of solvents, listed to help you become curious about when solvents may be in your household products.
— Dissolve, suspend, or disperse other substances to form a solution. Solvents help create a product that spreads easily and maintains its original balance of ingredients for the product's intended lifetime.
— Discourage clumping. Solvents may be designed to prevent other ingredients from clumping together.
— Speed up drying times. Since solvents evaporate relatively quickly, this trait makes them useful in the performance of many household products, such as paints and furniture polish. Using water as a solvent has its challenges, as it doesn't mix well with many chemicals and dries more slowly.
— Hollender and Davis's book *Naturally Clean: The Seventh Generation Guide to Safe & Healthy, Non-Toxic Cleaning*, explains that solvents disperse grease and oil and dissolve soil to help surfactants do their job in cleaning products. They are also used as a thickener or thinner in various products. Solvents have a unique and useful ability to quickly remove nearly everything. Often referred to as degreasers, hundreds of different kinds are used in more than 30,000 commercial combinations (Hollender et al. 2006).
— In paints, markers, pens, and nail products, solvents carry other ingredients, aid in the product's application, and evaporate quickly and cleanly.
— In *Planet Home*, Hollender and Zissu (2010) explain that solvents

make products like glass cleaners, dishwashing detergents, and all-purpose cleaners "fast-drying" and "streak-free."

POSSIBLE HEALTH EFFECTS

Many conventional solvents—natural or synthetic—can impair health if absorbed by the skin or inhaled. The US Department of Labor identifies health hazards associated with solvent exposure to include "toxicity to the nervous system, reproductive damage, liver and kidney damage, respiratory impairment, cancer, and dermatitis" (OSHA 2015). Even very short moments of contact with solvents can have negative health effects (Hollender et al. 2006). According to Tox Town, a National Library of Medicine project, some solvents are listed as human carcinogens (e.g., benzene) or "reasonably anticipated to be human carcinogens" (e.g., chloroform, 1,4-dioxane, perchloroethylene, and styrene). Tox Town also states that "exposure to glycol ethers may cause damage to a developing fetus and low fertility in men" (Tox Town 2014b).

POSSIBLE SOURCES OF EXPOSURE

Art Supplies
Inks, paint removers, paints, permanent and washable markers, photography and printing products, thinners, and varnishes.
Children's Stuff
Art supplies, and hand sanitizers.
Cleaning Products
Detergents, including all-purpose cleaners, dry cleaning from dry cleaning fluids, glass cleaners, odor removers, oven cleaners, and spot removers.
Construction and Home Improvement Materials
Adhesives, caulks and sealants, floor and metal polishes, glues, house paint and paint thinners, and paint removers and strippers.

In the Garage
Many automotive products, degreasers, gasoline, kerosene, and lighter fluids.
Interior Furnishings
Air fresheners, carpet and wallpaper backing adhesives, composite woods, furniture, furniture polishes and varnishes, mattresses, paints, and wood stains.
Personal Care Products
Colognes, facial toners, fragrances, nail polishes and nail polish removers, perfumes, and products that lather or foam (such as facial cleansers and shampoos).
Others
Aerosol spray products, dyed textiles, and leather goods.

HOUSEHOLD REPEAT OFFENDERS

Toxicants
— 1,4-dioxane
— Benzene
— Formaldehyde

ADDITIONAL OFFENDERS
— Toluene, an irritant and reproductive toxin (EPA 2013i)
— Xylene
— Others: Solvents suspected of being human carcinogens include carbon tetrachloride, chloroform, 1,4-dioxane, perchloroethylene, styrene, and trichloroethylene.

REPEAT ISSUES
— Endocrine disrupting chemicals, hazardous air pollutants (HAPs), and VOCs
— Lack of transparency in product ingredients
— Lack of unbiased safety reviews
— Petroleum-based ingredients
— Unintentional Potential Effects
— Unique vulnerabilities

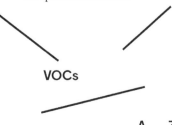

VOCs

TIPS: Be Strategic About Solvents

01. Reduce unnecessary exposures

The list of Possible Source of Exposure on the prior pages provides insight into which products commonly contain solvents. Review to see which ones you can easily avoid.

02. Pick your battles

Solvents can't be avoided entirely, so change product choices that provide chronic sources of exposures. Learning which household products may contain unhealthy solvents will help you focus your efforts.

01. For example, evaluate whether it's really worthwhile to use air fresheners and hair spray.

02. Consider chronic sources of solvent exposure in the bedroom, like mattresses and paint, where we generally spend one-third of our time.

03. Do you use perfume or cologne regularly? Consider finding healthier products, and reducing your use.

04. If pregnant or caring for young children, consider precautionary measures more seriously.

01. The EPA (2013j) considers 1,4-dioxane a probable carcinogen. Despite the agency's warning, it has been found in small amounts in a few major cleaning products. Ingredients that may combine to create 1,4-dioxane include certain detergents, foaming agents, emulsifiers, and solvents. These may be identified by finding the following on product labels: sodium laureth sulfate and polyethylene glycol (PEG) compounds such as polyethylene, polyethylene glycol, polyoxyethylene, and compounds ending in -eth-, or -oxynol-.

03. Start with cleaning products

02. Petroleum-based solvent products will be labeled "DANGER. Harmful or fatal if swallowed."

04. Identify healthier solvent-based products

While common among many household products, solvents are not necessarily disclosed on product labels. However, growing concern over the health effects of VOCs, as well as EPA regulations to protect the ozone layer, have led manufacturers to explore alternative formulas that may be safer.

When shopping, seek products from companies that are transparent about product ingredients. Safer solvents are water-based. Consider the Simple Solutions in chapter III.1.

Solvents: VOCs

VOCS OVERVIEW

Inherent in solvent formulas and sometimes unintentionally present, VOCs (or volatile organic compounds) are common among our consumer products. They are chemicals that evaporate into the air at normal room temperature and pressure. There are thousands of VOCs, including acetone, benzene, toluene, methylene chloride, formaldehyde, perchloroethylene, xylene, ethylene glycol, texanol, and 1,3-butadiene.

Certain VOCs contribute to greenhouse gases, smog formation, and ozone depletion. Some VOCs will also react with ozone to form secondary pollutants, including formaldehyde.

Although most VOCs have no discernible odor or color, there are people who can smell concentrated levels. According to the Minnesota Department of Health (2015), however, odor doesn't necessarily reflect health risks.

Certain products (e.g., paints and stains) disclose VOC information on product labels.

POSSIBLE HEALTH EFFECTS

Not all VOCs are necessarily harmful, but some have been linked to everything from minor irritations to serious complications.

Health effects depend on many factors, including the duration and level of exposure. Customers who make occasional visits to the nail salon will suffer fewer effects than will cosmetologists who work there for a substantial period.

According to the EPA, acute and immediate concerns include eye and respiratory tract irritation, headaches, dizziness, nausea, visual disorders, loss of coordination, and memory impairment. Over time, exposure to some VOCs can damage the kidneys, liver, and nervous system and may cause cancer. Some of these VOCs are known to cause cancer in animals, and some are suspected of causing, or are known to cause, cancer in humans. Because of potential high toxicity, VOCs are a major indoor air concern (EPA 2012b).

POSSIBLE SOURCES OF EXPOSURE

Building Materials
Adhesives, building insulation, caulks and sealants, plastics, pressed woods and wood preservatives, and vinyl.

Cleaning Supplies
Air cleaners that produce ozone, air fresheners, candles, cleaning and disinfecting chemicals, and dry-cleaned clothing.

Interior Furnishings
Carpets, curtains, furniture, lacquers, mattresses, paint strippers and varnishes, paints and stains, shower curtains, and textiles.

Office Supplies and Equipment
Adhesives, carbonless copy paper, copy machines and printers, correction fluid, permanent markers, and printing inks.

Personal Care Products
Aerosol sprays, conditioners and shampoos, cosmetics, perfumes, and underarm deodorants.

Others
Art and craft supplies, automotive products, fuels, gasoline, moth repellents, mothballs, newspaper, photographic solutions, tobacco smoke, and vehicle exhaust.

HOUSEHOLD REPEAT OFFENDERS

Toxicants
— Benzene
— Formaldehyde
— Methylene chloride

REPEAT ISSUES
— Endocrine disruption
— Hazardous air pollutants (HAPs)
— Petroleum-based ingredients

POTENTIAL SOURCES
— Cooking
— Dry cleaning
— Hobbies
— Newspapers
— Non-electric space heaters
— Photocopiers
— Smoking
— Stored paints and chemicals
— Wood burning stoves

TIPS: Minimize VOCs

Zero VOC may still emit toxicants
Products with labels that claim "zero VOC" (such as paints) may still emit VOCs and HAPs. The Paints section in chapter III.3 has more details.

Get to know solvents
Solvents can contribute to most of a product's toxic emissions, so learn about the solvents in your household products. Main product categories to focus on are cleaning products, paints, perfumes and cologne, and air fresheners.

Notice and respond to your body's reactions
Your body may send signals if exposed to unhealthy VOCs, such as dizziness, change in heart rate, and nausea.

Follow directions
Products containing VOCs and other HAPs have the greatest effect on indoor air quality while being installed, as well as immediately after, which makes the health hazard particularly acute for installers. It is vital to follow manufacturers' installation instructions.

Facilitate ventilation
Aside from providing warnings about solvents with well-known health concerns, such as benzene, toluene, or xylene, there is relatively little science to help consumers distinguish between acceptable and problematic VOCs. To be on the safe side, ventilate as much as possible, and if you are having any interior work done in your home, schedule it for when the family can be away for a few days.

Surfactants/Sulfates

OVERVIEW

Surfactants are a major class of ingredients found in a wide range of cleaning solutions and personal care products. In cleaning products, surfactants allow cleaners to easily penetrate stains and wash them away. In personal care products (like soaps or shampoos), they produce foam, disperse grease, and more. They help create thick, foamy lather and that squeaky-clean feeling.

Most surfactants are petroleum-based, making them practical for several reasons. They are inexpensive to make, do not leave a film after use, and are able to hold up against hard water. In personal care products, surfactants are often referred to as sulfates. They are also referred to as wetting agents and foamers.

POSSIBLE HEALTH EFFECTS

There are many surfactants (such as anionic, amphoteric, cationic, nonionic, and unspecified surfactants). Their adverse health effects are complicated and potentially wide ranging. In a study by EWG, 319 products were found to contain surfactants that have been linked to asthma and respiratory issues, skin allergies and irritation, and environmental issues (EWG 2015j). Below are some surfactants used in household products. The list suggests the complexity involved in understanding their safety.

Cancer from Unintentional By-products

— Alcohol ethoxylates, probable human carcinogens, may be formed from the manufacturing process.

— 1,4-dioxane, a probable human carcinogen, can penetrate skin.

— Alkyl ammonium chloride, used as a surfactant, releases formaldehyde, a recognized carcinogen.

— Sodium laureth sulfate (and other ingredients that have "-eth" in their name) may be contaminated by minute levels of dioxane.

— Nitrosamines, which cause cancer in laboratory animals and can be absorbed through the skin, can be unintentionally created when common ingredients—diethanolamine, triethanolamine, and monoethanolamine (DEA, TEA, and MEA)—react with another ingredient, nitrates, that are often used in preservatives (*National Geographic* 2008). The likelihood of contamination is higher if the end product also contains bronopol.

Hormone Disruption

— The alkylphenol ethoxylates found in some laundry detergents and some personal care products can disrupt hormones.

— Sodium lauryl sulfate (SLS), which can be seen on labels, removes moisture from the skin, so those with eczema or dry skin should be aware. It has been linked to hair loss, skin rashes, allergic reactions, and hormone disruption. It penetrates into tissue and is retained in the body for days.

— DEA, a possible hormone disruptor, depletes the body of choline, an essential nutrient for cell functioning and development.

POSSIBLE SOURCES OF EXPOSURE

Cleaning Products
Surfactants are in almost every kind of cleaning product because they're the key ingredient; most labels list only "surfactant." All-purpose and hard surface cleaners, bath and shower cleaners, carpet and upholstery cleaners, dishwasher detergents, dishwashing liquids, fabric softeners, floor cleaners, laundry detergents, toilet bowl cleaners, and window cleaners.

Diet
Several food-related applications, primarily food packaging.

Interior Furnishings
Adhesives, biocides, leather, paints and coatings, pesticides, and textiles.

Personal Care Products
Bath products, cosmetics, creams, hair care products, liquid soaps and body washes, lotions, shampoos, shaving products, sunscreens, and others.

Others
Paper, plastic additives, and wood pulp.

HOUSEHOLD REPEAT OFFENDERS

Toxicants
— 1,4-dioxane
— Formaldehyde

ADDITIONAL OFFENDERS
— Alcohol ethoxylates
— Alkyl ammonium chloride
— Alkyl benzene sulfonates (ABS) and linear alkyl benzene sulfonates (LAS), often referred to as "anionic surfactants"
— Alkylphenol ethoxylates
— Diethanolamine, triethanolamine, and monoethanolamine (DEA, TEA, and MEA)
— Sodium lauryl sulfate (SLS) and sodium laureth sulfate (SLES)
— Sodium myreth sulfate, ammonium lauryl sulfate, and ammonium laureth sulfate

REPEAT ISSUES
— Not planet-friendly: Most surfactants are made of petroleum-based ingredients, which generally make them slow to biodegrade.
— Unintentional Potential Effects: Some have the ability to cause hormone disruption and other illnesses in animals and humans.
— Unintentional By-products: Some ingredients in the environment break down into more harmful compounds; for example, nonylphenol, a breakdown product, harms the reproductive abilities and survival of fish (*National Geographic* 2008).

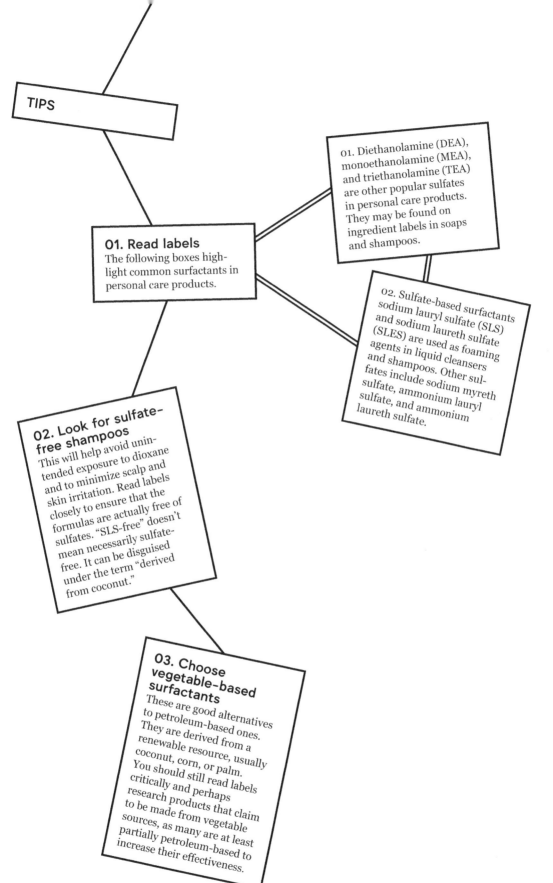

TIPS

01. Read labels
The following boxes highlight common surfactants in personal care products.

01. Diethanolamine (DEA), monoethanolamine (MEA), and triethanolamine (TEA) are other popular sulfates in personal care products. They may be found on ingredient labels in soaps and shampoos.

02. Sulfate-based surfactants sodium lauryl sulfate (SLS) and sodium laureth sulfate (SLES) are used as foaming agents in liquid cleansers and shampoos. Other sulfates include sodium myreth sulfate, ammonium lauryl sulfate, and ammonium laureth sulfate.

02. Look for sulfate-free shampoos
This will help avoid unintended exposure to dioxane and to minimize scalp and skin irritation. Read labels closely to ensure that the formulas are actually free of sulfates. "SLS-free" doesn't mean necessarily sulfate-free. It can be disguised under the term "derived from coconut."

03. Choose vegetable-based surfactants
These are good alternatives to petroleum-based ones. They are derived from a renewable resource, usually coconut, corn, or palm. You should still read labels critically and perhaps research products that claim to be made from vegetable sources, as many are at least partially petroleum-based to increase their effectiveness.

Synthetic Colors

OVERVIEW

Approximately 1,200 dyes are used to create desirable colors for household products (EPA 2014c).

POSSIBLE HEALTH EFFECTS

Certain FDA-approved coloring agents have had adverse health effects, ranging from irritation to cancer. They are listed on labels as FD&C or D&C colors, followed by a number. FD&C colors are approved for food, drugs, and cosmetics; D&C colors are approved for drugs and cosmetics only.
— FD&C Blue 1 and Green 3 have been found to be carcinogenic.
— D&C Red 33, FD&C Yellow 5, and FD&C Yellow 6 have been linked to cancer as well.
— Caramel: Contains impurities that may be carcinogenic.
(*National Geographic* 2008; EWG 2015a)

POSSIBLE SOURCES OF EXPOSURE

Children's Stuff
Fluoride rinses, medications, nail polishes, toothpastes, and toy jewelry.
Cleaning Products
Detergents, and soaps.
Food
Some beverages, candy, chewing gums, oranges, processed food, salmon, and sausages.
Home Furnishings
Paints, stains, and textiles.
Personal Care Products
Blushes, cold medicines, eye shadows, eyeliners, hair dyes, lipsticks, lotions, medications, mouthwashes, nail polishes, toothpastes, and vitamins.
Others
Art, office, and school supplies; cleaners; and clothing.

HOUSEHOLD REPEAT OFFENDERS

Toxicants
— Benzene
— Lead can be found in color additives or as a contaminant in many different kinds of products, including sunscreens, foundation makeups, nail polishes, whitening toothpastes, and lipsticks (EHANS 2011).
— Heavy metals are used in textile production and dyes. They include cadmium, a known carcinogen, as well as cobalt and antimony trioxide, both possible carcinogens.

Ingredients
— Nanoparticles

REPEAT ISSUES
— Lack of disclosure
— Lack of unbiased safety review
— Not planet-friendly: Most synthetic colors are derived from petroleum or coal tars. Many are resistant to biodegradation and are highly toxic to aquatic life.
— Trails of Contamination
— Unintentional Potential Effects

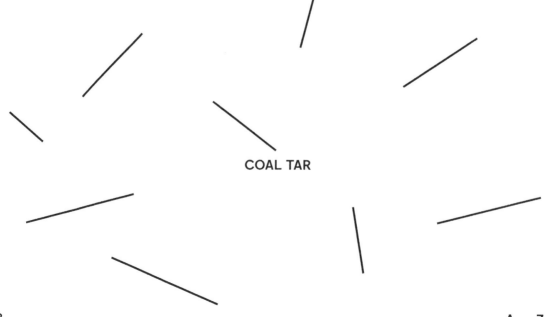

COAL TAR

Synthetic Colors: Coal Tar

OVERVIEW

Coal tar is used in a variety of consumer products. A petroleum-based product, coal tar can contain a variety of toxicants, such as benzene, xylene, naphthalene, phenol, and creosol. In Europe, many of these ingredients have been banned in hair dyes (EWG 2015k) and the US has banned some from use in cosmetics.

POSSIBLE HEALTH EFFECTS

Coal tars are recognized human carcinogens.

POSSIBLE SOURCES OF EXPOSURE

In the Kitchen
Food.
  Interior Furnishings
Paints, and textiles.
  Personal Care Products
Anti-itch creams, cosmetics, dandruff shampoos, deodorants, hair dyes, lotions, mouthwashes (FD&C Green 3), over-the-counter and prescription drugs, soaps, and toothpastes (FD&C Blue 1).

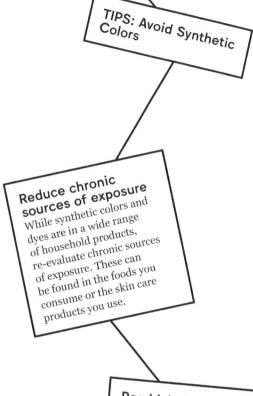

TIPS: Avoid Synthetic Colors

Reduce chronic sources of exposure
While synthetic colors and dyes are in a wide range of household products, re-evaluate chronic sources of exposure. These can be found in the foods you consume or the skin care products you use.

Read labels
Synthetic colors may be identified as "artificial colors," FD&C colors, or D&C colors. F indicates the color is approved for food use, D for drug use, and C for cosmetic use. The letters are followed by a color and a number.

Avoid coal tar
In hair coloring products, coal tar ingredients may be recognized with these names on the product label: naphtha, high solvent naphtha, naphtha distillate, benzin. naphtha, or petroleum benzin. B70, or petroleum benzin. Some coal tar ingredients can penetrate the skin (FDA 2014b). Other coal tar hair coloring ingredients include aminophenol, diaminobenzene, and phenylenediamine (EWG 2015k).

Synthetic Fragrance

OVERVIEW

"Fragrance" is in almost everything. Besides the obvious products like perfumes, candles, and shampoos, it's also in less obvious ones, like garbage bags and dolls. Synthetic fragrances are sometimes used to mask the chemical odor of other ingredients.

The concern is that most scents can be concocted from *any combination of thousands of chemicals* that companies can use (IFRA 2015). Most ingredients are not disclosed, not proven safe, and made of petrochemicals. Of the relatively few ingredients studied, the test results raise concern.

POSSIBLE HEALTH EFFECTS

A 1988 study by the US House Subcommittee on Business Opportunities cited the following in a 1989 report by the National Institute of Occupational Safety & Health (NIOSH): Of the 2,983 chemicals used in the fragrance industry, the NIOSH recognized 884 as toxic substances (Environmental Health Network 2008). One-third of fragrance compounds were found to be toxic by the NIOSH.

Chemicals in fragrance include potential endocrine disruptors (e.g., phthalates, Galaxolide, and Tonalide), irritants (e.g., benzophenones), neurotoxins (e.g., AETT, cyclohexanol, linalool, and benzene), immunotoxins (e.g., propylene glycol), and reproductive toxins and carcinogens (e.g., BHA, Tonalide). They have been linked to the following health effects: feminization of US male babies (Swan et al. 2005); respiratory distress (Lessenger 2001); central nervous system depression (EPA 2013i); diarrhea and earaches in infants (Farrow et al. 2003); hormone disruption that may be linked to birth defects and lifelong reproductive damage (Fisher et al. 2003); skin, eye, and lung irritation (EWG 2015i); allergic reactions (EWG and the Campaign for Safe Cosmetics 2010); head-

aches; nausea; shortness of breath; muscle weakness (Bader 2011); and even cancer (Sigurdson 2014; NTP 2014). One study found that 30.5 percent of Americans experience negative effects to scented products worn on others (Caress and Steinemann 2009).

One study found the following:

— 314 fragrance industry chemicals known to cause biological mutation
— 218 caused reproduction problems
— 778 caused acute toxicity
— 146 cause tumors
— 376 caused skin and eye irritations
(Environmental Health Network 2008)

POSSIBLE SOURCES OF EXPOSURE

The EWG found that 40 percent of all cosmetic products contain added fragrance (Houlihan 2015). Nearly every body lotion, conditioner, deodorant, shampoo, and soap contains it—even some labeled "unscented."

Children's Stuff
Baby wipes, diaper creams, diapers, dolls, lotions, markers, stickers, and stuffed animals.

Cleaning Products
Fabric softeners, and laundry detergents.

Personal Care Products
Antiperspirants, body oils, body washes, colognes, conditioners, deodorants, facial cleansers, feminine care products, lotions, perfumes, shampoos, skin care products, and soaps.

Others
Air fresheners, candles, drugs, garbage bags, oils, plastics, and solvents.

HOUSEHOLD REPEAT OFFENDERS

Toxicants
— Phthalates, such as diethyl phthalate (DEP) and dimethyl phthalate (DMP)

REPEAT ISSUES

— Allergens: Fragrances are among the top five allergens in the world (de Groot and Frosch 1997).
— Bioaccumulation: Synthetic musks have the ability to bioaccumulate (Campaign for Safe Cosmetics 2015). Fragrance compounds have been detected in human body fat, breast milk, and the umbilical cord blood of newborn American babies (EWG 2009).
— Confidential business information: Although manufacturers are required by law to list ingredients in cosmetics, they are not required to disclose proprietary fragrance mixtures.
— Complicated formulas: A single fragrance formula may use several hundred unique chemicals from among 2,600 compounds available as fragrance/flavor chemicals (Steinemann et al. 2010).
— Endocrine disruption
— Hazardous air pollutants: Fragrance generally includes solvents (such as benzene and toluene) and VOCs (including secondary air pollutants like benzenes and aldehydes).
— Hidden hazards: Fragrance tests have detected an average of 14 hidden compounds per formulation (EWG 2015g).
— Insufficient safety testing: 84 percent of ingredients used in fragrances have never been tested for human toxicity or have had only minimal testing (Hollender et al. 2006).
— Hazardous waste: According to the Green Guide, some compounds listed on the EPA's Hazardous Waste list are also commonly found in scented products, such as acetone (used in cologne and nail polish remover) and methylene chloride (used in shampoo and cologne) (*National Geographic* 2008).
— Lack of regulation: The CPSC doesn't regulate any of the specific ingredients included in the category of "artificial fragrance."

TIPS: Avoid Unhealthy Fragrance

— Neurotoxicity: In 1986, the House of Representatives' Committee on Science and Technology reported fragrance as an ingredient of concern given the potential neurotoxic effects (Fuqua 1986).

— Not planet-friendly: Some fragrance ingredients are petroleum-based, non-biodegradable, toxic to fish and animals, and are found in waterways throughout the US (EWG 2009).

— Prevalence: In a study of 204 cosmetic products and 97 detergents, "88 percent of the products contained fragrances" (Yazar et al. 2011).

01. Reduce unnecessary exposure
Read labels, especially when selecting cleaning supplies, personal care products, children's stuff, and even garbage bags! Be wary of the generic term "fragrance." Try to buy fragrance-free products.

01. Note that "unscented" products may not be free of fragrance compounds. Instead, they may contain fragrances designed to mask the smell of other natural and synthetic ingredients. "Fragrance-free," on the other hand, should be free of masking fragrance.

02. Look for full ingredient disclosure on product labels. Terms, such as "natural," are not necessarily defined or regulated by the FDA, so manufacturers have discretion as to their use. When in doubt, read labels closely and look for products with short, simple, readable ingredient lists. The more complex the formula, the more likely there are hidden fragrances.

02. Pregnant women and children should be extra protected
Due to the unique vulnerability of children (discussed in chapter I.3), children are especially vulnerable to the Unintentional Potential Effects (discussed in chapter I.8) of the hormone disruptors and other toxicants that may be in synthetic fragrance.

03. Consider essential oils
If you must have fragrance, then 100 percent pure—preferably those that are USDA-certified organic or Demeter-certified biodynamic—are ideal substitutes. They generally consist of plant-based oils blended with another natural oil, such as almond or olive oil.

04. Avoid air fresheners
These include aerosols and plug-in types. Since companies are not required to disclose all ingredients, it's hard to tell what toxicants may be in air fresheners. Usually they contain phthalate-containing fragrances. If you must have air fresheners, don't store them—or, for that matter, any cleaning agents or detergents—under the kitchen sink. It's best to keep them out of the reach of children.

05. Minimize use of candles
Most candles are made of petroleum-derived wax and may even contain lead wicks. For safer candles, look for those made with 100 percent beeswax or soy (preferably soy that has not been genetically modified), scented with essential oils (fragrance-free is ideal). Select wicks that are 100 percent cotton. Still, you should burn candles sparingly, as the burning pollutes the air.

06. Deodorize through natural ways

01. Scent your home with citrus peel, cinnamon, cloves, or any herb or flower petals. Add them to a small pot of water and simmer on the stove.

02. Light matches in the bathroom.

03. Vinegar is a natural deodorizer (the smell dissipates). Either place a small bowl of vinegar in the room or wipe down smelly or sticky areas with a vinegar solution.

04. Open windows, remove the source of the odor, or open a box of baking soda and set it in the smelly area.

Synthetic Fragrance: Essential Oils

OVERVIEW

Pure, organic essential oils can be a healthier alternative to conventional fragrances. According to the National Cancer Institute, some essential oils have antibacterial, antiviral, or antifungal effects. Studies on rats found different essential oils to be calming, energizing, and even to improve immune response (NCI 2014).

While organic essential oils are potentially safer than petroleum-based fragrance ingredients (and may even offer health benefits), keep in mind even pure essential oils may pose health risks and should be handled with caution, especially around children.

POSSIBLE HEALTH EFFECTS

Safety testing of essential oils showed "very few bad side effects or risks when they are used as directed," according to the National Cancer Institute (NCI 2014). However, some potential adverse effects include allergic reactions, skin irritations, sun sensitivity (from applying citrus or other oils before sun exposure), and hormone disruption (lavender and tea tree oils).

POSSIBLE SOURCES OF EXPOSURE

Children's Stuff
Body washes, bubble baths, conditioners, and shampoos.
Cleaning Products
Bar soaps, laundry detergents, and liquid soaps.
Interior Furnishings
Candles.
Personal Care Products
Body washes, bubble bath products, conditioners, fragrances, and shampoos.

TIPS: Beware of essential oils

02. Essential oils that have been exposed to air or sunlight or are simply old may contain more allergens than fresh, unexposed oils (EWG 2015d).

01. Chemicals called terpenes can be emitted from citrus or pine oil, which create formaldehyde when they react with traces of ozone in the air. They should be avoided, especially on smoggy days when the ozone level is high (EWG 2015d).

03. Some natural components of essential oils that can trigger allergic reactions include linalool, eugenol, and limonene.

Do your essential oils contain solvents?
Essential oils can contain a solvent, like alcohol. Choose ones with organic ingredients and without petroleum.

02. If you're allergic to a type of plant or flower, avoid any product containing its essential oil

04. Tea tree and lavender oils, two essential oils commonly recommended for homemade cleaning recipes for their antibacterial properties, can cause allergic skin reactions in sensitive individuals and may be endocrine disrupters. Both tea tree oil and lavender oil are also toxic to cats. They can also be poisonous if ingested. Children who have swallowed tea tree oil have experienced drowsiness, disorientation, rash, and lost balance and coordination from diminished muscle control. Use them cautiously.

03. Remember that the health effects from inhaling 100 percent pure essential oils have not been thoroughly studied
The following four examples illustrate why you should be cautious.

Triclosan

OVERVIEW

Triclosan is the main ingredient in most antibacterial and disinfectant soaps and sprays. It is added to reduce or prevent bacterial contamination.

A US FDA advisory committee concluded that household use of antibacterial products provided no advantage over plain soap and water. The American Medical Association advised that families should avoid using triclosan at home, because it could result in bacterial resistance to antibiotics (EWG 2015c). However, the FDA stated that for some consumer products, triclosan provided a clear benefit. In 1997, the FDA assessed extensive data on triclosan in a popular toothpaste, and found that triclosan was effective in preventing gingivitis (FDA 2000).

POSSIBLE HEALTH EFFECTS

In addition to being very toxic to the environment, triclosan disrupts thyroid function and reproductive hormones and may harm the liver. It is believed to be toxic to the immune system and to human sense organs. Overuse may promote the development of bacterial resistance against disease-causing germs like *E. coli* and salmonella. This common antibiotic, which has been detected in breast milk, interferes with testosterone activity in cells. The life cycle of triclosan can create harmful Unintentional By-products, such as dioxins. These can contaminate the environment and the end product in which the triclosan is used.

POSSIBLE SOURCES OF EXPOSURE

Cleaning Products
Antibacterial and disinfectant soaps and sprays to reduce or prevent bacterial contamination.

In the Kitchen
Cutting boards, kitchenware, and other products labeled "antibacterial," and products said to "fight odors" or "keep food fresher, longer."

Personal Care Products
Body washes, some cosmetics, nail products, toothbrushes, and toothpastes.

Others
Clothing, interior furnishings, and toys.

HOUSEHOLD REPEAT OFFENDERS

Toxicants
— Dioxins, among our deadliest pollutants, can form during the manufacture of triclosan and may contaminate the products in which these batches of triclosan end up. It can also form when triclosan is mixed with water and exposed to sunlight.

ADDITIONAL OFFENDER
— Triclocarban

REPEAT ISSUES
— Trails of Contamination: Wastewater treatment processes don't remove it entirely, so triclosan remains in our lakes, rivers, and other water bodies, disrupting aquatic systems.

ADDITIONAL ISSUES
— May contribute to resistance to antibiotics; and accumulates in breast milk and in animal tissue.

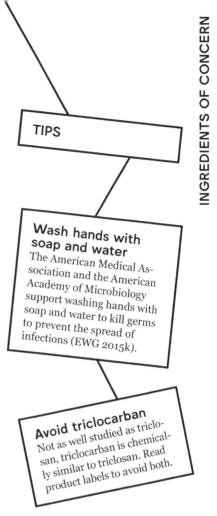

TIPS

Wash hands with soap and water
The American Medical Association and the American Academy of Microbiology support washing hands with soap and water to kill germs to prevent the spread of infections (EWG 2015k).

Avoid triclocarban
Not as well studied as triclosan, triclocarban is chemically similar to triclosan. Read product labels to avoid both.

Chapter II.3
Materials of Concern

In chapter II.3, I profile the most common materials in household products that can expose us to Household Ingredients of Concern and Household Toxicants of Concern as well as other threatening exposures (referred to as "Household Materials of Concern"). Materials of Concern can often be *physically identified* in the end product. For example, polyurethane foam, wood, textiles, and plastics are commonly found in furniture, mattresses, carpets, cars, car seats, and toys.

THE INTENTIONS OF CHAPTER II.3
— Briefly communicate the complexity of product formulations.
— Highlight key materials to investigate further when purchasing new products.
— Call attention to products that may contain these ingredients to help you "edit" your possessions.
— Provide details spotlighting why using fewer products helps all of our Homes.
— Identify healthy off-the-shelf products.
— Show why the Simple Strategies throughout part III are worth incorporating.

Name of the subject Material of Concern

OVERVIEW
This provides brief insight into the subject Material of Concern.

POSSIBLE HEALTH EFFECTS
Similar to prior chapters in part II: This section highlights reactions, disorders, and diseases to which the subject Material of Concern may contribute.

POSSIBLE SOURCES OF EXPOSURE
Similar to prior chapters in part II: This section lists products that may contain the subject material to quickly communicate its prevalence and to offer ideas on which of your household products you may want to re-evaluate.

REPEAT ISSUES
Discussed in other parts of the book.

HOUSEHOLD REPEAT OFFENDERS

Toxicants
This lists toxicants that may be in the subject material and that are profiled in chapter II.1.

Ingredients
This lists ingredients that may be in the subject material and that are profiled in chapter II.2.

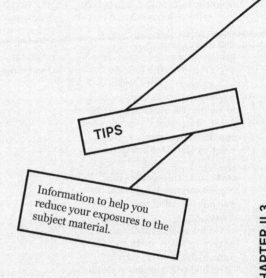

TIPS

Information to help you reduce your exposures to the subject material.

A CLOSER LOOK AT SOME MATERIALS OF CONCERN
Specifically of certain Conventional Textiles and Plastics.

Adhesives

OVERVIEW

Depending on the manufacturer, the terms *adhesive, caulk, sealant, stain,* and *paint* can mean the same thing. Sometimes caulk is used as an all-purpose term, and sealant is used by manufacturers to describe high-performance products. There are many types of adhesives, but most are based on SB (styrene-butadiene) latex—the same resin used in carpet backing.

They can serve various functions: fill in gaps (to protect from abrasion, water, and pests); keep certain things out and certain things in (such as minimizing formaldehyde evaporation from pressed wood); provide a protective barrier (e.g., to protect wood against stains and scratches); or affix one material to another (like linoleum tile to a floor). Since sealants can be used as a finishing step (as a sealer, paint, or stain) for a majority of building materials, they may cover more surface area than any other component and could be a significant influence on VOCs emitted.

Oddly, sealers made to protect against something like formaldehyde often contain formaldehyde themselves. While off-gassing diminishes significantly over time, chemicals can continue off-gassing for a year or two after application.

POSSIBLE HEALTH EFFECTS

Adhesives in carpets, wallpaper, and mattresses can be significant sources of VOC emissions if large amounts are used. Many VOCs are known carcinogens, and others are neurotoxins. In high concentrations or with prolonged exposure, all can cause respiratory irritation, dizziness, and headaches. The Urban Green Council, the New York Chapter of the US Green Building Council, believes that limiting VOC levels in adhesives, paints, coatings, and sealants will reduce exposure and avoid the health risks linked with indoor air contamination (Urban Green Council 2010).

POSSIBLE SOURCES OF EXPOSURE

Interior Furnishings
Adhesives used to fabricate foam for baby and children's products, mattresses, and upholstered furniture; to glue down carpeting and other flooring surfaces, such as cork and tile; to install cabinetry, countertops, decking, decorative plywood paneling, exterior siding, furniture, subflooring, wainscoting; and ones that are used on baseboards, moldings, sinks, tubs, windows, and anywhere wood comes in contact with plaster.

Others
Toys; and art, office, and school supplies.

HOUSEHOLD REPEAT OFFENDERS

Ingredients
— Solvents
— VOCs: Adhesive choices can significantly off-gas harmful chemicals and can be more dangerous than the materials they are bonding.

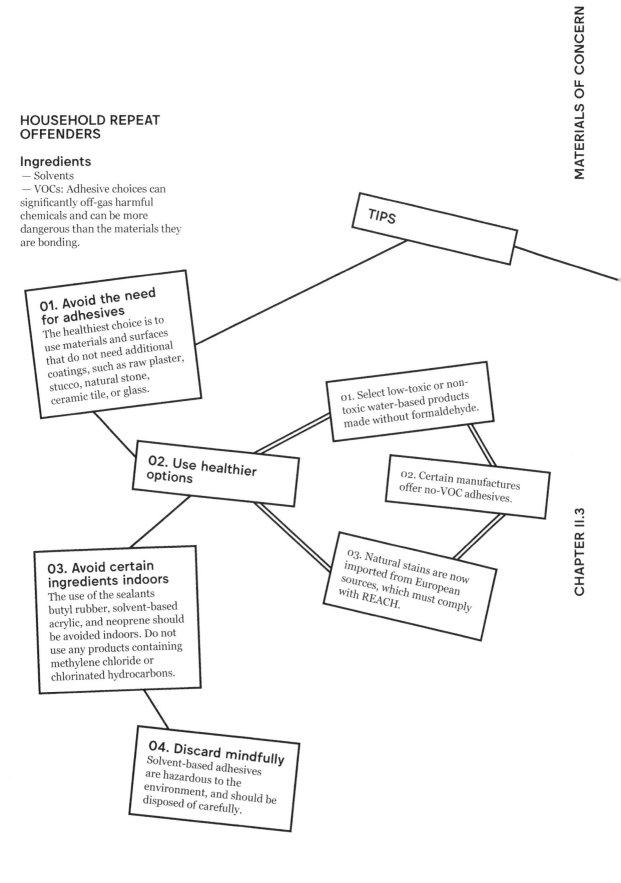

TIPS

01. Avoid the need for adhesives
The healthiest choice is to use materials and surfaces that do not need additional coatings, such as raw plaster, stucco, natural stone, ceramic tile, or glass.

02. Use healthier options

01. Select low-toxic or non-toxic water-based products made without formaldehyde.

02. Certain manufactures offer no-VOC adhesives.

03. Natural stains are now imported from European sources, which must comply with REACH.

03. Avoid certain ingredients indoors
The use of the sealants butyl rubber, solvent-based acrylic, and neoprene should be avoided indoors. Do not use any products containing methylene chloride or chlorinated hydrocarbons.

04. Discard mindfully
Solvent-based adhesives are hazardous to the environment, and should be disposed of carefully.

Conventional Textiles

OVERVIEW

Thousands of years before synthetic fibers were created, the four staples of the fabric industry were flax, wool, cotton, and silk. These were all created from natural, renewable, and abundant sources. These natural fibers, however, had limitations: cotton and linens are prone to wrinkling; silk is delicate; wool shrinks and can irritate the skin. That's where synthetic fabrics came in; by the mid-1960s they had a market share of over 40 percent (Silas, Hansen, and Lent 2007).

Synthetic fabrics tend to be made from petroleum-based ingredients. Some of the most common household synthetic fibers are polyester, rayon, acrylic, olefin, microfiber, and nylon.

Synthetic fibers offer many practical benefits. They are durable; more resistant to wrinkles, stains, liquids, and fading; easy to clean; antimicrobial; and relatively inexpensive. According to the *Green Guide*, however, many synthetic fabrics pose health risks to our Homes: pesticide residues, irritating dyes, unsafe fabric treatments, and potentially carcinogenic compounds that may off-gas or be absorbed through the skin (*National Geographic* 2008). To avoid toxic residues and reduce our demand of petrochemicals, we can reduce our demand of conventional textiles.

In this section, the following conventional textiles are spotlighted: nylon, polyester, acrylic, rayon, leather, and cotton.

Did You Know?

According to the NRDC (2012), it can take almost a one-third pound of synthetic fertilizers to grow the pound of raw cotton required to make a single cotton T-shirt in America. Now think about all the other products in your home that use conventional cotton.

HOUSEHOLD REPEAT OFFENDERS

Toxicants
— Formaldehyde
— Heavy metals
— Pesticides
— PFCs

Ingredients
— Synthetic dyes: Conventional textile dyes "fix" pigments to the fabric using carcinogenic heavy metals, such as cadmium (a known carcinogen), cobalt, antimony trioxide (both possible carcinogens), chromium VI, arsenic, mercury, and lead, which are known to damage the brain and nervous system. They may also use formaldehyde and petrochemicals. The EPA lists several dyes, including azo, triarylmethane, and anthraquinone, as hazardous waste materials. Many of these dyes may trigger contact dermatitis and asthma symptoms. Despite the known health risks of these substances, the textile-dyeing industry is notoriously lax about keeping them out of the environment.
— Nanoparticles

REPEAT ISSUES
— Fabric treatments
— Manufacturing may release pollutants like nitrogen and sulfur oxides, particulates, carbon monoxide, and heavy metals, which are lung-damaging (*National Geographic* 2008).
— Petroleum-based ingredients
— Toxic flame retardants
— Trails of Contamination

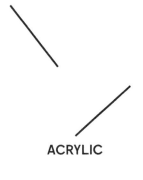

ACRYLIC

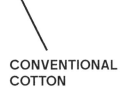

CONVENTIONAL COTTON

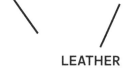

LEATHER

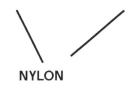

NYLON

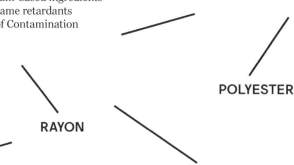

RAYON

POLYESTER

Conventional Textiles: Acrylic

Conventional Cotton

ACRYLIC OVERVIEW

Acrylic uses nonrenewable fossil fuels (Silas, Hansen, and Lent 2007).

POSSIBLE HEALTH EFFECTS

Acrylic is made using the industrial chemical acrylonitrile, a probable human carcinogen. Workers who make acrylic fiber are at greater risk of cancer. Effects from sleeping on or under acrylic are unknown.

POSSIBLE SOURCES OF EXPOSURE

Apparel
Hats and sweaters.
Home Furnishings
Blankets, mattresses, rugs, and upholstery.
Others
Awnings, boat covers, and knitting yarn.

CONVENTIONAL COTTON OVERVIEW

Both affordable and fairly easy to care for, conventional cotton is one of the most popular fibers. It is used in a wide range of household products, such as upholstered furniture, mattress coverings, mattress interiors, window treatments, carpets and area rugs, bed and bath linens, toys, and clothing.

However, conventional cotton is heavily sprayed with synthetic pesticides and fertilizers. Residues may remain. It's unclear whether these toxic residues escape their end products and threaten our health.

Regardless, it's clear many of these pesticides and fertilizers are harmful to cotton farmers, their families, and local communities. Since most cotton crops are grown in developing countries where farmers are not as aware of their toxicity or of safety precautions, consumers may want to avoid conventional cotton to protect the cotton farmers and to lower the environmental burden. Many of the pesticides and fertilizers are carcinogenic, contaminate groundwater, and add to the environmental burden our children will inherit.

HOUSEHOLD REPEAT OFFENDERS

Toxicants
— Pesticides: Conventional cotton is heavily sprayed with pesticides and fertilizers. The EPA considers seven of the top 15 pesticides used on cotton in the US in 2000 as "possible," "likely," "probable," or "known" human carcinogens (Bader 2011).

Ingredients
— Chemical flame retardants (and other chemical treatments)
— Synthetic colors
— Nanoparticles

ADDITIONAL ISSUES

— Insecticides: Insecticides are more hazardous to human and animal health than any other type of pesticide, and they are applied to cotton crops more than any other crop worldwide, including corn, rice, soybeans, and wheat. Some $1.31 billion is spent on insecticides for cotton each year (Environmental Justice Foundation 2007). Many insecticides impair biological processes such as the function of the nervous and reproductive systems.
— Synthetic Fertilizer: According to the USDA, more than 2.03 billion pounds (or 142 pounds per acre) of synthetic fertilizers were used on conventional cotton in 2000. This makes cotton the fourth most heavily fertilized crop, following corn, winter wheat, and soybeans (Bader 2011). Synthetic fertilizers containing nitrogen are considered the most detrimental to the environment. Impacts on human health include blindness among exposed workers, groundwater contamination, and methemoglobinemia (blue baby syndrome) in infants.
— Trails of Contamination: Approximately 23 million tons of cotton seeds and their derivatives are used as animal feed annually (Environmental Justice Foundation 2007). We ultimately eat the genetically modified substances as we eat the animals. Also, hazardous pesticides applied to cotton crops have been detected in cows' milk.

Our Appetite for Cotton
— 35 percent of total world fiber use
— 75 percent of the US apparel market
— 18 percent in US home furnishings
— 7 percent in US industrial products like medical supplies, industrial thread, and wall coverings
(USDA 2014; EPA 2013e)

Conventional Textiles:
Leather   Nylon   Polyester

LEATHER OVERVIEW

Making leather supple and durable involves a complex process; and tanning leather generally contaminates the environment. Tanneries use many toxic substances, including mineral salts (chromium, aluminum, iron, and zirconium), formaldehyde, coal-tar derivatives, and cyanide-based dyes and oils. More than 95 percent of leather produced in the world are chrome-tanned; the EPA considers all wastes containing chromium to be hazardous (*National Geographic* 2008).

POSSIBLE HEALTH EFFECTS

Since leather is made with-known and suspected carcinogens as well as chromium—an EPA hazardous waste—it's best to be wary of new leathers. A planet-friendly option is to buy used or vintage pieces.

POSSIBLE SOURCES OF EXPOSURE

Apparel
Belts, clothing, purses, shoes, and wallets.
Children's Stuff
Toys and sports equipment.
Home Furnishings
Upholstered furniture.

NYLON OVERVIEW

Nylon was among the first synthetic fibers made from petrochemicals. When it came to market in 1939, cotton was the most popular fiber, accounting for up 80 percent of all fiber production. Nylon soon became known as "the miracle fiber." By 1945, production of cotton had decreased to 75 percent as nylon grew in popularity (Silas, Hansen, and Lent 2007).

POSSIBLE HEALTH EFFECTS

Health concerns depend on the type of nylon used. For example, nylon 6, which can be found in various cosmetics (like mascara, nail polish, exfoliant scrubs, eye shadow, and brow liners) is not thought to be harmful to human or environmental health. Nylon 66, on the other hand, is thought to be harmful, though not bioaccumulative.

POSSIBLE SOURCES OF EXPOSURE

Apparel
Shoes, skirts, pocketbooks, raincoats, and wigs.
Home Furnishings
Carpets, draperies, and outdoor furnishings.
Personal Care Products
Artificial eyelashes, cosmetics, and hairbrush and toothbrush bristles.
Others
Knitting yarns, plastics, and surgical sutures.

POLYESTER OVERVIEW

Polyester is made by breaking down crude oil into petrochemicals and converting them into polyethylene terephthalate (PETE), a plastic used to make soda bottles and polyester fibers.

POSSIBLE HEALTH EFFECTS

Some polyesters contain chlorine, which pollutes the environment and harms wildlife and humans during its production and use and at the end of the product's life cycle. Polyester production can release nitrogen and sulfur oxides, particulates, carbon monoxide, carbon dioxide, and heavy metals, which are all considered lung-damaging pollutants (*National Geographic* 2008).

POSSIBLE SOURCES OF EXPOSURE

Apparel
Hats, jackets, pants, and shirts.
Children's Stuff
Backpacks, clothes, lunch bags, and toys.
Home Furnishings
Bedding, carpets, cushioning and insulating materials, furniture, and mattresses.
Personal Care Products
Diapers and sanitary napkins.

Conventional Textiles: Rayon

RAYON OVERVIEW

Commercially available in 1910, rayon was the first man-made fiber, which was produced to emulate silk. Highly absorbent, rayon is manufactured from wood pulp and is bleached with chlorine-containing substances.

POSSIBLE HEALTH EFFECTS

Rayon may contain residual chlorinated hydrocarbons, a class of chemicals that are often used as pesticides; two of the earliest ones were DDT and DDE. Rayon has been reported to also contain trace amounts of dioxin.

POSSIBLE SOURCES OF EXPOSURE

Apparel
Clothing.
Home Furnishings
Home furnishings, and towels.
Personal Care Products
Diapers, and feminine hygiene products.

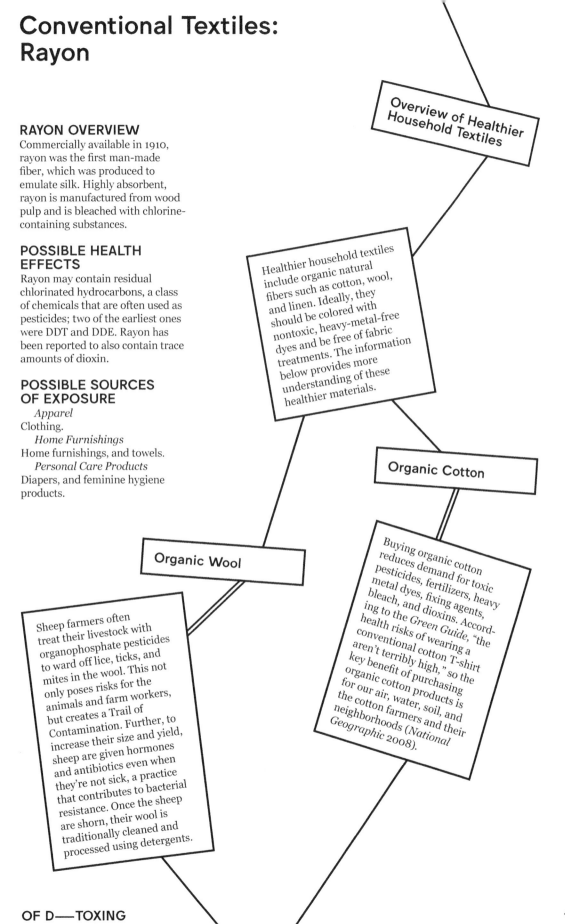

Overview of Healthier Household Textiles

Healthier household textiles include organic natural fibers such as cotton, wool, and linen. Ideally, they should be colored with nontoxic, heavy-metal-free dyes and be free of fabric treatments. The information below provides more understanding of these healthier materials.

Organic Cotton

Buying organic cotton reduces demand for toxic pesticides, fertilizers, heavy metal dyes, fixing agents, bleach, and dioxins. According to the *Green Guide*, "the health risks of wearing a conventional cotton T-shirt aren't terribly high," so the key benefit of purchasing organic cotton products is for our air, water, soil, and the cotton farmers and their neighborhoods (*National Geographic* 2008).

Organic Wool

Sheep farmers often treat their livestock with organophosphate pesticides to ward off lice, ticks, and mites in the wool. This not only poses risks for the animals and farm workers, but creates a Trail of Contamination. Further, to increase their size and yield, sheep are given hormones and antibiotics even when they're not sick, a practice that contributes to bacterial resistance. Once the sheep are shorn, their wool is traditionally cleaned and processed using detergents.

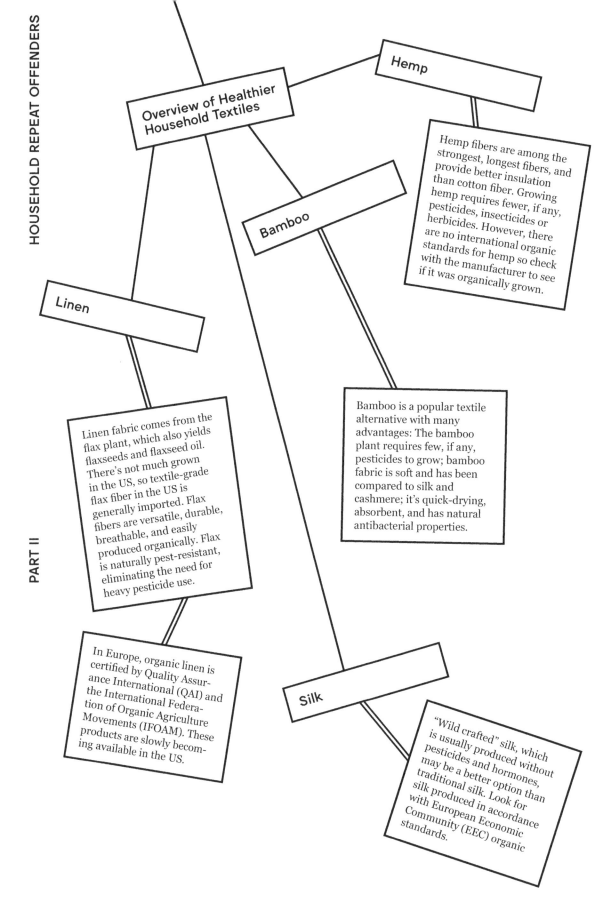

Overview of Healthier Household Textiles

Hemp

Hemp fibers are among the strongest, longest fibers, and provide better insulation than cotton fiber. Growing hemp requires fewer, if any, pesticides, insecticides or herbicides. However, there are no international organic standards for hemp so check with the manufacturer to see if it was organically grown.

Bamboo

Bamboo is a popular textile alternative with many advantages: The bamboo plant requires few, if any, pesticides to grow; bamboo fabric is soft and has been compared to silk and cashmere; it's quick-drying, absorbent, and has natural antibacterial properties.

Linen

Linen fabric comes from the flax plant, which also yields flaxseeds and flaxseed oil. There's not much grown in the US, so textile-grade flax fiber in the US is generally imported. Flax fibers are versatile, durable, breathable, and easily produced organically. Flax is naturally pest-resistant, eliminating the need for heavy pesticide use.

In Europe, organic linen is certified by Quality Assurance International (QAI) and the International Federation of Organic Agriculture Movements (IFOAM). These products are slowly becoming available in the US.

Silk

"Wild crafted" silk, which is usually produced without pesticides and hormones, may be a better option than traditional silk. Look for silk produced in accordance with European Economic Community (EEC) organic standards.

TIPS: Pure Organic Wool

USDA-certified organic wool comes from sheep raised without the use of synthetic hormones and on organic feed that wasn't grown with pesticides.

01. Avoid hormones and pesticides
Buy certified organic wool or "Pure Grow" wool.

02. Research wools that sound organic but are not certified
Check the manufacturer's website to investigate whether organic growing practices are followed. Look for strict guidelines indicating that the wool has been created and processed without animal cruelty, bleaches, formaldehydes, or dyes.

03. Choose wool for materials in your bedroom
If you aren't allergic to wool, it offers sleepers several benefits, such as the three noted in the following boxes.

04. Third-party certification of claims is ideal

01. Wool is good at regulating moisture and heat. Wool has the ability to absorb one third of its entire weight in moisture before it feels wet and moisture can evaporate quickly. So a wool pad is helpful against accidents on a mattress. Further, humans produce roughly a pint of water vapor while we sleep, and wool is the perfect material to keep skin dry during the night (Bader 2011).

02. Wool is naturally fire resistant. This takes away the need for chemical fire retardant treatments, which are often applied to cotton and synthetics. It's not moth-resistant, however, and is often treated with mothproofing insecticides (NRDC 2011a).

03. Wool is eco-friendly. Wool is a renewable resource when harvested without slaughtering the sheep. Sheep raised organically do not receive chemical treatments common in the industry. For example, conventional raising of sheep exposes them to pesticides, antibiotics, growth hormones, and vaccines, building healthy immune systems naturally. Sheep raised organically are bred for parasite resistance without using genetic engineering (Bader 2011). Furthermore, they don't graze on pastures sprayed with herbicides and are given only organic feed that helps them.

TIPS: Organic Cotton

01. Often organic cotton is unbleached, or is lightened using nontoxic peroxide, instead of dioxin-releasing chlorine (*National Geographic* 2008).

02. Dyes that are used are usually low impact, which means that they are free of dangerous and polluting heavy metal dyes and fixing agents. Be aware that this isn't the case for all organic clothing, however. As the demand for organic goods increases, some manufacturers are now using organic cotton as a raw material, but are still using chlorine bleach and conventional dyes (*National Geographic* 2008).

03. Historically, US labeling standards for organic clothing have not been well defined. Improvements are in process so research the latest guidelines, read labels, and consult the manufacturer.

04. Organic cotton can be much softer. However, it is not as durable as synthetic fibers.

How can you identify healthier cotton?

02. Organic cotton grows in shades of brown and green, so fabrics in these colors can be achieved without dyes.

01. Look for the USDA Organic seal. Organic farmers use biological pest control measures such as beneficial insects, rotate their crops to alleviate soil-borne pathogens, remove weeds by hand, and improve soil health and fertility by composting and other natural methods.

03. Look for a "Transitional Organic" seal. Cotton grown on fields free of chemicals for less than three years can get this certification.

TIPS: Fabric Finishes

"Finishing" broadly encompasses hundreds of processes and treatments used to achieve certain aesthetic and performance objectives, such as stain, water, wrinkle, and flame resistance and antimicrobial properties (Silas, Hansen, and Lent 2007). The chemicals involved vary, as do the related health issues. Some stain-guarding treatments contain the same perfluorinated chemicals used in nonstick cookware. As these are being phased out, new ones are now being made with silicones, among other things, which are less harmful.

Read labels
Beware of labels promising "permanent press," "no iron," "water repellent," and "flame retardant" properties. Formaldehyde, found in permanent press fabric and some fire-retardant clothes and home textiles, is an upper respiratory irritant and carcinogen.

Avoid unnecessary exposures
Think carefully about the risk versus reward of having these chemicals in your home. Some fabrics are treated with more than one finish, each applied at a different stage of production. Scientific studies of the chemicals used to enhance fabric performance show alarming links to a wide range of health effects, from asthma to cancer (Silas, Hansen, and Lent 2007).

TIP: Fabric Treatments

Avoid toxic residues
Most fabrics are treated with dyes and finishing agents (like wrinkle protectants, stain guards, and fire retardants) that can leave lingering residues on fabric. Instead, choose natural fabrics that are free of fabric "finishes."

TIPS: Textile Dyes

Historically, dyes were made of natural ingredients derived from plants, animals, or minerals. Today, most are made of synthetic chemicals and heavy metals. Some leave Trails of Contamination that persist in air and water, binds with soil, and becomes part of the food web. They are found in leafy vegetables, fish, dairy, meats, and poultry. Once in the body, metals remain for years (Silas, Hansen, and Lent 2007).

Research dyes

When a product is marked "low impact," be aware that the dyes used may contain the same petrochemicals and heavy metals as conventional dyes, which are generally toxic.

TIPS: Certifications for Healthier Textiles

Global Organic Textile Standard (GOTS)

This is the most stringent standard, so look for GOTS-certified fabrics. If you can't find certified GOTS, then request it or ask for other third-party-certified green fabrics.

The Oeko-Tex Standard 100

This is a globally uniform testing and certification system. It assigns specific tolerance levels of chemicals to clothing based on how much contact the clothing will have with skin. Products have been tested to ensure that formaldehyde, carcinogenic colors, phthalates, pesticides, and other potentially harmful residues are absent, or only minimally present.

Certified Organic

Marked by the USDA organic seal, this seal ensures that raw fibers have been produced through USDA-approved methods, which exclude the use of synthetic fertilizers, sewage sludge, irradiation, and genetic engineering. This certification relates to raw natural fibers, and not the treatment of those fibers to make products, nor the final products themselves. For that reason, many consumers turn to the GOTS for a better understanding of textile products.

Paths

OVERVIEW

Ingredients in paints vary with their formulas, which are designed to create different performance levels and aesthetics. However, most are made of four basic categories of ingredients: pigments, binders, solvents, and additives. Being mindful of solvents in your paint is a major filter against toxic fumes.

Solvents serve an important role in paints. A liquid component, solvents carry the pigment and binder and allow them to be spread onto its intended surface. Solvents also usually contain VOCs, which aid the drying of paint.

Different types of paint have different solvents:
— Water serves as the solvent for latex paints.
— Denatured alcohol is used for shellac-based primers and varnishes.
— Petroleum distillate is the solvent for most oil-based and alkyd paints.
— Various petrochemical products, most often a lacquer thinner, are used for clear and pigmented lacquers.

POSSIBLE HEALTH EFFECTS

As with any exposure, many factors determine the likelihood of certain adverse health effects, including the exposure level and duration, the individual's age and susceptibility, and any preexisting medical conditions. Some people experience eye, throat, or lung irritation; headaches; dizziness; and vision problems soon after exposure. Some chemicals in paint cause cancer or reproductive or developmental issues in laboratory animals. Those with unique vulnerabilities should avoid paint vapors (EPA 2000).

POSSIBLE SOURCES OF EXPOSURE

Art Supplies
Paint products.
Children's Stuff
Face paints, furniture, temporary tattoos, and toys.
Building Materials
Floors, walls, and windowsills.
Interior Furnishings
Cabinet doors, shelves, and other furniture.

HOUSEHOLD REPEAT OFFENDERS

Toxicants
— Formaldehyde
— Heavy metals
— Pesticides
— Unintentional Toxicants

Ingredients
— Inerts
— Nanoparticles
— Preservatives
— Solvents
— Surfactants
— Synthetic colors
— VOCs: One study concluded that less than 50 percent of the VOCs in latex paint are emitted within the first year (California Air Resources Board 2005). Some are known to persist for several years. The majority of petroleum-based products will take up to a year to fully oxidize, cure, and stabilize.

REPEAT ISSUES
— Additives, petrochemical ingredients, Unintentional Potential Effects, and unique vulnerabilities
— Hazardous air pollutants (HAPs): Paints can emit chemicals that the California EPA considers to be toxic air compounds; and emissions have the potential to continue for extended lengths of time (Urban Green Council 2015).

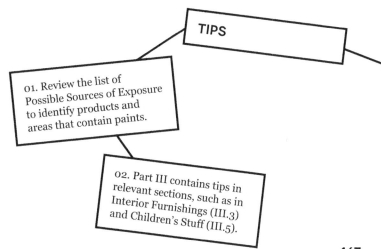

TIPS

01. Review the list of Possible Sources of Exposure to identify products and areas that contain paints.

02. Part III contains tips in relevant sections, such as in Interior Furnishings (III.3) and Children's Stuff (III.5).

Plastics

OVERVIEW

Although the first plastics were developed in the second half of the 19th century, it was not until World War II that plastic began to win broad acceptance in the marketplace. Plastics provided cheaper alternatives to their natural counterparts; for instance, vinyl was a less expensive substitute for natural rubber.

During the 1930s and 1940s, the plastics industry developed a host of new plastics for a broad variety of applications. In World War II, the military used these new materials to improve upon their weapons, protect existing equipment, and replace heavy components in various vehicles. After World War II, manufacturers applied plastics to a broad range of industries, including new consumer goods. Plastics steadily replaced wood and metal in many products and are now the most widely used manufacturing material in the world.

Plastics are popular as food containers and packaging for their lightweight and other conveniences. However, when you consider how plastics should be treated to prevent them from leaching toxic chemicals into food—washed by hand, and kept away from the heat of a microwave or dishwasher, especially when containing foods with a high fat content, like meat and cheese—then the convenience of plastics isn't that convenient.

POSSIBLE HEALTH EFFECTS

Cancer from vinyl chloride and dioxins, hormone disruption from phthalates, neurotoxicity from lead and mercury, reproductive toxicity from mercury.

POSSIBLE SOURCES OF EXPOSURE

Building Materials
Exterior housing, materials and pipes.
Children's Stuff
Car seats, lunch boxes, mattresses, toys, and utensils.
Food Packaging and Containers
Disposable beverage and water bottles, food containers, and packaging for processed and packaged foods.
In the Kitchen
Cutting boards, and utensils.
Others
Electronics, and storage containers.

WHAT ARE GOVERNMENTS DOING?

Many local, state, and national governments have started banning or charging for plastic and paper bags. These include Maui and Kauai counties in Hawaii; American Samoa; Portland, Oregon; South Padre Island, Texas; coastal North Carolina; and the California cities of Malibu, Palo Alto, Fairfax, San Jose, Santa Monica, and San Francisco. Marin and Los Angeles counties have also banned bags. California stands to be the first state to enact a bag ban, although SB270 is currently being appealed. Overseas, free plastic bags have been banned in China, Bangladesh, Australia, Italy, South Africa, Ireland, and Taiwan.

HOUSEHOLD REPEAT OFFENDERS

Toxicants
— Benzene
— BPA
— Chlorine: Of the more than 10 million tons of chlorine the US consumes each year, roughly one-third is used to produce 14 varieties of plastic (McGinn 2000).
— Dioxins
— Heavy metals, like lead and cadmium: They are not banned from plastics and are detected in various products including shopping bags and toys.
— Phthalates

Ingredients
— Endocrine disrupting chemicals: A study published in Environmental Health Perspectives tested 455 plastic items—from baby bottles to deli packaging—for the presence of estrogenic chemicals. More than 95 percent released these chemicals when exposed to microwaving, dish washing, or sunlight, including items advertised as BPA-free. According to the study, "In some cases, BPA-free products released chemicals having more estrogenic activity than did BPA-containing products" (Yang et al. 2011).
— Nanoparticles
— VOCs

VINYL

A—Z

ADDITIONAL OFFENDERS

— Other toxic chemicals released by the plastics industry include antimony, styrene, trichloroethane, sulfur oxides, nitrous oxides, methanol, ethylene oxide, and vinyl chloride.

REPEAT ISSUES

— Trails of Contamination: Of the 300 million tons of plastic produced globally each year, it is estimated that only 10 percent is recycled (Wassener 2011). The world's oceans contain at least five giant "garbage patches" that are changing marine life. For example, the midocean surface area they provide is allowing insects to breed like never before. Furthermore, plastics in our oceans both leach toxicants and absorb others; and are then ingested or absorbed by marine life and us.

TIPS: Handling Plastics Safely

Avoid plastics when you can. Review the list of Possible Sources of Exposure for ideas. As the EWG (2015e) suggests, when you do use plastics:

01. Do not microwave anything you intend to ingest in plastic containers, even if they are marketed as "microwave safe." Heat from the microwave can break down plastics, and release chemicals into food. Only use plastic containers for cool foods and liquids.

02. Do not reuse plastics that are intended for disposal. Repeated use can cause the breakdown of plastics and the release of chemicals. This includes old, scratched plastic water bottles!

03. Wash plastics by hand, or on the top rack of a dishwasher (far away from the machine's heat source). That will reduce the wear and tear that the plastics experience.

04. Do not permit young children to handle or chew on plastic electronics (including cell phones) because they may contain flame retardants.

05. Always wash children's hands before they eat.

Keeping Track of Plastics

Examples of common types

Type of Plastic	Found in	Helpful Information
Polyethylene terephthalate PET PETE	Bean bags; beverage containers for most bottled water and soda; combs; detergents and cleaning product containers; food containers for cooking oils, juices, medicine jars; microwavable meal trays; peanut butters, ropes, and salad dressings.	— Generally regarded as safe. Shown to leach antimony into the water in a couple of studies, but at levels considered safe by the EPA. — PET is one of the most easily recycled plastics. — Producing a 16-ounce PET bottle generates more than 100 times the toxic emissions to air and water than making the same bottle out of glass.
High-density polyethylene HDPE	Bottles for detergents, motor oils, and shampoos; some cereal box liners, milk and water jugs, and plastic grocery store and trash bags; and personalized toys.	— Generally regarded as safe. — HDPE is easily recycled.
Polyvinyl chloride PVC	Clear food packaging and cling wraps; bottles for various products, such as cooking oils, peanut butters, shampoos, detergents, and window cleaners; door and window frames, flooring products, home siding, pipes (including plumbing), and shower curtains; inflatable beach toys, raincoats, toys for children older than 12, and toys made before February 2009; and medical tubing. Not usually used for water bottles.	— Many harmful chemicals are produced (both intentionally and unintentionally) in the manufacturing, disposal, or destruction of PVC, including lead, DEHA (di(2-ethylhexyl) adipate), dioxins, ethylene dichloride, and vinyl chloride. PVC is one of the least recyclable plastics due to additives. Throughout its Life Cycle, it contaminates our Homes. — From contact with food and drinks, PVC can leach harmful chemicals into food and beverages.
Low-density polyethylene LDPE	Breads, frozen foods, and sandwich bags; grocery bags; shrink-wrap and most plastic wraps; squeezable bottles for condiments; and toys.	— Generally regarded as safe. However, when plastic containers made from recycled #4 (and #5) plastic become heavily worn or scratched, retire and recycle them. While no known health effects associated with the use of this plastic are known, organic pollutants are formed during its manufacturing. — #4 plastics are not as commonly recyclable.
Polypropylene PP	Disposable diapers; food containers: baby bottles, margarine containers, syrup bottles, takeout soup containers, yogurt cups; house wrap; medicine bottles; outdoor carpets; plastic bottle caps; and straws.	— Generally regarded as safe. — PP is not easily recycled. Differences in the varieties of type and grade mean achieving consistent quality during recycling is difficult. — When reusable plastic containers made from #5 plastic become heavily worn or scratched, retire and recycle them.

Type of Plastic	Found in	Helpful Information
Polystyrene (commonly known as Styrofoamt)	Compact disc cases; disposable bowls, coffee cups, cutlery, egg cartons, food containers, grocery store meat trays, and plates; packing peanuts and foam; and other applications.	— Polystyrene can leach styrene, a chemical that can damage the nervous system and is listed as a possible human carcinogen (IARC 2002). Over the long term, it can act as a neurotoxin. Studies on animals report harmful effects of styrene on red blood cells as well as the liver, kidneys, and stomach. — Styrene can be absorbed by food; once ingested, it can be stored in body fat. It is thought that repeated exposure can lead to bioaccumulation. — The manufacture of polystyrene is harmful to the ozone layer (EJNet 1996). — Recycling is possible, but it requires a lot of energy and is not normally economically viable.
Polycarbonate	— "7" indicates plastic other than those listed above; the letters PC under the recycling symbol specify polycarbonate. — Polycarbonate is a hard, durable plastic typically used to make 5-gallon water bottles, clear plastic sippy cups and some plastic cutlery, electronics, food can linings and lids, lunch boxes, medical storage containers, most plastic baby bottles, reusable food containers, "sport" water bottles," thermoses and other travel containers, and water bottles.	— Polycarbonate plastic is manufactured with BPA. In 2008, the National Toxicology Program raised concerns that exposure to BPA during pregnancy and childhood could impact the developing breast and prostate and affect brain development and behavior in children (NTP 2008). — A study from Harvard found that college students drinking from polycarbonate bottles had 69 percent more BPA in their bodies than they did during the weeks they drank from other containers (Carwile et al. 2009). — Mixed-resin plastics like #7 are difficult, if not impossible, to recycle. — Health effects vary, depending on the resin and plasticizers. For example, polycarbonate plastic can leach BPA.
Acrylonitrile butadiene styrene (ABS)	ABS wasn't part of the original plastics ID system, so it doesn't have a number. It is often used in automotive body parts, musical instruments, piping, toys, and wheel covers.	— This plastic is manufactured with styrene, a possible human carcinogen that is discussed above. Other key chemicals used in its manufacture include acrylonitrile, which is listed as a possible human carcinogen, and butadiene, which is probably carcinogenic to humans (IARC 1999).

Plastics: Vinyl

VINYL OVERVIEW

PVC, or vinyl, has been described as one of the most toxic plastics made. The PVC industry is one of the largest consumers of mercury, chlorine, and phthalates, as part I explained. Other ingredients include lead, vinyl chloride, and ethylene dichloride (a probable human carcinogen). During its manufacturing and incineration, vinyl can create highly toxic dioxins as an Unintentional By-product. The US Green Building Council's Technical Science Advisory Committee report on PVC in building products confirmed "dioxin emission puts PVC consistently among the worst materials studied for human health impacts" (Green Building Council 2007).

From 1988 to 2009, global production of PVC expanded from 12.8 million tons to 32.3 million tons. Growth is projected to continue to 55.2 million tons by 2020 (Business Wire 2011; Worldwatch Institute 2000).

Since manufacturing and disposing of PVC produces dioxins, some companies are trying to shift away from PVC. Examples include Hewlett-Packard, Microsoft, Honda, Walmart, Target, and Nike. However, there's still plenty of vinyl waste.

Is there any regulation?

Since 2009, child care products (for children under three) and children's toys (for children under 12) containing concentrations of certain phthalates (DEHP, BBP, and DBP) greater than 0.1 percent have been banned as hazardous materials. An interim ban on DINP (diisononyl phthalate), DnOP (di-n-octyl phthalate), and DIDP (diisodecyl phthalate) in concentrations greater than 0.1 percent has been established for toys that can be placed in a child's mouth (CPSC 2015b). This restriction does not apply to other PVC products. Some manufacturers have chosen to eliminate PVC entirely, others just in teething toys, and some just in toys for children under three. Since kids tend to put almost anything in their mouth, it's best to avoid products made with PVC altogether.

The CHEJ is focused on getting schools to stop using PVC in construction. You can find great tips on avoiding PVC in schools and in school supplies on the CHEJ website (chej.org).

POSSIBLE HEALTH EFFECTS

The various toxicants and Unintentional Toxicants that are related to vinyl pose health risks through the seemingly immortal Life Cycle of vinyl, as part I explained. Health risks include cancer from vinyl chloride and dioxins, hormone disruption from phthalates, neurotoxicity from lead and mercury, and reproductive toxicity from mercury.

HOUSEHOLD REPEAT OFFENDERS

Toxicants
— Chlorine
— Dioxins
— Lead
— Mercury
— Phthalates

Ingredients
— HAPs
— VOCs

ADDITIONAL OFFENDERS
— Ethylene dichloride: a probable human carcinogen
— Vinyl chloride

REPEAT ISSUES
— Trails of Contamination
— Unintentional By-products
— Unintentional Potential Effects
— Unique vulnerabilities

POSSIBLE SOURCES OF EXPOSURE

Apparel
Aprons, bags, backpacks (PVC waterproof coating), bibs, boots, children's umbrellas, diaper covers, lingerie, luggage, rain pants, raincoats, shoes and shoe soles, skirts, t-shirts with PVC prints, and watchbands.

Automotive
Auto-related product containers, components, car interiors, car seats for children, dashboards, door panels, traffic cones, underbody coatings, upholstery treatments, and wire coatings.

Building Materials
Cavity closure insulations, door frames, door gaskets, fencing, flooring, gutters, molding, pipes, roofing membranes, shutters, siding, tiles, wall coverings, window frames, and wire/cable insulations.

Children's Stuff
Children's rain gear, crib bumpers, crib rail teething guards, strollers, and toys (e.g., flexible bath toys, plastic dolls).

In the Kitchen
Commercial food wraps, dish drying racks (coating) and dry pans, dishwashers, refrigerators, and freezer racks, drinking straws, food containers, plastic tablecloths, plastic utensils, and plastic wraps.

Interior Furnishings
Imitation leather furniture, mattress covers, shelving, shower curtains, textiles, and water beds.

Medical Supplies
Bed liners, blood bags, catheters, colostomy bags, gloves, IV bags, mattress covers, and tubing.

Outdoor Items
Balls, children's swimming pools, flower bed edging, garden hoses, greenhouses, inflatable furniture, outdoor furniture, pond liners, and tarps.

Office Supplies
Binders, cellular phones, clipboards, coated paper clips, computer keyboards, computer monitor housing, credit cards, and mouse pads.

Personal Care Items (packaging)
Aloe vera gels, baby oils, bubble bath products, face washes, hair gels, liquid soaps, lotions, massage oils, mouthwashes, shampoos, and suntan lotions.

Others
Checkbook covers, cleaning product containers, clothes racks (covers metal to prevent rusting), credit cards, electrical cords, pet care product containers, photo album sheets, and self-adhesive labels/stickers.

(Liu, Schade, and Simpson 2008)

TIPS: Reduce PVC-Free in Your Home

01. Scan the list of Possible Sources of Exposure to select items that are easy for you to avoid. Of higher priority is the avoidance of foods and beverages packaged in PVC materials as well as PVC products in general. Make special efforts to buy PVC-free baby products and toys.

02. For home remodeling projects, consider PVC-free building materials.

03. See chapter III.6 for tips on how to avoid PVC in art, school, and office supplies.

Polyurethane Foam

OVERVIEW

Created as a substitute for natural rubber, polyurethane foam has many practical purposes since it's inexpensive, durable, and light weight.

While various chemical formulas are used to produce polyurethane foam with various traits (such as densities), the general components are petroleum-based chemicals, used in the roles of catalysts, additives, flame retardants, and others. Therefore, polyurethane foam is highly flammable.

Your upholstered sofa could "engulf an entire living room in flames, filling the home with thick, dark smoke and toxic gases," according to the National Association of State Fire Marshals (2015). Polyurethane foam cushioning is the most flammable part of a mattress or couch (Betts 2008). Depending on what it's made of, the fabric covering of a couch could make the fire even worse.

According to the National Association of State Fire Marshals (2015), this could happen in "just minutes" because of the presence of polyurethane foam. In fact, fire marshals refer to polyurethane foam as "solid gasoline."

Two types of foam, which are on extreme ends of the natural-to-synthetic spectrum (and are discussed more in figure #09), are 100 percent petroleum-based foam and 100 percent natural latex foam. There are also many variations in between those two. The next few pages discuss key considerations that should help you formulate questions before you purchase polyurethane foam products.

POSSIBLE HEALTH EFFECTS

Chemicals from polyurethane foam that evaporate into the indoor environment or leach into household dust may contribute to asthma; eye, nose, and throat irritation; headaches; loss of coordination; nausea; and damage to the liver, kidneys, and central nervous system. VOCs have been linked to cancer after prolonged exposure. Some companies certify that products emit low or no EPA-listed VOCs (Clean and Healthy New York 2011).

POSSIBLE SOURCES OF EXPOSURE

Children's Stuff
Car seats, diaper changing pads, high chairs, nursing pillows, playpens, portable cribs, and stuffed toys.

Construction Materials
Building insulation materials.

Interior Furnishings
Carpet backings, cushions, mattresses (including crib mattresses), pillows, and upholstered furniture (sofas and chairs).

HOUSEHOLD REPEAT OFFENDERS

Toxicants
— Benzene
— Chlorine
— Formaldehyde
— Methylene chloride
— PFOS

Ingredients
— Chemical flame retardants: penta-, octa-, and deca-PBDEs; Tris flame retardants; and boric acid
— Solvents
— VOCs

ADDITIONAL REPEAT OFFENDERS

— 4,4' methylene diphenyl diisocyanate (MDI): MDI is another key ingredient that's made from formaldehyde, aniline, and various other chemicals, including benzene (Healthy Building Network 2008).

— Additional toxic chemical additives: They can come in the role of stabilizers, catalysts, surfactants, fire retardants, emulsifiers, pigments, blowing agents, and Unintentional Toxicants. These include formaldehyde, benzene, and toluene.

— Petroleum-based ingredients: Examples include crude oil, natural gas, and sodium chloride.

— Toluene diisocyanate (TDI): A potential carcinogen, TDI is a key raw material for polyurethane. It is made from chlorine, toluene, phosgene, sulfuric acid, and nitric acid, all of which are considered hazardous VOCs.

REPEAT ISSUES

— Lack of disclosure of ingredients and potential toxicity

— Safety of substitutes? Used to produce softer, lower-density foams, chlorofluorocarbon was an ingredient in polyurethane foam until it was banned for its ozone-depleting characteristics. In 1992, the EPA required the industry to phase out its production completely by 1995. Methylene chloride became a common replacement. The EPA has listed methylene chloride as a probable human carcinogen, and it is linked to nervous system damage, as well as decreased visual and auditory acuity. Each year, US production of polyurethane foam releases about 24 million pounds of this chemical into the atmosphere (Bader 2011). High levels of methylene chloride may build in indoor air if there is inadequate ventilation.

— Toxicants contaminate air and dust: Foams contain chemicals that escape into household dust. Children can ingest these toxic chemicals as they crawl on the floor, touch everything in sight, and put things into their mouths.

— Trails of Contamination throughout our Homes

— Unintentional By-products: The manufacture of a key ingredient in some formulas, polyether polyols, creates hazardous air pollutants that are known to cause or are suspected of causing cancer and other serious health concerns.

— Unique vulnerabilities

— Unknown Potential Effects

TIPS

Follow my D-Tox Strategy

Petrochemical ingredients from polyurethane foam can off-gas and leach from their products. Follow the tips in part IV to improve indoor air quality, fight the dust, and wash hands frequently.

Critically assess your products

For products that contain polyurethane foam, look for "TB 117-2013" on the label. Since there's no ban on chemical flame retardants on any part of the sofa, ask the manufacturer if the product is free of chemical flame retardants and fabric treatments.

Review part III

Other tips to reduce exposure to polyurethane foam are included in relevant products of concern in part III (e.g., upholstered sofas, mattresses, and children's products).

TIPS: Healthier Alternative to Polyurethane Foam

TIPS: Greenwashing

Navigating marketing claims is challenging. The information in the boxes below should provide helpful perspective.

100 percent natural latex or natural rubber

Made from the sap of rubber trees, natural rubber latex is a good substitute to polyurethane foam. It is a renewable resource, as opposed to synthetic latex, which is made from petroleum derivatives. Natural latex was a popular material used for cushioning until the invention of the cheaper and lighter polyurethane foam.

02. Disadvantages

01. Although most latex allergies are related to synthetic versions, natural latex allergies do occur.

02. Natural latex mattresses are more expensive, with cost increasing along with purity and certifications. They're also extremely heavy.

Organic products vary in their "purity"

"Organic" products may still contain polyurethane foam. Just as an "organic" mattress may have one organic component and many more toxic ones, mattresses made of "green" foam may contain meaningful amounts of petroleum-based components that contribute to harmful indoor contamination.

01. Advantages

01. Natural latex is not highly flammable and does not require fire retardant chemicals to pass the California TB 117 test.

02. Little or no off-gassing is associated with it.

03. Natural latex is resistant to mold, mildew, bacteria, and dust mites.

04. It is recyclable and biodegradable.

03. Shopping tips

01. There are no labeling requirements obligating a manufacturer to disclose what percentage of the latex is natural and what percentage is synthetic. "Latex" on the label may represent synthetic latex, which generally is made of about 70 percent polyurethane and 30 percent natural latex. A mattress label can say "Made from Natural Rubber" and contain only 10 percent natural rubber, along with 90 percent synthetic materials. Read labels critically and question what information may be missing.

Avoid Household Repeat Offenders

In seeking healthier products, you need to understand the components of certain products to get the purity you desire.

"In the [US], a typical modern housing unit of 1,800 square feet of floor space, including furniture, carpet underlay, and bedding, contains 306 pounds of flexible polyurethane foam" (NTP 2014).

05. Natural rubber is durable, elastic, and provides great support. Its elastic properties give mattresses the ability to keep their shape and firmness after years of use. They also offer excellent heat and moisture regulation, air circulation, and a metal-free environment for sleep. Natural rubber latex mattresses have the largest share of the organic mattress market (Bader 2011).

02. Natural latex is usually "washed" to remove potential allergens. This can involve any number of processes. It may be worth asking which process was used.

Potential Adverse Health Effects from Different Types of Foam

100 PERCENT NATURAL INGREDIENTS

Natural Rubber Latex
Made from the sap of rubber trees, natural rubber latex is a renewable resource. Those with latex allergies should take precautions. It is heavy.

Soy- or Plant- Based Foam
These could be a blend of petroleum- and plant- based ingredients from soy or castor beans. The advantage is that fewer petroleum-based ingredients are used. However, since a portion of ingredients may be petroleum-based, adverse health effects may be present. Also, conventional soybeans are often grown with harmful pesticides or genetically modified seeds and are energy-intensive to farm.

Polyethylene Foam
A low-density, food-grade polyethylene still contains petrochemical ingredients, but it can be of low toxicity if it's tested to ensure absence of contaminants. It is lightweight.

Polyurethane Foam
100 percent polyurethane foam is made of petroleum-based ingredients. Inexpensive and lightweight, it may also off-gas and leach toxic chemicals.

Memory Foam
Memory foam, aka viscoelastic foam, may contain the same chemicals as those in polyurethane foam, or similar ones, and may, therefore, pose similar health risks.

100 PERCENT PETROLEUM-BASED INGREDIENTS

(Source: Bader 2011)

FIGURE #09

177

Woods

OVERVIEW

Wood options include solid hardwoods and composite (also known as pressed) woods, such as plywoods, particleboards, and medium-density fiberboards (MDF). Most furniture is constructed of pressed woods because they're less expensive. Pressed woods consist of wood or other components bonded with adhesives, which can emit formaldehyde and pollute your indoor air for years. Therefore, pay attention to wood adhesives used in your floors, furniture, mattresses, dressers, tables, children's toys, etc.

POSSIBLE HEALTH EFFECTS

Please see Possible Health Effects in the Solvents profile. Solvents are used in the chemical adhesives that bind wood particles, and they are found in finishing products such as paints, stains, and sealers.

POSSIBLE SOURCES OF EXPOSURE TO PRESSED WOOD

Interior Furnishings
Hardwood plywood paneling (cabinets, decorative wall coverings, and furniture); MDF (cabinets, drawer fronts, and furniture tops); and particleboard (used as shelving and subflooring, and in cabinetry and furniture). MDF has a higher resin-to-wood ratio than any other UF (urea-formaldehyde) pressed wood product, and it is considered to be the highest formaldehyde-emitting pressed wood product (CA EPA 2015).
Toys
Figures, playsets, and wooden puzzles.

HOUSEHOLD REPEAT OFFENDERS

Toxicants

— Formaldehyde: The Formaldehyde Standards for Composite Wood Products Act, signed into law in July 2010, establishes limits for formaldehyde emissions from composite wood products: hardwoods, plywoods, medium-density fiberboards, and particleboards. The regulation should finalize by the end of 2015.
— Heavy metals: These, including lead, are used as drying agents.
— Pesticides: These, like biocides, protect against mold and fungi.

Ingredients

— Solvents: These may be in the wood adhesives, paints, or other wood treatments. They can off-gas formaldehyde, heavy metal drying agents, and biocides.

TIPS: Adhesives

01. To avoid adhesives, solid wood is ideal. Recycled wood is best for our planet.

02. While pressed wood products are often covered by a layer of plastic laminate that limits the release of formaldehyde, it can still be released from exposed edges (*National Geographic* 2008). Be aware of wood products with veneers, as they may be applied with a variety of chemical adhesives.

03. Particleboards, fiberboards, and plywoods are manufactured with adhesives that contain urea-formaldehyde (UF) or phenol-formaldehyde (PF) resin. PF resin generally emits formaldehyde at considerably lower rates than UF resin.

Avoid toxic solvents

Wood products are often finished with wood stains and surface sealers. Oil-based stains that use mineral spirits as a solvent are unhealthy for consumers and contaminate our water supply. Rags soaked in it can spontaneously combust.

Ventilate

Surface coatings using toxic ingredients, such as polyurethane, are produced through condensation and a reaction among various chemicals. The end result is a host of potentially carcinogenic and irritating compounds that you could inhale as you sleep.

TIPS: Finishing Products (surface stains, paints and sealers)

Healthier Wood Products

Solid wood, rather than composite wood, reduces the level of formaldehyde in the air since it doesn't use adhesives. If you purchase furniture that was made from pressed wood products, follow the precautionary steps in this section.

02. Avoid toxic solvents

Finishes often applied to wood include fillers, caulk, sealants, stains, sealers, wax, oils, lacquer, varnish, and paints. While these products contain proprietary ingredients, solvents are a key ingredient that can also be a key source of contamination.

03. Check with the manufacturer

Consult the manufacturer about the product's formaldehyde levels and whether any limits are placed on the chemical's use. Composite wood can be found in building materials, cabinetry, and furniture.

04. Look for products made with phenol-formaldehyde resin

Phenol-formaldehyde is less volatile than urea-formaldehyde.

05. Research exterior-grade pressed wood products, if available

"Exterior-grade" pressed wood products release less formaldehyde as they contain phenol resins, and not urea resins (CPSC 2015a).

06. Buy from informed retailers

Shop at stores that are committed to helping the issue. You can search for retailers of formaldehyde-free pressed-wood furniture on the Forest Stewardship Council (FSC) website (us.fsc.org).

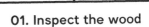

TIPS: When Shopping

01. Inspect the wood

01. Consumers can determine if the wood is pressed by inspecting exposed wood, and looking for a bumpy texture and visible layers.

02. A certain piece may look like it is made of hardwood, but may in fact be composite wood that is covered by thin wood veneers (*National Geographic* 2008).

03. Unlaminated or uncoated panels of pressed wood products typically emit more formaldehyde than those which are laminated or coated (CPSC 2013). If purchasing furniture made of pressed wood, then choose those that are laminated with coated edges, and that is not made with urea-formaldehyde glues, lumber, or metal.

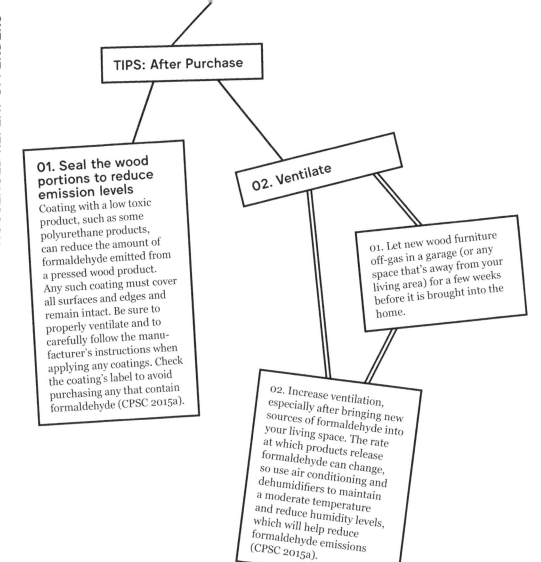

TIPS: After Purchase

01. Seal the wood portions to reduce emission levels

Coating with a low toxic product, such as some polyurethane products, can reduce the amount of formaldehyde emitted from a pressed wood product. Any such coating must cover all surfaces and edges and remain intact. Be sure to properly ventilate and to carefully follow the manufacturer's instructions when applying any coatings. Check the coating's label to avoid purchasing any that contain formaldehyde (CPSC 2015a).

02. Ventilate

01. Let new wood furniture off-gas in a garage (or any space that's away from your living area) for a few weeks before it is brought into the home.

02. Increase ventilation, especially after bringing new sources of formaldehyde into your living space. The rate at which products release formaldehyde can change, so use air conditioning and dehumidifiers to maintain a moderate temperature and reduce humidity levels, which will help reduce formaldehyde emissions (CPSC 2015a).

Part III

Tips for Products of Concern

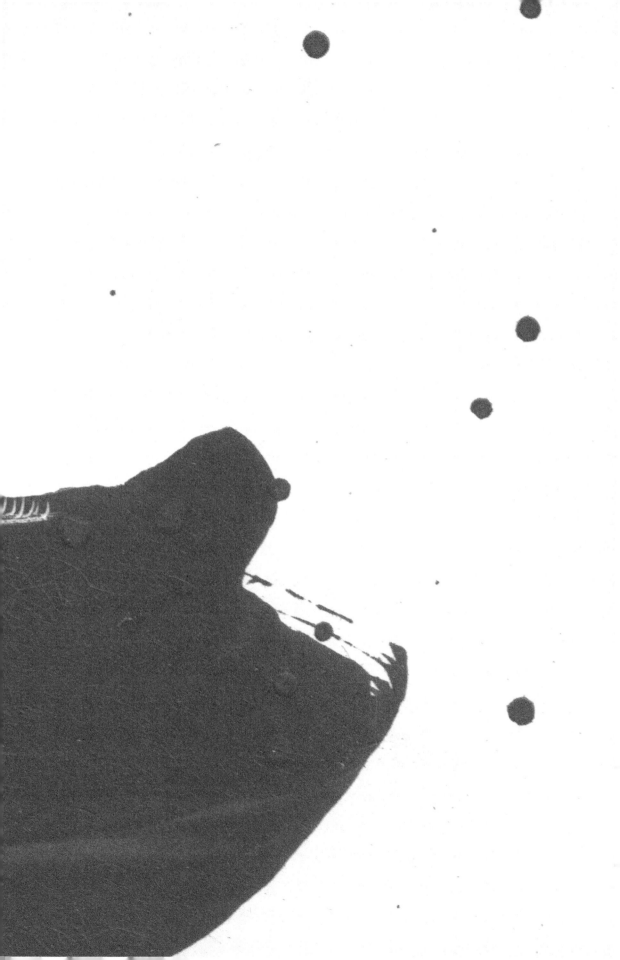

Part III Introduction

As you clear up your *avidya* and break old habits, part III can help you form healthier ones that suit your unique budget, circumstances, and preferences.

Part III contains profiles of popular end products. These profiles include both a list of Household Repeat Offenders that may be in the subject product and tips for healthier Homes. This is meant to further develop the informational framework introduced in part II, which should help you navigate the uncertainty and confusion that surround our household products.

Products are organized into the following chapters: Cleaning Products, In the Kitchen, Interior Furnishings, Personal Care Products, Children's Stuff, and Miscellaneous.

Part III has three main intentions. First, when I began learning about everyday toxic exposures, I was determined to do everything I could to purify my children's environment. I wished for something like part III: a comprehensive list of tips from which I could select what I wanted to adopt. If you have a similar reaction, I hope that part III helps soothe your concerns by empowering you with actions to pursue.

Second, the details in part III communicate, as concisely as possible, the complexity of finding "off-the-shelf" products that are truly safe. From these notes, you can appreciate the Simple Strategies that end each chapter as well as the D-Tox Strategy in part IV. Turns out that the safest solutions are the most basic and timeless approaches.

Last, part III is a reference section that you can revisit as you are ready to incorporate more change. You can also visit my website, NontoxicLiving.tips, to learn more about my favorite products. Since new products and better information will continue to surface, subscribing to my email newsletter is the best way to stay current.

All of us have unique health issues, homes, circumstances, budgets, and environments. So independent research and critical thinking should be pursued!

PLEASE NOTE THAT YOU WILL ENCOUNTER THE TERMS BELOW IN PART III

Off-gassing and VOCs

Many consumer products are made of petroleum-based ingredients, which can vaporize over time (a process known as off-gassing), and emit volatile organic compounds (VOCs), semi-volatile organic compounds (SVOCs), and hazardous air pollutants. These toxicants can also settle into dust (Blanchard et al. 2014; Roberts et al. 2009). Off-gassing is more common in environments with higher humidity and temperature.

Hazardous air pollutants

According to the EPA (2012a), hazardous air pollutants (HAPs), or toxic air pollutants, are a group of chemicals that are known or suspected to cause serious health conditions, like cancer, birth defects, and reproductive abnormalities. They also pollute our environment. HAPs include formaldehyde, benzene, methylene chloride, toluene, asbestos, perchloroethylene, dioxins, and heavy metals like lead and cadmium.

Secondary air pollutants

These are formed from the reactions of other, primary pollutants. Examples include ozone, formaldehyde, and smog.

Profiles of Consumer End Products

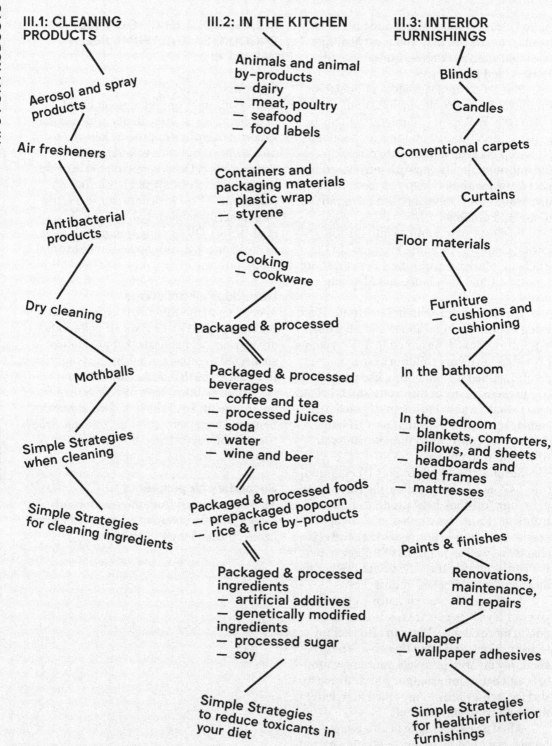

III.1: CLEANING PRODUCTS

Aerosol and spray products

Air fresheners

Antibacterial products

Dry cleaning

Mothballs

Simple Strategies when cleaning

Simple Strategies for cleaning ingredients

III.2: IN THE KITCHEN

Animals and animal by-products
— dairy
— meat, poultry
— seafood
— food labels

Containers and packaging materials
— plastic wrap
— styrene

Cooking
— cookware

Packaged & processed

Packaged & processed beverages
— coffee and tea
— processed juices
— soda
— water
— wine and beer

Packaged & processed foods
— prepackaged popcorn
— rice & rice by-products

Packaged & processed ingredients
— artificial additives
— genetically modified ingredients
— processed sugar
— soy

Simple Strategies to reduce toxicants in your diet

III.3: INTERIOR FURNISHINGS

Blinds

Candles

Conventional carpets

Curtains

Floor materials

Furniture
— cushions and cushioning

In the bathroom

In the bedroom
— blankets, comforters, pillows, and sheets
— headboards and bed frames
— mattresses

Paints & finishes

Renovations, maintenance, and repairs

Wallpaper
— wallpaper adhesives

Simple Strategies for healthier interior furnishings

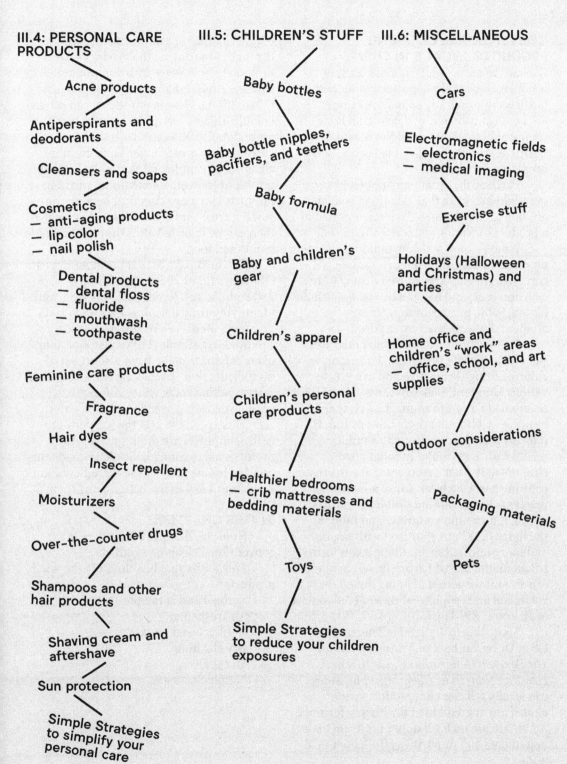

Chapter III.1
Cleaning Products

CONVENTIONAL CLEANING PRODUCTS: WHAT'S IN THEM?

It's hard to know what's in our cleaning products. Federal laws protect confidential business information, so manufacturers are not legally bound to disclose all their chemical ingredients or all the potential health problems that they may cause (EWG 2015j), as part I explained.

Further, there isn't any unbiased oversight ensuring that cleaning products are safe for our Homes. Federal approval of a product's formula is not even required.

What is known of conventional cleaning products raises concern. For example, corrosive cleaners can cause burning of the skin and eyes; and a popular one, household bleach, is the most common cleaner accidentally swallowed by children.

Furthermore, unintentional mixtures can create toxic by-products. For example, chlorine is highly reactive and can create various Unintentional Toxicants: Mixed with ammonia (e.g., from some glass cleaners, or urine in a training potty bowl or toilet), it forms toxic gases called chloramines; mixed with acid (found in toilet bowl cleaners and other detergents), it can create chlorine gas, which can cause adverse reactions like breathing problems, blurred vision, nausea and vomiting, and fluid in the lungs (CDC 2013); mixed with organic and inorganic matter in water, it can form trihalomethanes, which are linked to bladder cancer and suspected of being linked to colorectal and esophageal cancer (Villanueva et al. 2004; EWG 2013b).

According to Jeffrey Hollender and Geoff Davis, authors of *Naturally Clean: The Seventh Generation Guide to Safe & Healthy, Non-Toxic Cleaning,* companies can legally sell cleaning products with almost any ingredient and with any formula. And there are no legal upper limits on toxic ingredients and impurities (Hollender et al. 2006).

These toxic ingredients have several opportunities to enter our bodies: ordinary use, accidental ingestion, absorption through skin (during the product's use or upon later contact with contaminated surfaces), and inhalation of polluted air. Conventional cleaning products can off-gas volatile organic compounds and hazardous air pollutants. EPA studies found that cleaning fumes can linger long after the cleaning is completed (*National Geographic* 2008). Moreover, conventional cleaning products can leave chemical residues on surface areas and contaminate dust, which then can be ingested after they contaminate hands and food.

The next page lists Household Repeat Offenders that I encountered in my research. As you'll see, the list is long, and identifying truly harmless cleaning products is complicated! As a result, my cleaning solutions are simple. I have peace of mind using mixtures made from a short list of ingredients that have a long track record of safety: baking soda, white vinegar, castile soap, hydrogen peroxide, and hot water.

This approach gets the job done and really simplifies my shopping list. A few professional cleaning ladies have made the point of telling me, "These ingredients work great, and I feel much better using them!"

IN THIS CHAPTER:

— Household Repeat Offenders in conventional cleaning products
— Tips for buying healthier off-the-shelf products
  — Aerosol and spray products
  — Air fresheners
  — Antibacterial products
  — Dry cleaning
  — Mothballs
  — Simple Strategies

A—Z

HOUSEHOLD REPEAT OFFENDERS

Toxicants
— Chlorine
— Formaldehyde
— Heavy metals, like arsenic
— Pesticides
— Phthalates
— Unintentional Toxicants. For example, in late 2011, the environmental group Women's Voices for the Earth discovered small amounts of 1,4-dioxane in popular laundry products, including those that were labeled "fragrance free" and "sensitive" (Scranton 2011). Activists persuaded the manufacturer to reformulate the products to drastically reduce levels of 1,4-dioxane.

Ingredients
— Fragrance: Fragrances in four laundry products were found to contain 18 to 20 chemicals in each product. Toxicants detected included likely human carcinogens (acetaldehyde and 1,4-dioxane), developmental toxicants (methyl ethyl ketone and chloromethane), and allergens (linalool; Steinemann et al. 2010).
— Inerts
— Nanoparticles
— Petroleum distillates (naphtha): There are numerous petroleum-based possibilities, so it's hard to assess their risks.
— Solvents
— Surfactants: There is a wide range of surfactants. Some may release formaldehyde or create other carcinogenic compounds like dioxane.

ADDITIONAL OFFENDERS
— Ammonia: When mixed with chlorine, it can create a deadly gas. Ammonia is also an irritant.
— Essential oils: Beware of potential health risks, as there is some concern that lavender and tea tree oil may cause hormone disruption.
— Glycol ethers: Can produce harmful VOCs, including HAPs (EPA 2013d).
— Lye: Used in soap, metal polish, drain cleaners, and pool cleaners, lye (potassium hydroxide) fights grease and drain clogs. Made from ash, lye can irritate skin and eyes, and lye fumes can corrode respiratory passages.
— Optical brighteners: These are synthetic chemicals that are added to laundry detergents to make clothes appear brighter and whiter. Designed to remain on our laundry, optical brighteners may irritate the skin, creating a sunburn appearance (*National Geographic* 2008; Seventh Generation 2010). These chemicals can survive wastewater treatment and don't completely biodegrade. They bioaccumulate in fish.
— Phosphates: Phosphates are minerals that soften water. Once widely used, they are now less common since they harm aquatic environments. Major manufacturers have pledged to phase out phosphates from their laundry detergents; hand-washing and dish-washing liquids tend to not contain them (but some dishwasher detergent and cleaning formulas are still found with phosphates). Products with phosphates tend to have higher levels of heavy metals, especially arsenic. Chemicals that replaced phosphates in laundry detergents (polycarboxylates and EDTA [ethylenediaminetetraacetic acid]) are considered safer. However, they are petroleum-based and do not biodegrade.

REPEAT ISSUES
— Difficulty determining which off-the-shelf cleaning products are safe
— Health risks: Some ingredients are known respiratory irritants, carcinogens, hormone disruptors, and neurotoxins and are linked to chronic and long-term effects. Cancer, asthma, birth defects, and respiratory impairment have been linked to cleaning products.
— Insufficient regulation of toxic ingredients in consumer products
— Lack of disclosure of ingredients and potential toxicity
— Lack of required safety testing by an objective third party
— Misleading/confusing label claims
— Trails of Contamination throughout our Homes
— Unintentional By-products that can persist beyond their intended useful life
— Unique vulnerabilities
— Unintentional Potential Effects

ADDITIONAL ISSUES
— Accidental poisonings of children is an obvious concern.

TIPS: Buying Off-the-Shelf Cleaning Products

Labels — Key Terms to Understand

"Danger," "Poison," "Warning," "Caution," and "Use in well ventilated area"
Avoid or be cautious of products with these terms on the labels.

"Active" ingredients
In cleaning products, this term may include pesticides added to kill bacteria, viruses, or molds. They are not necessary. In fact, overuse of antimicrobial pesticides may contribute to antibiotic-resistant bacteria that have their own adverse health effects.

The EWG
The EWG has a database (ewg.org/guides/cleaners) that ranks the toxicity/safety of the most common cleaning products. Seek labels that are transparent about their ingredients and about health and safety concerns.

"Inert" ingredients
Do not have to be disclosed on product labels. While "inert" implies that the ingredients are harmless, in cleaning products they can include petroleum-based solvents, preservatives, and fragrances. Potential health effects include irritation to the skin and respiratory system as well as neurotoxicity.

Research manufacturers' online information
While all ingredients are rarely provided on product labels, manufacturers may share more information online. However, according to the EWG (2015b), "even online, most companies provide vague or incomplete information."

Items that are vegetable-based, certified organic, and biodegradable are ideal
Remember that natural products can be harmful too, but third-party certifications can help identify safer options. According to the EWG (2015e), the Green Seal or EcoLogo are the best third-party certifications that can help identify healthier cleaning products. These organizations provide third-party certification that certain toxic chemicals are absent.

Bleach or "color safe" detergents
Hydrogen peroxide (also called oxygen bleach) is the key ingredient in many products marketed as "color safe" or containing "natural" bleach. This sanitizes and whitens without producing chlorinated by-products.

Labels —
Unsubstantiated
Claims

"Nontoxic"
No standard definition
or regulation of this term
exists in the cleaning
products industry. Products
so labeled can contain
hazardous ingredients.

"Safe"
No standard definition
or regulation of this term
exists in the cleaning
products industry. Products
so labeled can contain
hazardous ingredients.

"Organic"
No standard definition or
regulation of this term exists
in the cleaning products
industry, except for USDA
Certified Organic. Some
manufacturers use this term
to mean that ingredients
are made mostly of
carbon (petroleum-based)
ingredients.

"Natural"
No standard definition or
regulation of this term exists
in the cleaning products
industry.

"Green"
No standard definition
or regulation of this term
exists in the cleaning
products industry. Products
so labeled may contain
hazardous ingredients.

**"Fragrance-free" or
"unscented"**
These terms can mean that
no fragrances have been
added, but it can also mean
that a masking agent or
"neutral" fragrance has been
added to hide the smell of
other ingredients.

"Fresh"
This can indicate that a synthetic fragrance like lemon
or citrus was used to mask
other odors in the product.
This could suggest the presence of harmful fumes.

"Free" and "Clear"
Products with these labels
are probably the best option,
but they still could contain
synthetic scents to mask the
smells of other ingredients.

"Biodegradable"
While this implies that
ingredients will break down
into less harmful substances,
the term is not regulated.
Most modern cleaning
products are designed to
biodegrade relatively quickly,
but it is hard for consumers
to evaluate the biodegrad-
ability of a product.

**TIPS: Natural
Ingredients are
Potent Too**

Enzymes
Natural enzymes are added
to some cleaning products
that remove or break down
grime and stains (e.g., drain
cleaners and spot removers).
These products may cause
irritation and should be
handled according to instructions provided on the label.

Essential oils
Don't assume that these are
safe either. Some may cause
irritation, allergies, and
other adverse health effects.
For example, tea tree oil and
lavender are suspected of
causing hormone disruption.
The evidence is inconclusive
however.

TIPS: Storage and Handling Warnings to Heed

Whether homemade, organic, or conventional, keep in mind that many cleaning products can be harmful when ingested. Please store all your cleaning products in spots that are inaccessible to children and pets to avoid accidental poisonings or other harm.

"Flammable"

Since a product with this warning may ignite and burn easily, store products according to the manufacturer's advice.

"Corrosive"

Keep these products away from children since they can burn delicate skin. The biggest hazards include acidic toilet bowl cleaners, oven cleaners, and corrosive drain cleaners.

"Do not induce vomiting"

Read product labels for this warning, and respond according to manufacturers' directions. Some products may contain ingredients that can cause harm to the throat if vomited and damage the lungs if aspirated (EWG 2015e).

Never mix

Warnings to keep products away from certain other products should be taken seriously because mixtures can create even more toxic by-products.

The mixture of bleach and ammonia releases chloramine gas, which is highly toxic. These ingredients can accidentally mix when bleach is put into a toilet that is concurrently being scoured with a cleaner containing ammonia. Bleach and vinegar can produce deadly gases as well. In one study of injuries caused by cleaning products, bleach was most common culprit of injury (McKenzie et al. 2010), and the results of other studies do not indicate that antibacterial cleaners, like bleach, reduce the risk of sickness in the home (EWG 2015f). Hydrogen peroxide is an effective replacement for chlorine (and ammonia). It is a popular active ingredient in green products.

Think twice about what you spray

Cleaning solutions from spray bottles are a common source of harmful exposure (McKenzie et al. 2010).

Store products out of reach of children

Children aged one to three years accounted for 72 percent of injuries from household cleaning products (McKenzie et al. 2010). The American Academy of Pediatrics suggests that toxic substances be stored in their original containers and put in locked cabinets that are inaccessible to children; products that are ready to be disposed, should be done so properly (AAP 2015). Consider not buying conventional products, since safer, healthier, and effective alternatives exist.

Consider all manufacturers' warnings

Read product labels and follow all warnings.

Aerosol and Spray Products

OVERVIEW

The chemical formulas in aerosol and spray products contain toxicants that can be inhaled, which can damage lungs, and settle onto surface areas, including the skin (EWG 2015e). Further, cleaning products in spray bottles are common sources of accidental poisonings of children.

HOUSEHOLD REPEAT OFFENDERS

Toxicants
— Formaldehyde
— Methylene chloride

Ingredients
— Nanoparticles

ADDITIONAL OFFENDERS
— Nitrous oxide
— Propane
— Trichloroethylene: A carcinogen that can impair the central nervous and immune systems, kidneys, liver, and the male reproductive system

REPEAT ISSUES
— Potential unknown VOCs and HAPs
— Unintentional Potential Effects
— Unique vulnerabilities

ADDITIONAL ISSUES
— Accidental poisonings

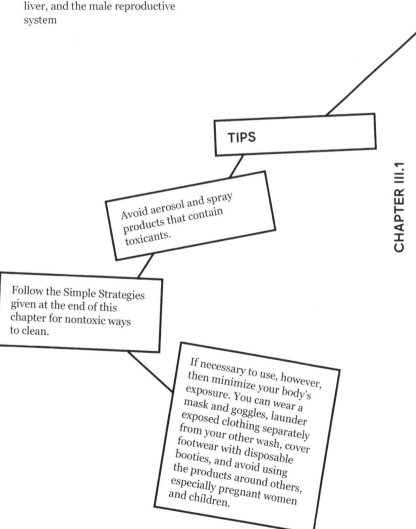

TIPS

Avoid aerosol and spray products that contain toxicants.

Follow the Simple Strategies given at the end of this chapter for nontoxic ways to clean.

If necessary to use, however, then minimize your body's exposure. You can wear a mask and goggles, launder exposed clothing separately from your other wash, cover footwear with disposable booties, and avoid using the products around others, especially pregnant women and children.

Air Fresheners

OVERVIEW

Air fresheners are used often in residential homes as well as in places of business. I also encounter them in taxi cabs and cars from various car service companies. However, just because they are popular doesn't mean they are safe. Air fresheners contain Repeat Offenders as well as additional offenders, and we can inhale these toxicants easily.

For example, air fresheners can be a source of hormone disruptors, such as phthalates. In 2007, a NRDC study found that 12 of 14 air fresheners from a popular drugstore chain had phthalates (Cohen, Janssen, and Solomon 2007). Even air fresheners called "organic" or "green" (Steinemann et al. 2010) and some labeled "all-natural" or "unscented" emitted hazardous chemicals, particularly phthalates. And none of these air fresheners listed phthalates as an ingredient anywhere on the label (Cohen, Janssen, and Solomon 2007).

Many other types of toxicants can be found in air fresheners too. All laundry products and air fresheners tested in one study emitted chemicals considered toxic or hazardous under federal law (Steinemann 2008).

HOUSEHOLD REPEAT OFFENDERS

Toxicants
— Benzene
— Formaldehyde
— Phthalates

Ingredients
— Fragrance
— Nanoparticles
— Petroleum distillates
— Solvents

OTHER OFFENDERS
— Alcohols
— Aldehydes
— Ammonia
— Bleach
— Esters
— Ketones
— Phosphates
— Propane
— Styrene
— Terpenes, such as limonene

REPEAT ISSUES
— Potential unknown VOCs and HAPs
— Unintentional Potential Effects
— Unique vulnerabilities

ADDITIONAL ISSUES
— Can trigger asthma attacks and allergies (EWG 2015c)
— Increased risk of eye sensitivity, respiratory tract irritation, headaches, depression, and dizziness (Walsh 2011; EWG 2015c)
— Possible heart stress (EWG 2015c)

Antibacterial Products

OVERVIEW

Antibacterial products are found everywhere—in homes, schools, children's play spaces, day care centers, bathrooms, kitchens, and much more. Since they generally contain a registered pesticide, triclosan, avoid them and talk to your schools about doing the same.

The American Medical Association advises against using antibacterials in consumer products. Overuse could lead to antibiotic-resistant bacteria, or "superbugs" (Tan et al. 2002). Moreover, killing all bacteria—the bad and the good—may weaken the immune system, since some bacteria contribute to a healthy body's ecosystem.

In late 2013, the FDA announced that manufacturers would have until late 2016 to prove that their antibacterial soaps are more effective than ordinary soap and water (Perrone 2013). The CDC (2014a) recommends washing with plain soap and water.

HOUSEHOLD REPEAT OFFENDERS

Toxicants
— Pesticides: Some 275 active ingredients in antibacterial products are classified as pesticides (Gavigan 2008).

Ingredients
— Nanoparticles
— Triclosan

REPEAT ISSUES
— Lack of disclosure: Not all ingredients in hand soaps are necessarily disclosed.

ADDITIONAL ISSUES
— Alcohol from hand sanitizers: May be absorbed through skin or ingested as children put their fingers in their mouths and eat with their hands.
— Antibacterial products: May weaken the immune system.

TIPS: Avoiding Antibacterial Products

Make sure your kids wash their hands often with plain soap and water, especially before they eat, after they use the bathroom, and during cold and flu season.

Clean your home regularly. Cleaning often will reduce germs' opportunity to thrive.

Periodically microwave your damp kitchen sponge for two minutes to discourage germs.

If you use cloth to clean the toilet, discard immediately or set aside for laundering. Keep the toilet brush in an area where it cannot easily contaminate other objects.

Remember that if the label says "triclosan," it's an antibacterial product.

Tea tree oil is a natural disinfectant that can fight mold and serve as an alternative to antibacterial products. However, beware that while tea tree oil is generally considered safe for humans, some studies indicate that it may disrupt hormones, so be cautious around children. It's also toxic to cats.

Disinfect with 3 percent hydrogen peroxide in one spray bottle and undiluted white vinegar in another. Spray the two on whatever needs disinfecting, alternating one right after another. Lab tests show this kills salmonella, shigella, and E. coli just as well as harsher chemicals.

Alcohol-based hand sanitizers are sometimes worthwhile when soap and water aren't available, like after petting animals at the zoo.

Dry Cleaning

OVERVIEW

Avoid or minimize dry cleaning. The EPA (2015c) says that perchloroethylene (perc), the chemical most widely used for dry cleaning, has proven to be carcinogenic in laboratory animals and is likely to cause cancer in humans. While the agency believes that wearing dry-cleaned clothes isn't cause for concern, if you dry clean, traces of dry cleaning fluid may off-gas into your indoor air and pose a risk.

ADDITIONAL OFFENDERS
— Perc

REPEAT ISSUES
— Trails of Contamination: Perc has been detected in our food supply.
— Unintentional Potential Effects
— Unique vulnerabilities
— VOCs

TIPS

01. Few items labeled "Dry Clean Only" truly require it
Silk, rayon, and wool, while often bearing that label, can actually be washed by hand. Research the proper techniques to avoid shrinking or ruining the texture of your garments. Wool and silks are generally fine with hand-washing or can be gently machine-washed and line-dried.

01. Consider wet and liquid CO_2 cleaners. If you must dry clean, seek a cleaning company that uses safer methods like "wet cleaning" or liquid CO_2 technology. Inquire about the solvents they may use (check out nodryclean.com).

02. Consider wet cleaning. It entails a combination of hand washing, spot cleaning, steaming, and pressing to clean delicate garments. Wet cleaners use specialized washing machines that clean delicate fabrics without stressing them, and the cleaning agents used can be less harmful.

03. Consider liquid carbon dioxide cleaning. It is a professional cleaning method that forgoes perc, and instead uses pressurized liquid CO_2 (a natural, nontoxic, and nonflammable gas) in conjunction with other cleaning agents.

02. Steer clear of hydrocarbon and GreenEarth cleaning
While these options are better than perc, they also use toxic solvents.

04. Let dry-cleaned items off-gas away from people
If there are no alternative cleaners near you, then let dry cleaned clothes off-gas either outdoors (anywhere from several hours to a day or two, or even a week), or in a closet that's away from bedrooms and away from children.

03. Does it pass the smell test?
Check if your dry-cleaned clothes have a strong chemical odor, and if they do, don't take them home from the cleaners until they have been adequately dried.

Mothballs

OVERVIEW
Avoid conventional mothballs, which are often stored with wool clothes to ward off moths. Conventional mothballs may off-gas toxicants that are carcinogenic and can irritate the nervous system.

ADDITIONAL OFFENDERS
— Naphthalene: The main ingredient in mothballs, naphthalene has been associated with hemolytic anemia (a condition in which red blood cells are damaged and removed from the bloodstream) in infants and is categorized by the EPA as a possible human carcinogen (EPA 2013c).
— Paradichlorobenzene: Listed by the California Environmental Protection Agency as a known carcinogen (CA EPA 2015).

REPEAT ISSUES
— Unique vulnerabilities
— Unintentional Potential Effects
— VOCs

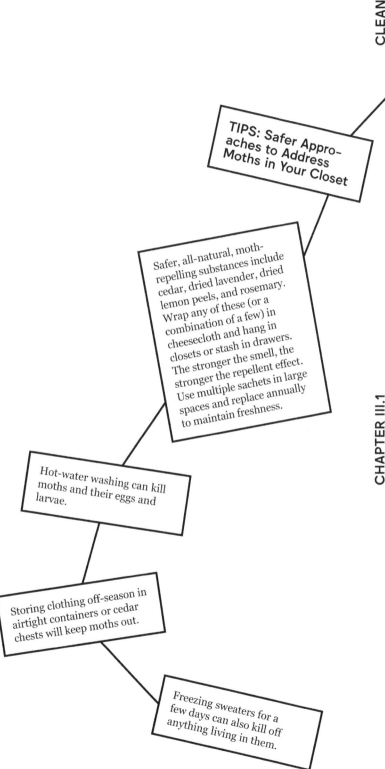

TIPS: Safer Approaches to Address Moths in Your Closet

Safer, all-natural, moth-repelling substances include cedar, dried lavender, dried lemon peels, and rosemary. Wrap any of these (or a combination of a few) in cheesecloth and hang in closets or stash in drawers. The stronger the smell, the stronger the repellent effect. Use multiple sachets in large spaces and replace annually to maintain freshness.

Hot-water washing can kill moths and their eggs and larvae.

Storing clothing off-season in airtight containers or cedar chests will keep moths out.

Freezing sweaters for a few days can also kill off anything living in them.

Simple Strategies: When Cleaning

01. Make your own cleaning solutions
Use ingredients that have a long track record of little or no controversy. These ingredients are listed on the next page.

02. Vacuum frequently
Using a vacuum cleaner with a HEPA (high efficiency particulate air) filter, is best for trapping finer particles that often contain pollutants and allergens. Conventional vacuums can miss these small particles, and recirculate them into the air. Remember to change the filter according to the model's directions, and to thoroughly vacuum upholstered furniture.

03. Wet mop
Wipe surfaces with a wet cloth. Micro-fiber cloths tend to capture more dust. Dry mopping can recirculate dust. Wet with water. Skip synthetic sprays and wipes. Pass this job to someone else if you are sensitive to dust exposure.

04. Give more attention
Prioritize areas where children spend a lot of time. Younger children are often closest to the floor and are most exposed to the toxicants in dust.

05. Consider ventilating
Ventilate mindfully when cleaning! Does it make sense to open windows? Evaluate the outdoor situation: Is there a lot of traffic generating exhaust fumes? Is a neighbor spraying pesti-cides? Avoid opening windows on days when smog and ozone levels are high, which can trigger symptoms in those who suffer from asthma.

Simple Strategies: Cleaning Ingredients

The ingredients below have a track record of safety and are multipurpose, which streamlines my shopping list.

01. Baking soda

Baking soda effectively cuts through grime and grease, and lifts away dirt.

— Use alone to scrub. Baking soda can be used as an abrasive for cleaning sinks, tubs, and toilets.

— Add a little to liquid soap to boost cleaning powers; add a lot to make a scouring paste. A little baking soda on a sponge cleans up most countertop stains.

— Baking soda also absorbs odors, softens water, and neutralizes minerals.

— Use one-half cup to three-quarters cup to a laundry wash to leave clothes soft and fresh-smelling.

— Leave in the refrigerator or in rooms to absorb odors.

02. Castile soap

Soap can dissolve oil that causes dirt and grime to stick to a surface. Castile soap is my favorite type since it is effective and multipurpose. Incorporate into cleaning solutions.

03. White vinegar

It has a strong smell, but the smell disappears soon after drying. Available by the gallon at the supermarket, distilled white vinegar can serve several purposes.

— Kills mold and bacteria, so it's good for sinks and bathrooms.

— Fights unpleasant odors.

— Dissolves soap scum and mineral buildup from toilets.

— Improves laundry. Add a cup of vinegar to a load of laundry to brighten white sheets. Add a half cup of white vinegar while your clothes are in the rinse cycle to soften fabrics.

— Cleans glass. Dilute 1:1 with water.

04. Hydrogen peroxide

A natural bleaching agent and antimicrobial, hydrogen peroxide is the active ingredient in many natural kitchen and bathroom cleansers. Use as a replacement for bleach.

Note: Borax (sodium borate) is popular in many homemade cleaning recipes. The EWG rated it of "some concern" for asthma, respiratory issues, skin allergies, and irritation; and of "high concern" for developmental and reproductive toxicity (EWG 2015a). The EU considers it toxic to human reproductive systems (ECHA 2010).

Chapter III.2
In the Kitchen

WHAT'S IN OUR FOOD?

Generally, we think a lot about food: Which diet or balance of foods will help us lose weight; which foods will help our bodies heal, detox, or even defy aging; and whether to buy organic or nonorganic or something in between. After decades of trying to understand how best to eat, I'm still learning, experimenting, and tweaking. Since junior high school, I have tried a variety of diets—low fat/high carb, high animal protein/low carb, whole foods, macrobiotic, and raw. Only in recent years have I begun to assess healthy eating in terms of the toxicants in our food supply.

Turns out, food is a major source of exposure to some toxicants. For example, diet is thought to provide up to 90 percent of a person's PCB and DDT body burden (Furst 2006). Nutritional biochemist T. Colin Campbell PhD and his son Thomas M. Campbell II MD, write in their book *The China Study* that avoiding animal products may reduce one's exposure to environmental toxins by as much as 95 percent (Campbell and Campbell 2006). Family physician and best-selling author Joel Fuhrman MD agrees. He states that "animal products, such as dairy, fish and beef, contain the most toxic pesticide residues" (Fuhrman 2015). In addition, the materials that touch our foods—food containers and cookware—can contaminate our diet too.

This section spotlights how to minimize exposure to toxicants in what you eat and drink, an overlooked consideration in healthy eating.

IN THIS CHAPTER:

— Household Repeat Offenders that are found in the standard American diet (SAD)
— Animals and animal by-products
— Containers and packaging materials
— Cooking
— Packaged and processed foods
— Simple Strategies to reduce the toxicants in your diet

HOUSEHOLD REPEAT OFFENDERS: THE STANDARD AMERICAN DIET (SAD)

Toxicants
— BPA
— Chlorine
— Dioxins and dioxin-like compounds
— Formaldehyde
— Heavy metals, like lead, mercury, and arsenic
— PBDEs
— PCBs
— Pesticides, including those banned decades ago, like DDT
— PFCs, like C8
— Phthalates
— Unintentional Toxicants, like PAHs

Ingredients
— Chemical flame retardants
— Nanoparticles
— Preservatives such as sodium benzoate
— Synthetic colors
— Synthetic fragrance
— Triclosan

Materials
— Plastics
— Woods

OTHER OFFENDERS
— Antibiotics
— Artificial additives, such as sweeteners, flavor enhancers, and preservatives, including sodium nitrite, and sulfites
— Growth hormones
— Pathogens
— Perc

REPEAT ISSUES
— Bioaccumulation and biomagnification of toxicants in our diet
— Hidden hazards, such as POPs, EDCs
— Lack of disclosure of toxicity (or potential toxicity) in food, beverages, or the packaging materials
— Our choices contribute to Trails of Contamination
— Unintentional By-products
— Unintentional Potential Effects
— Unintentional Toxicants

ADDITIONAL ISSUES
— Animal cruelty is a concern.
— Even without toxicants, the standard American diet is unhealthy.
— It is estimated that 90 to 95 percent of our exposure to environmental toxins is from consuming animal products (Campbell and Campbell 2006).
— Nutritional density supports the body's natural immunity and other mechanisms.
— Nutritional value is highest among fresh, homemade foods and drinks.
— Our current demand for consumption of animals and their by-products stresses and pollutes the environment.

ON PROBATION
— Genetically modified ingredients
— Soy

Animals and Animal By-products

OVERVIEW

Since animals and their by-products are higher on the food chain than are plants, they tend to have higher concentrations of persistent, fat-soluble toxicants. As you can see from the extensive roster of Household Repeat Offenders, the list of contaminants is long. Limiting consumption of animals would significantly reduce your exposure to toxicants.

Common contaminants include pesticides, antibiotics, growth hormones, phthalates, and unhealthy food that is fed to animals raised for human consumption. When excreted, these compounds, as well as other pollutants (such as nitrates and ammonia), contribute to the toxic waste from agricultural operations, eventually contaminating our Homes. According to the *Green Guide*, "hormones used in livestock (which come through in their manure) have been found downstream from factory farms and are linked to altered sexual traits in fish and other wildlife" (*National Geographic* 2008). According to the 2010 PCP report, *Reducing Environmental Cancer Risk: What We Can Do Now*, "the impact on human cancer [from the unintentional contamination of veterinary pharmaceuticals, such as antibiotics and growth hormones] is unknown at this time, but there is speculation that the growth hormones may contribute to endocrine disruption in humans."

Minimizing processed meat products is also healthier. A study published in the journal *Circulation* in April 2010 found that eating one daily serving of processed meats like bacon, sausage, and deli meats was linked to a 42 percent increased risk of heart disease, as well as a 19 percent higher risk of diabetes. However, there was no association found between the consumption of unproccessed red meat and an increased risk for these diseases (Micha, Wallace, and Mozaffarian 2010).

While physicians and other health experts tout the nutritional benefits of eating more vegetables, fruits, nuts, seeds, and whole grains, researchers are also discovering more evidence that a plant-based diet will reduce your exposure to toxicants. Unprocessed foods are great, and if they're organic, local, and seasonal, all the better. Hard to do? Absolutely. Worth doing? Absolutely! But even if you only increase your intake of plant-based foods, you can pat yourself on the back for trying to get on, and stay on, a healthier path.

HOUSEHOLD REPEAT OFFENDERS

Toxicants

— DDT: Diet is a major source of exposure.
— Dioxins: Diet is a major source of exposure. Dioxins are found predominantly in fatty foods: meats, dairy fat (cheese, butter, and ice cream) as well as some seafood (catfish, lobster, and mollusks; Fuhrman 2006). After analyzing US meat and poultry products between May 2002 and May 2003 for the presence of dioxins and dioxin-like compounds including PCBs (collectively, DLCs), the USDA's Food Safety and Inspection Service confirmed that "dioxin accumulates in the fatty tissues of humans and food animals consumed by humans. It is generally believed that the most significant exposure to DLCs by humans is from the dietary intake of animal and fish products" (FSIS 2009). The FDA (2014a) says that some of these DLCs "may be carcinogens at low levels of exposure over extended periods of time." In June 2003, the Institute of Medicine of the National Academy of Sciences published a report about food containing dioxin and other PCBs, warning the public that they posed a cancer risk (Institute of Medicine 2003). These toxic chemicals have been associated with an increased

risk of cancer, birth defects, and reproductive damage.
— PAHs: Found in grilled or charred meats, and smoked foods
— PBDEs
— PCBs: Diet is a major source of exposure, especially foods like fish, meat, and dairy.
— Pesticides: Diet is a major source of exposure. In 2006 and 2007, the US used over 1 billion pounds of pesticides (Grube et al. 2011). Animals are exposed to pesticides through their environment and diet. In any given year, an estimated 167 million pounds of pesticides are used in the US on animal-feed crops (Hamerschlag 2011). In addition, pesticides are sometimes sprayed directly onto animals to ward off parasites, insects, rodents, and fungi. These pesticides are inhaled and absorbed and then stored in the animals' fat tissues.
— Phthalates: Attracted to fat, phthalates are commonly found in meat, dairy, and processed foods. Contamination may occur from a variety of sources and stages, such as food preparation and packaging. Ted Schettler MD MPH, an expert on phthalates, suspects that phthalates may be found in milk not only because of their presence in the diet of dairy animals, but also because of leaching from the flexible vinyl tubing used in milking machines (Smith and Lourie 2009).
— Heavy metals: Diet is a major source of exposure. The FSIS National Residue Program for Cattle is a program under the USDA that aims to protect the nation's food supply from residual veterinary drugs, pesticides, and heavy metals. A March 2010 audit report expressed "growing concern" over the potential effects of these residues on humans. The report states, "Not only does overuse of antibiotics help create antibiotic-resistant strains of diseases, but the residues of certain drugs and heavy metals can have potentially adverse health consequences if they are consumed

in meat." Further, the report notes that heat used to control microbiological pathogens like *E. coli* and salmonella can't destroy drug, pesticide, and heavy metal residues. In fact, heat can sometimes break down residues into more harmful by-products (USDA 2010).

Materials
— Plastics: A popular material to wrap and contain foods and drinks. Plastics leaves a Trail of Contamination during and after a product's useful life, contaminating both our diets and our environment.

OTHER OFFENDERS
— Antibiotics: In September 2012, the *New York Times* reported that "80 percent of the antibiotics sold in the [US] goes to chicken, pigs, cows and other animals that people eat, yet producers of meat and poultry are not required to report how they use the drugs—which ones, on what types of animal, and in what quantities" (Tavernise 2012). In December 2013, the FDA began restricting the use of certain antibiotics on farm animals due to concern that they contribute to the increase in antibiotic-resistant bacteria (FDA 2013c). Some consumer advocates believe that the restrictions are not protective enough.
— Bovine Growth Hormone (BGH): Used in the US since it was approved by the FDA in 1993, BGH is a hormone given to cows to have them mature more quickly and increase their milk production. BGH is also called bGH, rBGH, GE, or BST. While its use is not permitted in the EU, Canada, Japan, New Zealand, Australia, and other countries, it has never been restricted in the US. Studies have shown that BGH causes adverse health effects in cows. However, evidence of the effect on humans remains inconclusive. As debate over its safety continues, demand for BGH in the US has decreased. Both the World Trade

Organization and the United Nations Food Safety Agency have refused to endorse the hormone's safety. In 1989, the EU fully banned imports of meat and meat products from animals treated with growth-promoting chemicals, citing concerns.
— Unintentional Toxicants, including Unintentional By-products and banned substances
— Veterinary medications

REPEAT ISSUES
— Biomagnification or bioconcentration
— Contaminated food: According to David Acheson MD, former managing director for Food and Import Safety at the FDA, a shipment of beef from the US was rejected by Mexican officials in 2008 because the copper levels in the beef exceeded Mexican standards. It's unclear what happened to the contaminated beef but the US didn't have a standard that would have protected American consumers against that same shipment. (Claiborne, Childs, Siegel 2010).
— Industries' Webs of Influence, as explained in chapter I.12: There are claims that industries' influence has led to the introduction and popularity of unhealthy foods and drinks.

ADDITIONAL ISSUES
— Animals may be raised on contaminated land: Free-range chickens in both the US and the EU have been found to have higher levels of PCBs, probably because the chickens were roaming and pecking in contaminated space. According to an article in *Time* in July 2010, "a study in California of a free-range or organic farm with a wood-processing facility nearby" found "the chickens there had 100 times the PCB level of battery-cage chickens. A Brazilian study found something similar with DDT, even though the pesticide, which is slow to degrade, hadn't been used in the area in nine years" (Kluger 2010).

— Eating too much animal protein is not healthy: In addition to higher concentrations of toxicants in animals and animal by-products, there is a strong body of evidence linking higher levels of animal protein consumption and higher incidences of a long list of illnesses, including heart disease and cancer (Campbell and Campbell 2006).
— Farming practices may be unsanitary: This can lead to pathogens and other illnesses infecting the animals.
— Testing and standards are insufficient: An audit that took place in 2007 and 2008—the National Residue Program for Cattle Audit Report—determined that in the US, the testing of beef for hazardous contaminants was inadequate (USDA 2010).
— Animals may be subject to cruelty: Some farm practices are cruel to animals. Some people believe animals simply shouldn't be eaten, or that they should be eaten more consciously. About 65 billion land animals are killed per year for food; some are sent to slaughter within weeks or months of being born.
— Animal farming takes an environmental toll: Animal agriculture is a major source of carbon dioxide, methane, and nitrous oxide emissions. Several studies from the United Nations (Steinfeld et al. 2006) and the Worldwatch Institute (Goodland and Anhang 2009) have found that raising animals for food creates more greenhouse gases than all the cars and trucks in the world combined. Their analyses estimated that raising animals for food accounts for 18 percent (Steinfeld et al. 2006) to 51 percent (Goodland and Anhang 2009) of all greenhouse gas emissions.

Animals and Animal By-products: Dairy Products

HOUSEHOLD REPEAT OFFENDERS

Toxicants
— BPA and phthalates: From food or beverage manufacturing and packaging
— Dioxins
— Pesticides

Ingredients
— Nanoparticles: May be added to enhance color and texture.

Materials
— Plastics

ADDITIONAL OFFENDERS
— Antibiotics
— Artificial growth hormones
— Perc: California's agriculture department tested 32 samples of milk and found that half contained perchlorate levels deemed unsafe in drinking water (EWG 2004).

REPEAT ISSUES
— Bioaccumulation and biomagnification

TIPS: Healthier Dairy

Avoid unnecessary fat
Although young children may benefit from drinking whole milk because of their unique biological development, older children and adults whose nutritional requirements are different can reduce consuming dioxins in milk by drinking skim (nonfat) milk, which contains virtually no dioxins because it contains no fat.

Choose dairy products that are as close to what nature designed
Buy milk certified as organic or labeled "BGH-free." Organic dairy products are free of bovine growth hormone and antibiotics. The cows' feed, whether grass or grain, is grown without pesticides. The cows are required to have access to pasture, but the current standard does not require a specific length of time in pasture. In the meantime, drinking organic milk may also be healthier: It's associated with lower rates of allergies, asthma, and eczema in children. When pregnant and breast-feeding women and their children consumed organic dairy products, their children had 36 percent lower rates of asthma, eczema, and allergies by age 2, according to a study published in the *British Journal of Nutrition* (Kummeling et al. 2008). According to the Organic Consumers Association (2015), "levels of antioxidants in milk from organic cattle are between 50 percent and 80 percent higher than [in] normal milk."

Animals and Animal By-products: Meat, Poultry, and Eggs

Eat less of it, and increase your intake of fresh fruits, vegetables, beans, nuts, and seeds (barring any allergies).

TIPS: Meat & Poultry

TIPS: Eggs

Efforts to reduce dioxins exposure should begin in pregnancy and childhood, as the contaminants accumulate in the body throughout one's life (Institute of Medicine 2003). This goes one step further for girls, who will eventually pass some of their bodily dioxin burden on to their children (Olson 2003).

Are brown eggs healthier than white ones? No. Color varies only by the breed of chicken laying it. Also, since brown-egg-laying chickens eat more feed, which keeps production costs higher, brown eggs typically cost more.

Best label to buy for eggs: USDA Certified Organic. Bonus: "Pasture-raised" (though this claim isn't verified by a third party), and eggs from local chickens.

TIPS: Turkey

Avoid fatty cuts of meat and high-fat dairy products since toxins tend to settle in fat. Opt for lean meats and fat-free milk.

Turkeys labeled "basted" or "self-basting" are typically filled with added fat, broth, water, and flavor enhancers.

Reduce intake of processed, charred, and well-done meats, as they can be a source of exposure to carcinogenic heterocyclic amines and polyaromatic hydrocarbons (Reuben 2010).

TIP: Raw Meat and Poultry

See Food Labels in this chapter.

Raw meat and poultry food items are sometimes marinated or injected with salt water, flavorings, and various additives. Read the fine print on packages for clues.

Animals and Animal By-products: Seafood

HOUSEHOLD REPEAT OFFENDERS

Toxicants
— BPA
— Chlorine: Used in processing so unintentional contamination may occur; historically, chlorine was widely used as a disinfectant in the seafood-processing industry, and may still be used on seafood such as shrimp (Andrews et al. 2002).
— Dioxins
— Heavy metals, such as mercury. Unlike dioxins, mercury accumulates in the fish's muscle meat rather than in its fat, so it cannot be trimmed away.
— PBDEs
— PCBs: These accumulate in fatty fish, farmed fish, oysters, and other shellfish. Studies conducted in 2002 (Easton, Luszniak, and Von der Geest 2002) and 2004 (Hites et al. 2004) determined that levels of PCBs are much higher in farmed salmon than they are in wild Pacific salmon. Wild salmon have fewer PCBs because they eat lower on the food chain, meaning they consume fewer PCBs from other fish. They are also more active than farmed fish and therefore have less fat in which to store PCBs.
— Pesticides, such as DDT

Ingredients
— Preservatives

REPEAT ISSUES
— Antibiotics
— Biomagnification and bioconcentration: Contaminants found in seafood include PCBs, PBDEs, mercury, hormone-disrupting chemicals (from plastic garbage, detergents, and pesticides), excreted by-products of birth control pills, and other industrial chemicals. Some wild male fish have become so feminized that they produce eggs. Some of these toxicants are found in greater concentrations in predators that are larger and older, like tuna and swordfish.
— POPs

TIPS: Healthier Seafood Consumption

Seafood offers many health benefits, such as omega-3 fatty acids that help our hearts and brains. However, seafood should be consumed mindfully and in moderation due to the bioaccumulation of toxicants.

01. Eat lower on the food chain

01. Seafood that are less contaminated include sardines, wild salmon, mackerel, tilapia, pollock, and farmed striped bass.

02. Avoid predator fish. This is especially important for women and children. Predator fish include swordfish, tuna, wild bass, shark, king mackerel, and tilefish. Those higher on the food chain are more likely to contain higher levels of pollutants, such as mercury, PCBs, DDT, and dioxins.

03. Tuna is consistently contaminated with mercury. Canned tuna tends to be less contaminated than tuna steaks, since it comes from smaller tuna. Canned salmon is better than canned tuna. However, most cans are lined with a protective coating that has historically leached BPA, and the safety of substitute materials is unknown.

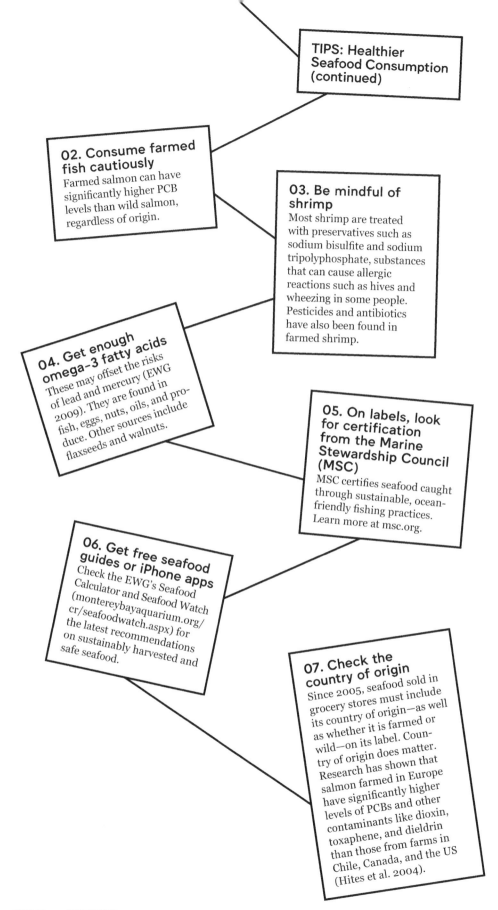

TIPS: Healthier Seafood Consumption (continued)

02. Consume farmed fish cautiously
Farmed salmon can have significantly higher PCB levels than wild salmon, regardless of origin.

03. Be mindful of shrimp
Most shrimp are treated with preservatives such as sodium bisulfite and sodium tripolyphosphate, substances that can cause allergic reactions such as hives and wheezing in some people. Pesticides and antibiotics have also been found in farmed shrimp.

04. Get enough omega-3 fatty acids
These may offset the risks of lead and mercury (EWG 2009). They are found in fish, eggs, nuts, oils, and produce. Other sources include flaxseeds and walnuts.

05. On labels, look for certification from the Marine Stewardship Council (MSC)
MSC certifies seafood caught through sustainable, ocean-friendly fishing practices. Learn more at msc.org.

06. Get free seafood guides or iPhone apps
Check the EWG's Seafood Calculator and Seafood Watch (montereybayaquarium.org/cr/seafoodwatch.aspx) for the latest recommendations on sustainably harvested and safe seafood.

07. Check the country of origin
Since 2005, seafood sold in grocery stores must include its country of origin—as well as whether it is farmed or wild—on its label. Country of origin does matter. Research has shown that salmon farmed in Europe have significantly higher levels of PCBs and other contaminants like dioxin, toxaphene, and dieldrin than those from farms in Chile, Canada, and the US (Hites et al. 2004).

Animals and Animal By-products: Food Labels

OVERVIEW

There are dozens of food claims made on food labels: certified organic, organic, pasture-raised, grass-fed, free-range, free-farmed, free-roaming, cage-free, natural, no antibiotics, no antibiotics administered, raised without antibiotics, antibiotic-free, no hormones administered, hormone-free, natural, no chemicals, omega-3-enriched, and many more. "And there are also literally dozens of certifications, such as Certified Humane Raised and Handled, Certified Organic, Inc., and USDA–Organic.

How is a consumer supposed to make sense of these claims? To begin, don't assume that everything a label implies is true. Remember that, generally, manufacturers are trying to sell goods produced at the lowest cost for the highest price. Getting to the truth is complex. First, you have to determine if standards have been set, and if so, by whom? Were they established by an objective third party, such as the USDA, or by those with self-interests, such as a manufacturer or an industry? Are manufacturer claims verified by a third party?

In general, USDA Certified Organic is the safest selection, since objective verification is required.

REPEAT ISSUES
— Lack of regulation
— Lack of transparency

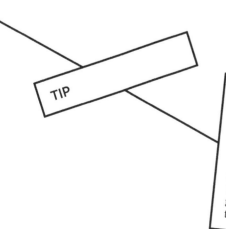

TIP

Identify farms and companies that you trust

Bypass the confusion of food labels by finding farms and companies whose practices you trust. This is a long-term project so, in the meantime, get to know the key labels on the next page.

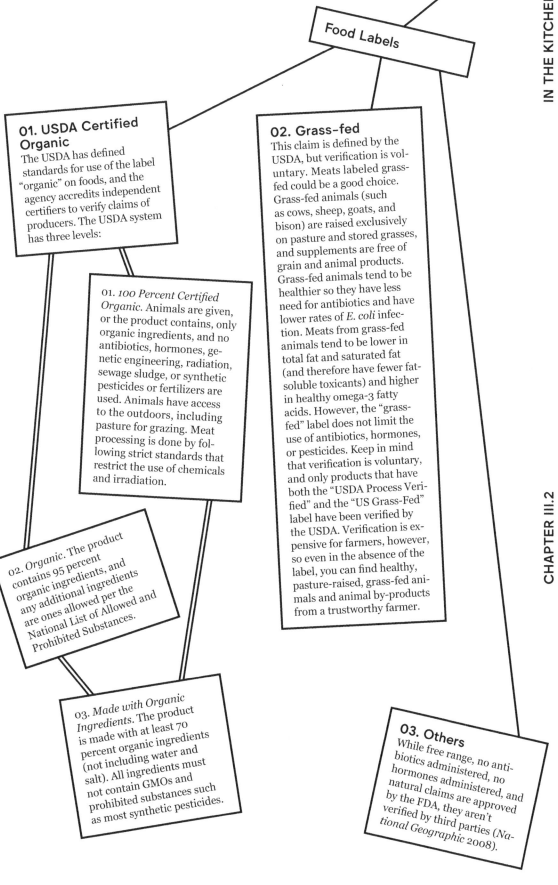

Food Labels

01. USDA Certified Organic
The USDA has defined standards for use of the label "organic" on foods, and the agency accredits independent certifiers to verify claims of producers. The USDA system has three levels:

01. *100 Percent Certified Organic*. Animals are given, or the product contains, only organic ingredients, and no antibiotics, hormones, genetic engineering, radiation, sewage sludge, or synthetic pesticides or fertilizers are used. Animals have access to the outdoors, including pasture for grazing. Meat processing is done by following strict standards that restrict the use of chemicals and irradiation.

02. *Organic*. The product contains 95 percent organic ingredients, and any additional ingredients are ones allowed per the National List of Allowed and Prohibited Substances.

03. *Made with Organic Ingredients*. The product is made with at least 70 percent organic ingredients (not including water and salt). All ingredients must not contain GMOs and prohibited substances such as most synthetic pesticides.

02. Grass-fed
This claim is defined by the USDA, but verification is voluntary. Meats labeled grass-fed could be a good choice. Grass-fed animals (such as cows, sheep, goats, and bison) are raised exclusively on pasture and stored grasses, and supplements are free of grain and animal products. Grass-fed animals tend to be healthier so they have less need for antibiotics and have lower rates of *E. coli* infection. Meats from grass-fed animals tend to be lower in total fat and saturated fat (and therefore have fewer fat-soluble toxicants) and higher in healthy omega-3 fatty acids. However, the "grass-fed" label does not limit the use of antibiotics, hormones, or pesticides. Keep in mind that verification is voluntary, and only products that have both the "USDA Process Verified" and the "US Grass-Fed" label have been verified by the USDA. Verification is expensive for farmers, however, so even in the absence of the label, you can find healthy, pasture-raised, grass-fed animals and animal by-products from a trustworthy farmer.

03. Others
While free range, no antibiotics administered, no hormones administered, and natural claims are approved by the FDA, they aren't verified by third parties (*National Geographic* 2008).

Containers and Packaging Materials

OVERVIEW

Reducing your diet's contact with certain materials can reduce your body burden: In one study, participants reduced the amount of various chemicals in their bodies by 50 to 95 percent after just three days (Rudel et al. 2011). What did they do? Participants ate mostly fresh foods; didn't eat anything from a can; avoided using plastic utensils or nonstick cookware; stored food and drinks in glass or stainless steel containers and avoided having the contents touch lids; and made coffee in a French press or ceramic drip so that no plastic was involved (*Discovery News* 2011).

HOUSEHOLD REPEAT OFFENDERS

Toxicants
— BPA: In an analysis of 204 samples of fresh, frozen, and canned foods that were gathered in 2010, BPA was detected in 73 percent of the canned food, while only being detected in 7 percent of non-canned samples. (Lorber et al. 2015).
— PFCs or C8
— Phthalates

Ingredients
— Nanoparticles

Materials
— Plastics

ADDITIONAL OFFENDERS

— BHA: Used to preserve fats and oils in food, butylated hydroxyanisole (BHA) is "reasonably anticipated to be a human carcinogen" (NTP 2014). It can also cause skin depigmentation. In animal studies, BHA causes liver damage and stomach cancers and interferes with normal reproductive system development and thyroid hormone levels. The EU considers it unsafe in fragrance. It is found in food, food packaging, and personal care products sold in the US.
— Styrene: Found in Styrofoam cups and plates.

REPEAT ISSUES

— Trails of Contamination throughout our Homes, both during and after a product's useful life

TIPS: Utensils

Avoid unnecessary use of plastic utensils. Stainless steel, enamel-coated metal, and even shatterproof glass are preferable. Children may enjoy antique silver baby spoons or small stainless steel utensils, easily found at kitchen-supply stores.

If you need disposable utensils or dinnerware, look for the bio-based kind made with polylactic acid (PLA) or polyhydroxyalkanoates (PHA) plastics.

TIPS: Appliances

Coffee makers
Consider brewing coffee the old-fashioned way: using a French press. Automatic, plastic coffee makers can contain BPA and phthalates in water reservoirs and tubing (Silent Spring Institute 2015).

Blenders
The containers for most blenders are made of plastic. Remember that chemicals in plastics can be released through normal wear and tear such as scratching or dishwashing. In the meantime, sign an online petition asking appliance companies to make stainless steel containers for their blenders.

TIPS: Materials that Touch Your Food

Chemicals commonly found in the linings of metal cans and in plastic containers can migrate into food and drinks. Heat, harsh detergents, and time all promote the breakdown of plastics and the leaching of their compounds. The nine tips can help you further reduce your exposure to toxicants from plastics and canned goods.

02. Do not microwave cling wrap or plastic containers; and assume that "microwave safe" only means the product will not be destroyed (and means nothing about health). Heat-resistant glass, stoneware, or ceramic containers are safer choices (you can cover food in the microwave with a paper towel). You can also reheat food on the stove, starting with a small amount of water for moisture.

01. Avoid buying, serving, or storing hot, acidic, or fatty foods in plastic containers. Plastics are the suspected source of phthalates that have been detected in a range of foods, and especially in foods with high fat content, like eggs, milk, cheese, margarine, seafood, infant formulas, and baby food (Steingraber 2010).

03. Do not put plastics in the dishwasher. Instead, hand wash with warm water and mild dish liquid.

04. Don't reuse food and beverage containers that weren't designed for repeated usage.

05. With BPA-free containers, remember that substitute chemicals may not be safer. The claim "BPA-free" is not regulated. If you must have plastic, then avoid PVC, polystyrene (PS), and polycarbonate (PC) plastics. Alternatives to canned foods: dried, fresh or frozen foods; and those in glass jars.

09. Beware of PFCs in nonstick coatings for pots and pans. Better choices: cast iron or stainless steel (EWG 2015g).

08. Avoid greasy and fatty packaged/fast foods. They usually come in treated wrappers which may contain PFCs. Microwaveable popcorn bags are typically coated with these chemicals as well (EWG 2015g). Candy bar wrappers may also have PFCs.

07. Favor foods that are stored in glass, stoneware, ceramic, stainless steel, and biodegradable storage containers. Choose soups and milks that come in cardboard cartons. Beware of nonstick coatings in disposable containers though.

06. Use glass or stainless steel for drinking cups, without any plastic or epoxy lining.

TIPS: Dinnerware

Use real plates instead of paper (to avoid PFCs) and plastics (to avoid EDCs). Healthier options include dinnerware made of glass and stainless steel. Other products can be safe too. However, test your dinnerware (and crystal) for lead.

TIPS: Be Mindful of Lunch Boxes

In 2007, canvas lunch boxes from China that had been given away at health fairs in California tested positive for lead; the Department of Public Health warned parents to discard them (CDPH 2007).

Without label warnings, lead can be found in a variety of pottery glazes: brightly colored dishware from other countries, and dinnerware made from major manufacturers and sold in major department stores. Lead in levels higher than 2,000 ppb can cause lead poisoning, and exceedances are prohibited in dinnerware. The state of California mandates warning labels for any dishware that releases lead in levels higher than 224 ppb (Dadd 2011). You can purchase a lead-testing kit at a hardware store to assess what you have.

Many plastic lunch boxes are manufactured with PVC, or have PVC coating on its inside panels (Liu, Schade, and Simpson 2008). Avoid lunch boxes and hot-food containers made from #3, #6, and #7 plastic. For guidance on safer plastics, check out the table in chapter II.3.

If your dinnerware contains lead and you must keep them, then a few tips: women of child-bearing years and children should avoid them; limit use to special occasions; don't store food and beverages in them (especially acidic juices, vinegar, and alcoholic beverages).

Healthy alternatives include tin or stainless steel food containers and certified organic cotton canvas lunch sacks. Or make your own out of cloth.

Containers and Packaging Materials: Plastic Wrap

HOUSEHOLD REPEAT OFFENDERS

Toxicants

— BPA and other chemicals that soften plastics: Can leach into foods.

— Phthalates: Manufacturers strongly assert that phthalates are not used in cling wrap in the US. Some studies reveal that phthalates exist in plastic wrap in other parts of the world (Smith and Lourie 2009).

Ingredients

— Nanoparticles

Materials

— Plastics

ADDITIONAL OFFENDERS

— In a study conducted by the Consumers Union (1998), 19 pieces of prewrapped cheese were studied for DEHA, a plasticizer that has been of toxicological concern. The seven that were packaged in #3 PVC cling wrap had levels of DEHA that ranged from 51 to 270 ppm, averaging 153 ppm. This was far higher than the 18 ppm limit on DEHA migration into food set by the European Commission (Burros 1999). Currently, the US has not established any limits for DEHA in food.

TIPS: Reduce Ingesting Toxic Chemicals from Plastic Wraps

Whenever you can, wrap your food in PVC-free butcher paper, parchment paper, unbleached wax paper, wood-based cellulose bags, low density polyethylene (LDPE), or paper bags. Or store it in glass or stainless steel containers. Ideally, for wax paper, choose a brand that uses non-genetically-modified soy wax instead of petroleum-derived wax (petroleum-based paraffin or wax is FDA-approved for food storage use) (*National Geographic* 2008).

If you must use plastic wrap, avoid putting it in direct contact with food.

Do not reuse plastic sandwich and food storage bags. Although they are typically made from polyethylene, which is considered non-toxic, the safety of washing and reusing such bags is not fully established, and this practice could make them prone to leaching.

01. Use a cheese slicer to take a millimeter off the surface of meat or cheese to help reduce your exposure.

02. Remove food from plastic wrap as soon as possible, especially from cheese or meat, since leaching may continue over time.

Typical deli (and grocery deli) meats, cheeses, and other foods are packaged in #3 PVC cling wrap (*National Geographic* 2008). Avoid this. If you can't, then you can reduce your exposure to EDCs with the three steps described further:

Do not microwave or heat plastic cling wraps. According to the NRDC (2011), microwave-safe plastic wrap should not touch food, but instead be loosely placed over it, which will allow steam to escape. An even healthier choice, however, is to cover food with a dish, or microwave your food uncovered.

03. Contact your grocery store to request that their deli use PVC-free products to wrap deli meats and cheeses.

Containers and Packaging Materials: Styrene

OVERVIEW

Products made of polystyrene, a possible human carcinogen that can also act as a neurotoxin, may expose you to small doses of it.

In addition, the styrene products can contaminate our environment after the product's useful life. In 2009, *National Geographic* reported that 100 percent of water samples collected from the US, Europe, India, Japan, and elsewhere by a Japan-based team contained derivatives of polystyrene (Barry 2009).

HOUSEHOLD REPEAT OFFENDERS

Materials
— Plastics

ADDITIONAL OFFENDERS
— Styrene

REPEAT ISSUES
— Developmental neurotoxicity
— Global contamination
— Presence in household dust, breast milk, sewage sludge, wildlife
— Reproductive toxicity
— Thyroid hormone disruption

NOTES
— The IARC has classified styrene as a "possible human carcinogen."
— It is a proposed POP under the Stockholm Convention.

TIPS: Avoid Styrene

Polystyrene can be identified by the number 6 inside the recycling symbol.

Semi-soft and lightweight, it is used to make Styrofoam, coffee cups, egg cartons, takeout food boxes, and disposable bowls, plates, and trays. A hard version of polystyrene is used to make DVD cases, plastic cutlery, yogurt and cottage cheese containers, cups, and clear takeout food containers.

Cooking

HOUSEHOLD REPEAT OFFENDERS WHEN COOKING

Toxicants
— BFA and phthalates: From food packaging
— PAHs: From cooking
— PFCs: From nonstick surfaces like pots and pans and certain food packaging

REPEAT ISSUES
— Carcinogens in smoke and charred food
— Gases from composite wood cabinets, and other construction materials

ADDITIONAL ISSUES
— Carbon monoxide emissions from a gas stove
— Pollution from self-cleaning ovens
— Toxic compounds created in cooking oils that are heated beyond certain temperature thresholds

TIPS: Ventilation

Use a stove vent. Ideally, your range will be vented outside.

Open windows to create an air exchange.

If you burn something like plastic—a pot handle, for instance—remove the ruined item from the kitchen (ideally taking it outside) so it doesn't continue to pollute your indoor air. Then use fans to get the bad air out of the room.

Clean oven hood filters according to manufacturer instructions. Most can be washed with soap, water, and baking soda. Reducing grease on filters offers less opportunity for dust to stick.

TIPS: When Cooking

Eat home-cooked meals: Not only can you control the quality and purity of your food but you can also reduce toxicants from food packaging (e.g., BPA) and cookware (e.g., PFOA).

Do not char foods. Charred or well-done meat may contain carcinogenic heterocyclic amines and polyaromatic hydrocarbons.

Consider using iodized salt. Iodine can help guard against the hazards of chemicals like perchlorate, which can disrupt the thyroid system and affect brain development during pregnancy and the months after birth (EWG 2009).

Get to know the heat thresholds, or smoke points, of the oils you cook with, to avoid releasing toxic compounds. (See the table on the next page.)

Avoid food aerosol spray cans (e.g., cooking oils), which can deposit chemicals like propane, butane, and dimethyl ether on food (Varlet, Smith, and Augsburger 2014). Those around may also inhale toxicants.

Buy certified organic cooking oils, which signals that these products were made without genetically engineered ingredients and were grown without pesticides.

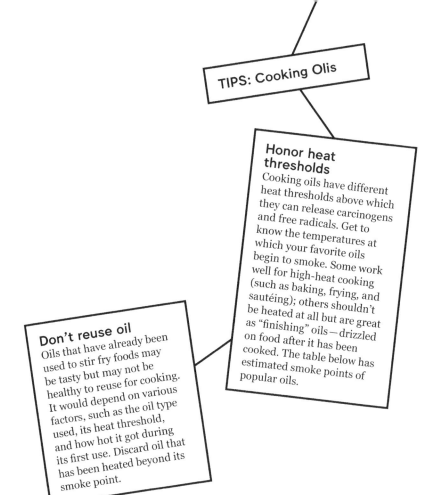

Honor heat thresholds

Cooking oils have different heat thresholds above which they can release carcinogens and free radicals. Get to know the temperatures at which your favorite oils begin to smoke. Some work well for high-heat cooking (such as baking, frying, and sautéing); others shouldn't be heated at all but are great as "finishing" oils—drizzled on food after it has been cooked. The table below has estimated smoke points of popular oils.

Don't reuse oil

Oils that have already been used to stir fry foods may be tasty but may not be healthy to reuse for cooking. It would depend on various factors, such as the oil type used, its heat threshold, and how hot it got during its first use. Discard oil that has been heated beyond its smoke point.

PART III

(Source: Spectrum Organics)

ESTIMATED SMOKE POINTS OF POPULAR OILS

Purpose	Oil Type	Smoke Point
High-heat sauteing, frying, and other high-heat cooking.	Canola (super-high heat)	460° F
Sauteing at medium heat or baking.	Canola Grapeseed Coconut	425° F 425° F 365° F
Sauteing at medium heat, adding to sauces and salad dressings.	Sesame* Toasted Sesame* Olive* Coconut*	350° F 350° F 325° F 280° F
Drizzling for flavor or nutrients, adding to salad dressings and sauces.	Flaxseed*	225° F

*Unrefined oil

Cooking: Cookware

HOUSEHOLD REPEAT OFFENDERS

Toxicants
— Lead
— PFCs, like C8: A key ingredient in nonstick coatings. While it is being phased out, the safety of replacement formulas is not known.

Ingredients
— Nanoparticles

ADDITIONAL OFFENDERS
— Chromium
— Copper
— Iron
— Nickel

ADDITIONAL ISSUES
Leaching of cookware materials into food:
— Aluminum: It can react with certain foods (like acidic or salty ones) to create a metallic taste.
— Cast iron: Iron can leach into food, but cast iron is still considered to be among the safest cookware.
— Copper: Copper cookware can leach copper.
— Stainless steel: Acidic foods, such as tomato sauce, can cause stainless steel to leach nickel and chromium into food.

TIPS: Cooking with Nonstick Cookware

Scratched nonstick pans facilitate the leaching of cookware chemicals. They are unsafe to use and should be thrown away (they cannot be recycled).

Never heat nonstick cookware on high or place it under the broiler. Elevated temperatures (500° F) may release fumes that can sicken humans and even kill birds.

If you must have them, then treat nonstick pans carefully and according to manufacturer instructions.

Healthier Cookware Materials

01. Cast Iron

Used for thousands of years, cast iron is generally regarded to be safe. It is extremely durable (cast iron pots and pans get handed down through generations) and energy efficient, retaining heat well and distributing it evenly. It can also be transferred from stovetop to oven, and is quite inexpensive.

Cast iron also releases iron, which the body needs to produce red blood cells, into what you are cooking. There is some controversy over whether this is safe: Some say it is harmless, while others say it is toxic. Mostly, it is considered among the safest options.

If you buy new cast iron, avoid those that are "preseasoned" in China. They tend to be seasoned with paint that can chip off and contaminate food. Among good alternatives is Lodge, an American-made brand. Also, cooking acidic foods in cast iron that hasn't been properly seasoned (or "cured") might produce a metallic flavor.

Season your cast iron periodically following the manufacturer's instructions.

02. Enamel-coated cast iron

This is cast iron covered with a fused hard coating of glass particles. Glass is inert so it should be safe. Anything can be cooked in enameled cast iron; it shares the heat distribution properties of cast iron but doesn't require the seasoning process. It is also dishwasher-friendly and easier than cast iron to clean, and it will last a lifetime if treated well (helping to offset its cost, which is substantially more than uncoated cast iron).

03. Stainless steel

Corrosion-resistant and lighter than cast iron, which makes it easier to work with. Some pans have cores made of other metals, but 100 percent stainless is safer. The least likely to leach their components into food, however, are designated as 18/8 or 18/10. While the manufacturing of stainless steel (mainly iron, chromium, and nickel) creates a hefty carbon footprint, stainless steel is long-lasting and recyclable.

01. While it's fine to cook acidic foods, like tomato sauce, in stainless steel, don't store acidic foods in it. The acids can cause the stainless steel to leach.

02. Scratched stainless steel can leach amounts of nickel and chromium, which poses health risks. Minimize leaching by using only wooden cooking tools with stainless steel to avoid scratching as a result of using metal.

Healthier Cookware
Materials (continued)

04. Glass
A safe material for cooking and storing food. It is non-reactive (made mainly from sand), inexpensive, reusable, and recyclable. I like multipurpose glass that is safe in the freezer, oven, and microwave (but remember that extreme temperature changes can cause the glass to break). Ovenproof glass dishes can be used for baking cakes, cookies, pies, and breads and for roasting vegetables. Keep in mind that most glass cannot be used on a stovetop. Beware of leaded glass, however, which can leach lead.

05. Aluminum
Relatively inexpensive but not very durable. There are better options. Aluminum has the capability to react with various foods or leave behind a metallic taste, so only use it to store foods that are not acidic or salty.

06. Lead-free ceramic
Safe for baking and roasting. However, some ceramic can contain lead (particularly if it is painted). Make sure yours does not.

07. Copper
Conducts heat well and is long lasting, but is expensive. Since copper can leach into food, choose cookware that is lined with stainless steel; too much copper in our diets isn't healthy.

Packaged and Processed

OVERVIEW

Packaged and processed foods are popular for their convenience, taste, and affordability. We Americans value them so much that we spend about 90 percent of our total food budget on processed foods (Schlosser 2001). In fact, we consume more packaged foods than anyone else in the world (Fairfield 2010).

One overlooked drawback are the chemicals involved in not just preserving them for a long shelf life but also from unintentional contamination.

Starting with the ingredients, toxicants can be intentionally added, unintentionally created, and unintentionally absorbed. For example, a study from Japan showed that the vinyl gloves worn by people handling and packaging food was a source of phthalate contamination (Tsumura et al. 2001).

Furthermore, toxicants in the packaging materials can leach into the foods, as has already been discussed.

HOUSEHOLD REPEAT OFFENDERS

Toxicants

— Arsenic: Diet, including fruit juices (Rock 2011) and rice (*Consumer Reports* 2012), is a main source of exposure to arsenic.
— BPA and phthalates
— PFCs including C8

Ingredients

— Nanoparticles: Can be in food packaging materials and could be present in food ingredients.
— Preservatives
— Synthetic colors

Materials

— Plastics

ADDITIONAL OFFENDERS

— Artificial additives: Nearly 4,000 chemicals are added to color, stabilize, emulsify, bleach, texturize, soften, sweeten, flavor, de-odor, and preserve processed "foods" (FDA 2013a). The human immune system treats chemical food additives as toxic foreign agents and attempts to rid the body of them, thus causing biochemical reactions that are sometimes severe and can stress the immune system.
— Genetically modified ingredients
— Sodium: The CDC estimates that 90 percent of Americans ingest more sodium than is suggested for health (CDC 2012b). Also, according to the CDC, almost 77 percent of our daily salt intake is from processed and restaurant-prepared foods. In contrast, approximately 10 percent of salt is added during cooking and meals (Gunn et al. 2010).
— Trans fats (partially hydrogenated vegetable oil): Used for deep-frying food and in baked goods, including those served in restaurants. Trans fat is linked to increased risk of heart disease and type II diabetes. The American Heart Association (2015) suggests that you get less than 1 percent of your total daily calories from trans fats.

REPEAT ISSUES

— Lack of disclosure: Typically, the FDA does not require food manufacturers to specify additives if those ingredients are classified as "generally regarded as safe" (GRAS). In these cases, you will may see "artificial flavor" or "artificial coloring" or "natural" on labels.
— Leaching of chemicals from packaging and storage materials into food and drinks.

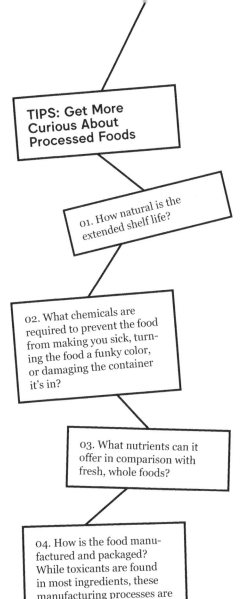

TIPS: Get More Curious About Processed Foods

01. How natural is the extended shelf life?

02. What chemicals are required to prevent the food from making you sick, turning the food a funky color, or damaging the container it's in?

03. What nutrients can it offer in comparison with fresh, whole foods?

04. How is the food manufactured and packaged? While toxicants are found in most ingredients, these manufacturing processes are likely to add more toxicants.

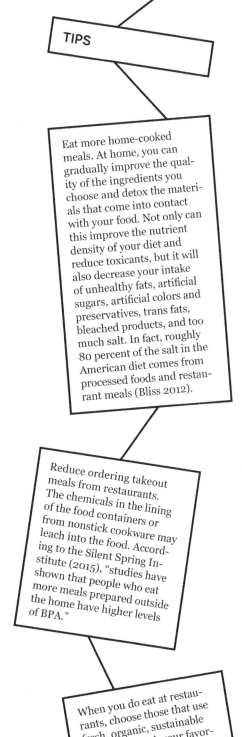

TIPS

Eat more home-cooked meals. At home, you can gradually improve the quality of the ingredients you choose and detox the materials that come into contact with your food. Not only can this improve the nutrient density of your diet and reduce toxicants, but it will also decrease your intake of unhealthy fats, artificial sugars, artificial colors and preservatives, trans fats, bleached products, and too much salt. In fact, roughly 80 percent of the salt in the American diet comes from processed foods and restaurant meals (Bliss 2012).

Reduce ordering takeout meals from restaurants. The chemicals in the lining of the food containers or from nonstick cookware may leach into the food. According to the Silent Spring Institute (2015), "studies have shown that people who eat more meals prepared outside the home have higher levels of BPA."

When you do eat at restaurants, choose those that use fresh, organic, sustainable ingredients. Ask your favorite establishments where their food comes from and which types of cookware are used. Let them know that you care.

Packaged and Processed Beverages: Coffee and Tea

OVERVIEW

Plants grown to produce coffee and tea thrive more when pesticides and fertilizers are used. For coffee, although great amounts of pesticides and chemical fertilizers may be used to grow the plants, most pesticide residues are burned away during the roasting process. The key health concerns, then, are the contamination of the environment from the agricultural practice, the health of the workers, and local residents who are more immediately exposed to the toxic pesticides on their coffee plantations; and the Trails of Contamination that ultimately end in our bodies.

As for tea, a lot of it comes from China and India, where pesticides that are barred in the US may still be used. Pesticide residues can linger longer in tea than in coffee. For example, tests of Chinese green tea have detected high levels of both lead and DDT.

Further, removing caffeine to create decaffeinated coffee and tea involves a chemical process that may contaminate the end product. Common chemicals used to extract caffeine include methylene chloride and ethyl acetate. Other processes use water or carbon dioxide.

HOUSEHOLD REPEAT OFFENDERS

Toxicants
— Methylene chloride
— Pesticides: From a contaminated environment or intended use, a variety of pesticides have been detected in coffee and tea, including DDT, lead, chlorpyrifos, ethion, dicofol, paraquat, and dalapon. Some that have been banned in the US are still used overseas, such as in India and China.

Ingredients
— Solvents. Methylene chloride is sometimes used to decaffeinate coffee. Trace amounts of this suspected carcinogen may remain from the decaffeination process (ATSDR 2000). The FDA says that consuming it in the low doses found in decaffeinated coffee is safe (although inhaling it may cause cancer). However, we are exposed to other sources of methylene chloride in other products, in drinking water, and in air, so an individual's cumulative exposure is an issue. If you're pregnant, you may want to take precautionary measures given the unique vulnerability of the fetus.

Materials
— Plastics

ADDITIONAL ISSUES
— Ethyl acetate: This is a solvent commonly used to remove caffeine. It's also used as a solvent in industrial products such as lacquers, paints, inks, and pesticides and as a flavoring aid in pharmaceuticals (EPA 2006).

TIPS: Healthier Coffee and Tea

Coffee: Buy coffee and tea labeled "Certified Organic," or "Fair Trade Certified."

Tea: Drink organic to avoid unnecessary pesticides.

Decaffeinated products: Consider the process of removing caffeine. Did it involve a chemical solvent, like methylene chloride? If not, then how was the caffeine removed? If drinking decaf coffee, seek organic brands processed with Swiss water, carbon dioxide, or sparkling water.

Packaged and Processed Beverages: Processed Juices

HOUSEHOLD REPEAT OFFENDERS

Toxicants

— Arsenic: As part I explained, inorganic arsenic, the kind that can cause cancer, has been found in apple and grape juice samples (Rock 2011), including in some of the nation's best-known brands of apple juice.

— Lead: In 2010, an EPA-certified lab in Berkeley detected high amounts of lead in over 85 percent of 146 fruit products tested. These products included apple and grape juice, packaged pears and peaches (including baby food), and fruit cocktail mixes. The results warranted California's Proposition 65 warning label for the products (Black 2010).

— Pesticides: Our international economy interconnects us to our global environment. For example, carbendazim, a fungicide that was banned in the US in 2008, has been detected in popular brands of orange juice. Contamination may occur on overseas soil, especially in Brazil. The FDA monitored the situation but didn't find the fungicide at levels that warranted recalling the products or barring them from entering the US (Juice Products Association 2012).

Ingredients

— Nanoparticles
— Preservatives
— Synthetic colors

Materials

— Plastics

TIPS: Healthier Juices

Reduce consumption. For example, my kids don't have juice boxes at home but they can enjoy them at parties.

Make your own juice or smoothie. Use organic ingredients or those that tend to have fewer residual pesticides (Check out the EWG's Clean 15/Dirty Dozen lists at ewg.org/foodnews/). You can even sneak in veggies like spinach and the kids may not notice. You'll enjoy the nutritional benefits that can get lost in the processing and shipping of commercially produced juice.

The Environmental Law Foundation published a list of baby and children's foods, including juice boxes, that they tested for lead. You can find the results at envirolaw.org/documents/FoodList.pdf.

Dilute your juices with water.

Diversify the types of juice you offer your children (such as apple, grape, and orange).

Buy apple juice made with apples from the US only. Choosing organic apple juice helps ensure that you get the purest products.

Be aware that products made with juice concentrate can be made of ingredients grown in many different locations worldwide. As an example, Asia and South America are predominant suppliers of apple juice concentrate. When a company purchases juice from a sole supplier, they could be getting concentrate from dozens of different farms. If enough samples of a supplier's juice are tested, varying amounts of arsenic (perhaps due to different soils or pesticide policies) will be detected (FDA 2013d).

Websites that share more information include those of the FDA, Consumer Reports, and DoctorOz.com.

Buy orange juice made only with oranges grown in the US. Look for 100 percent USDA-certified organic orange juice.

Eat organic whole fruit instead of juice. It offers more fiber and no additives.

Packaged and Processed Beverages: Soda

HOUSEHOLD REPEAT OFFENDERS

Ingredients

— Chemical flame retardants, like brominated vegetable oil (BVO). BVO, a flame retardant intended for plastics that Europe and Japan have banned in food, has been added to some sodas in North America for decades, as an emulsifier that prevents the flavoring ingredients from separating. Studies suggest that BVO may accumulate in human tissues. In mouse studies, large doses caused reproductive and behavioral problems (Israel 2011).
— Synthetic colors

Materials

— Plastics

ADDITIONAL ISSUES

— Artificial additives, such as sweeteners
— Caffeine
— Health issues, including obesity; high blood pressure, which can lead to strokes and other cardiovascular disease; type II diabetes, which can cause a number of health problems, including cataracts, high cholesterol, nerve damage, stroke, reproductive problems, and blindness; kidney damage; and dental damage.

TIPS

Avoid or reduce consumption of soda.

Try organic juice (preferably homemade) mixed with sparkling water.

Try cut-up fruits, vegetables, or herbs (berries, cucumbers, mint, lemons, limes, pineapple, etc.) in sparkling or still water. It also makes a pretty display.

Packaged and Processed Beverages: Water

OVERVIEW

The FDA regulates bottled water while the EPA regulates tap water. Which is better? The answer depends on your local water supply and the bottled water that you choose.

Drinking water in the US comes from groundwater and rain that fills streams, reservoirs, rivers, lakes, and oceans. As businesses and individuals contaminate these natural sources, water purity becomes challenged. Some contaminants are not hazardous to health in trace amounts, but others may cause or contribute to adverse health effects.

Water screening varies among local water companies. Regardless, filtered tap water tends to be a great choice. Filtering allows you to reduce contamination by avoiding plastic bottles that leach chemicals into our Homes throughout their Life Cycle, including during and after their useful life. More than 80 percent of recyclable plastics accumulate in landfills each year.

Plus, filtered tap water is cheaper. Globally, we spend $100 billion a year buying bottled water. The US alone buys about 50 billion bottles of water a year (Karlstrom and Dell'Amore 2010), and in 2012, Americans spent $11.8 billion dollars on bottled water, a 6.5 percent increase from 2011 (Boesler 2013). So drinking more filtered tap would save us a lot of money, provide us with water quality that is usually at least as good as bottled water, and significantly alleviate our planet's burden (Karlstrom and Dell'Amore 2010).

HOUSEHOLD REPEAT OFFENDERS

Toxicants

— Arsenic: Has the capacity to enter water through soil deposits or industrial and agricultural pollution.
— Benzene and dioxins: Manufacturing plastics used to make bottles may produce toxic by-products, such as dioxin and benzene, which are released into the environment.
— BPA
— Chlorine
— Lead: Can leach into drinking water from lead-containing pipes in your home and in public water systems.
— Pesticides
— Phthalates
— Unintentional Toxicants: For example, trihalomethanes (THMs) can form when chlorine (often used in water as a disinfectant) reacts with organic matter like treated sewage, animal waste, leaves and soil. THMs can contribute to cancer risk and may damage the liver, kidneys, and nervous system.

Materials

— Plastics

ADDITIONAL OFFENDERS

— Atrazine: Can cause organ and cardiovascular damage and is a suspected hormone disruptor. It's a weed killer used on most corn crops.
— Fluoride: The benefits of fluoride in drinking water and how much is safe for adults and kids continues to be debated.
— Ingredients from drugs, detergents, disinfectants, insect repellents, and personal care products: Have been found in drinking water supplies.

REPEAT ISSUES

— Trails of Contamination throughout our Homes if buying plastic water bottles
— Unintentional By-products

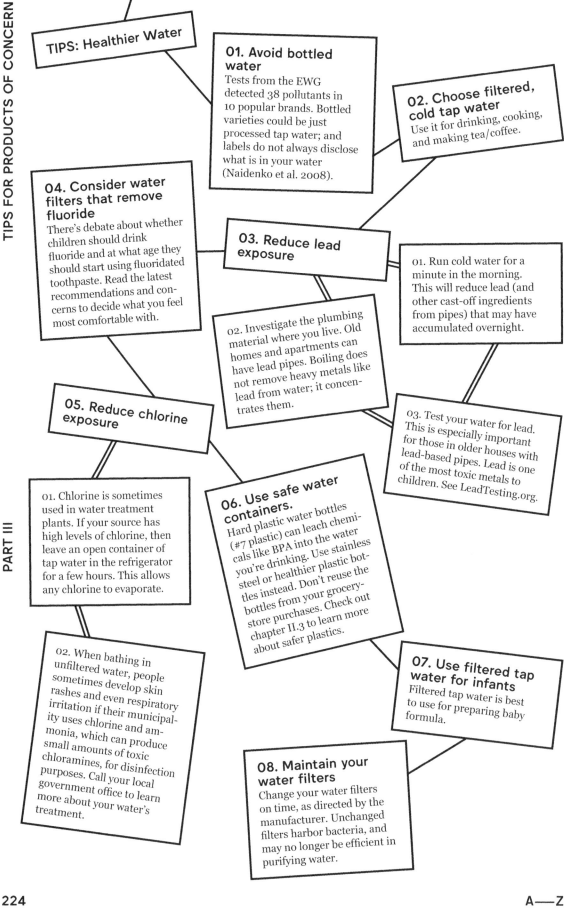

TIPS: Healthier Water

01. Avoid bottled water
Tests from the EWG detected 38 pollutants in 10 popular brands. Bottled varieties could be just processed tap water; and labels do not always disclose what is in your water (Naidenko et al. 2008).

02. Choose filtered, cold tap water
Use it for drinking, cooking, and making tea/coffee.

04. Consider water filters that remove fluoride
There's debate about whether children should drink fluoride and at what age they should start using fluoridated toothpaste. Read the latest recommendations and concerns to decide what you feel most comfortable with.

03. Reduce lead exposure

01. Run cold water for a minute in the morning. This will reduce lead (and other cast-off ingredients from pipes) that may have accumulated overnight.

02. Investigate the plumbing material where you live. Old homes and apartments can have lead pipes. Boiling does not remove heavy metals like lead from water; it concentrates them.

05. Reduce chlorine exposure

03. Test your water for lead. This is especially important for those in older houses with lead-based pipes. Lead is one of the most toxic metals to children. See LeadTesting.org.

01. Chlorine is sometimes used in water treatment plants. If your source has high levels of chlorine, then leave an open container of tap water in the refrigerator for a few hours. This allows any chlorine to evaporate.

06. Use safe water containers.
Hard plastic water bottles (#7 plastic) can leach chemicals like BPA into the water you're drinking. Use stainless steel or healthier plastic bottles instead. Don't reuse the bottles from your grocery-store purchases. Check out chapter II.3 to learn more about safer plastics.

02. When bathing in unfiltered water, people sometimes develop skin rashes and even respiratory irritation if their municipality uses chlorine and ammonia, which can produce small amounts of toxic chloramines, for disinfection purposes. Call your local government office to learn more about your water's treatment.

07. Use filtered tap water for infants
Filtered tap water is best to use for preparing baby formula.

08. Maintain your water filters
Change your water filters on time, as directed by the manufacturer. Unchanged filters harbor bacteria, and may no longer be efficient in purifying water.

Water Filter Systems

There are two types of water filters: point-of-use and point-of-entry. When used properly, they can reduce toxicants and significantly improve the taste and odor of tap water.

Point-of-use systems

Most kitchen water filters are point-of-use, which can filter water in a specific area only, such as the kitchen sink. They may use a container (pitcher or larger dispenser) that stores water in a refrigerator, or they may be mounted more permanently on a faucet or under a sink. Point-of-use water filters typically absorb impurities (including odors) by using carbon.

Point-of-entry systems

Point-of-entry systems, usually installed in basements or outside, filter an entire household's water supply. Whole-house filters not only improve your drinking water quality but will also reduce contaminated vapors that can be inhaled while bathing, showering, and cleaning dishes. Effectiveness varies widely, so research manufacturers' details. Point-of-use filters may still be necessary to remove parasites and other contaminants.

The Most Common Types of Water Filters

Different filters remove different contaminants, so it is important to know what's in your tap water in order to choose the best filter.

Carbon filters

Carbon filters can be relatively inexpensive and are sufficient for most needs. They are used in countertop pitchers, faucet-mounted and under-sink models, and whole-house or point-of-entry systems (which are typically installed outside or in the basement). Carbon-activated filters absorb impurities as the water passes through. These include lead and some other heavy metals, chlorine by-products (chloramines and trihalomethanes), pesticides and herbicides, some organic chemicals, PCBs, certain parasites, radon, MTBE (an additive in gasoline), trichloroethylene (a solvent used in dry cleaning), various volatile organic compounds, bacteria (like cryptosporidium and giardia), a small number of pharmaceuticals, and intrusive odors and tastes. They won't remove dissolved inorganic contaminants or metals such as arsenic, fluoride, or mercury, nor will they pick up nitrates, most bacteria, or sediments (use a reverse osmosis filter for help with these pollutants).

Reverse osmosis filters

Reverse osmosis water filters are usually used in conjunction with a carbon filter but add the filtering capability of a semi-permeable membrane. This additional filter can trap certain harmful contaminants that carbon filters cannot catch, such as nitrates, perchlorate, and arsenic. They effectively remove industrial chemicals, heavy metals, and asbestos, and usually also remove sulfates, fluoride, industrial chemicals, heavy metals (including lead), chlorine by-products, chlorides (which are responsible for making water taste salty), and pharmaceuticals. They do not filter out radon, certain volatile organic compounds, or certain pesticides. Moreover, reverse osmosis systems waste water as a result of its filtration process, which flushes away a few gallons of contaminated water. They also filter water slowly, occupy a lot of space, and can remove good minerals like calcium and fluoride that your body may need. Typically expensive and difficult to install, experts find them unnecessary for most households. They are good choices, however, for individuals with weak immune systems or particularly contaminated water.

TIPS: Locations for Water Filters

Water in the kitchen

Investing in filtered water for drinking and cooking is a high-impact change, especially if you are pregnant or have young children.

Water in the bathroom

Exposure to potentially harmful chemicals as you brush your teeth is pretty low. However, if you frequently drink water from your bathroom tap, or if your tap water contains high levels of a contaminant that may be of concern in the shower or bath, then consider a whole-house filter. One reason I chose a whole-house filter is because my young kids enjoy long, leisurely baths, and our municipal water has a high level of chlorine, which they could inhale and absorb.

Showerheads

An inexpensive and easy solution for showering is a removable charcoal filter that you can place on your showerhead. This helps reduce your risk of inhaling vaporized disinfecting agents (like chlorine) and whatever else might be in your water. Absorption through the skin is less of an issue than exposure via drinking or inhaling vapors.

TIPS: Well Water

Test water from a private well every two to three years for nitrates and other contaminants such as volatile organic compounds; test annually for coliform bacteria (and more frequently for radon or pesticides if those are problems in your area).

To find out which pollutants are typical for your area, check with your local health department or contact National Testing Laboratories, which performs water tests by mail. State-certified water laboratories are listed on the EPA's Drinking Water website as well.

If you can, install a reverse osmosis filter, which can remove pollutants that carbon filters can't, such as arsenic and perchlorate.

Consider using a whole-house water filter, which can remove contaminants from the steam generated from the shower and dishwashing. Models vary in effectiveness, so be sure to research and consult the manufacturer for details.

TIPS: Research Your Local Water Supply

See if your local water supplier provides an annual water-quality report, also known as a consumer confidence report. If you have trouble interpreting the report, consult a guide for understanding them, which are available from the Campaign for Safe and Affordable Drinking Water's website.

Learn more information regarding your tap water and water filters at EWG's National Tap Water Database: ewg.org/tap-water.

Packaged and Processed Beverages: Wine and Beer

HOUSEHOLD REPEAT OFFENDERS

Wine

— Pesticides: In 2008, the Pesticide Action Network Europe found 24 different pesticides in 40 bottles of conventionally produced wine purchased within the EU (including wines made by world-famous vineyards). Five were classified by the EU as being carcinogenic, mutagenic, or hazardous to the reproductive system. All bottles were found to contain pesticides, including one bottle that was found to have 10 different varieties. Each sample of wine contained an average of more than four pesticides (Pesticide Action Network 2008).

Beer

— Pesticides and other toxic chemicals: Herbicides, insecticides, fungicides, and fossil fuel-derived fertilizers are used in the commercial production of the grains (barley and wheat) that go into beer.

ADDITIONAL OFFENDERS IN WINE

— Perc in wine (and beer too)
— Sulfites: Naturally occurring, sulfites are added to foods and beverages as a preservative and even as a bleaching agent. Some people are sulfite-sensitive. Reactions can range from mild to severe. Possible signs of sensitivity include headaches, nausea, diarrhea, and sometimes allergic reactions. There is concern that cumulative, long-term exposure to inorganic chemicals like sulfites can strain the immune system, which renders the body vulnerable to other stressors.

TIPS: Healthier Beer

"Certified Organic" beers are made with 95 percent organic ingredients, which follow the standards created by the USDA.

Beers "Made with Organic Ingredients" have been brewed with at least 70 percent organic ingredients.

To earn the organic label, both types of beer must be processed in breweries that are cleaned without using harsh acids or chemicals. Both are made with products supplied by organic farmers.

When wines are organically processed, it means that the winemaker avoided adding synthetic agents in the clarifying process and that hot water or steam was used to sterilize the equipment, instead of chemical agents. Further, little or no manipulation of the wine occurs during the winemaking process in the way of reverse osmosis, excessive filtration, or added flavoring.

Organic winemaking may improve taste. It is growing in popularity, so it's easier to find than ever before.

"Organic Wine" is made from 95 percent organic ingredients and may have added sulfites up to 100 ppm.

Bottles marked "100 percent Organic Wine" are made from organic ingredients and do not have any added sulfites (although small amounts of sulfites occur naturally in wine).

Wine labeled "Made with Organic Grapes" is made from at least 70 percent organic ingredients and could have added sulfites up to 100 ppm.

Evaluate the winemaking process

Evaluate the ingredients

TIPS: Healthier Wine

Packaged and Processed Foods: Prepackaged Popcorn

HOUSEHOLD REPEAT OFFENDERS

Toxicants
— PFCs: PFOA or other potentially harmful chemicals from the lining of the popcorn bag.

Ingredients
— Synthetic colors

Materials
— Plastics

REPEAT ISSUES
— Substitute chemicals are not necessarily safer

ADDITIONAL ISSUES
— According to the CDC (2012a), "The flavorings industry has estimated that over a thousand flavoring ingredients have the potential to be respiratory hazards due to possible volatility and irritant properties."
— Artificial butter flavoring, such as diacetyl (discussed in chapter I.12)

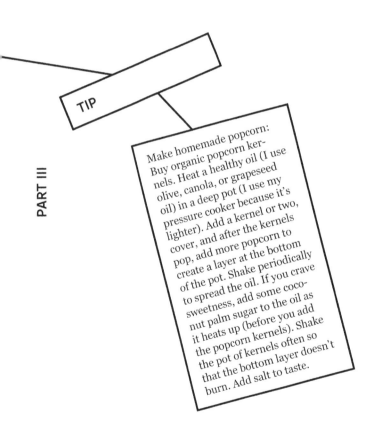

TIP

Make homemade popcorn: Buy organic popcorn kernels. Heat a healthy oil (I use olive, canola, or grapeseed oil) in a deep pot (I use my pressure cooker because it's lighter). Add a kernel or two, cover, and after the kernels pop, add more popcorn to create a layer at the bottom of the pot. Shake periodically to spread the oil. If you crave sweetness, add some coconut palm sugar to the oil as it heats up (before you add the popcorn kernels). Shake the pot of kernels often so that the bottom layer doesn't burn. Add salt to taste.

Packaged and Processed Foods: Rice and Rice By-products

OVERVIEW

Rice accumulates arsenic from its growing environment since arsenic pervades our soil and water. It's then stored in the rice grain's outer layer, which is polished off when brown rice is processed into white rice. So brown rice tends to have higher levels of arsenic than white rice does. In fact, according to *Consumer Reports* (2014), "Brown rice has 80 percent more inorganic arsenic [the cancer-causing type] on average than white rice of the same type."

In 2012, the FDA tested over 1,300 samples of rice and rice by-products. It found that "among the rice grain categories, the average levels of inorganic arsenic ranged from 2.6 to 7.2 micrograms of inorganic arsenic per serving, with instant rice at the low end of the range and brown rice at the high end. Among the rice product categories, of which there was a wide variety, the average levels of inorganic arsenic ranged from 0.1 to 6.6 micrograms of inorganic arsenic per serving, with infant formula at the low end of the range and rice pasta at the high end. These amounts of detectable arsenic are not high enough to cause any immediate or short-term adverse health effects." *(FDA 2013b)*

HOUSEHOLD REPEAT OFFENDERS

Toxicants
— Arsenic

PRODUCTS OF CONCERN
— Organic brown rice syrup: Products with organic brown rice syrup may introduce significant concentrations of arsenic into the diet.
— Rice by-products: Rice pasta, rice cakes, infant and toddler cereals; teething biscuits; grain-based bars; pie and pizza crust; snacks, such as cookies, brownies, pastries, and puddings; and beverages, including rice milk, beer, rice wine, and rice water.

TIPS: Reducing Your Arsenic Exposure from Rice

Below are tips on how to reduce arsenic when cooking rice, as reported by the FDA (2013b), *Consumer Reports* (2014) and the Chicago Tribune (Eng 2012).

Diversify
Diversify the types of rice in your diet, and the geographies from which they were grown. Safer options include white rice (but those from Texas tend to have high levels of arsenic; those from California tend to have 38 percent less inorganic arsenic than those from other parts of the US); aromatic rice, such as basmati and jasmine rices (Brown basmati from California, India, or Pakistan tested about a third less inorganic arsenic than other brown rices); quinoa; buckwheat; amaranth; polenta; grits; and millet. Options that tend to have higher levels of arsenic include brown rice (Brown basmati from California, India, or Pakistan is the best choice; rice from Southern US regions had higher levels of arsenic).

Know your water
Check with your water source (such as a municipal water report) on whether arsenic levels are below 10 ppb. If so, then rinse the rice until the water becomes clear. This can take 4-6 cycles. Studies show that this can reduce total arsenic levels by 25-50 percent. If your water source contains high levels of arsenic then rinsing rice won't reduce its arsenic content so check your water supply.

Cook with awareness
Cook your rice with six parts water to one part rice. Then discard the excess water after the rice has finished cooking (like you do with pasta). The FDA estimates that rinsing, cooking with excess water, and then draining the water can diminish levels of arsenic by 50-60 percent.

Stay updated
Check in with the websites of the FDA and *Consumer Reports*. New information, including guidelines, will evolve as this topic is pursued.

Packaged and Processed Ingredients: Artificial Additives

HOUSEHOLD REPEAT OFFENDERS

Ingredients
— Nanoparticles
— Preservatives

ON PROBATION

— Monosodium glutamate (MSG): An ingredient that commonly serves as a flavor enhancer in Chinese food, canned vegetables, soups, and processed meats (Mayo Clinic 2015). The FDA (2012) considers MSG an ingredient that is generally recognized as safe in food, and a lot of research has found no cause for concern for the general population. Still, some believe that it may be a neurotoxin.

ADDITIONAL OFFENDERS

— Artificial colors
— Processed sugars
— Sodium benzoate: Often used as a preservative in a wide range of processed foods and drinks. It may increase hyperactivity in some children (McCann et al. 2007).
— Sodium nitrite: Used as a preservative, coloring, flavoring, and curing agent in meat products like bacon, ham, hot dogs, luncheon meats, corned beef, and smoked fish. There is conflicting evidence on whether high sodium nitrite exposure is linked to cancers in adults and children (EPA 2007a).

REPEAT ISSUES

— Unintentional By-products. For example, in soft drinks, sodium benzoate can react with vitamin C to create benzene, which is carcinogenic (Downs 2008); sodium nitrite can interact with other chemicals in food or in the body to form carcinogens called nitrosamines.
— Unintentional Potential Effects

TIPS: Read Labels to Avoid Artificial Sugars, Colors, and Preservatives

Avoiding processed foods can help reduce exposures to artificial colors, flavors, and preservatives.

Avoid any products that contain the artificial sweeteners aspartame or neotame, keeping in mind that they can turn up where you might least suspect them. Neotame, the newest artificial sweetener, may affect MSG-sensitive people the same way aspartame does.

Avoid unnecessary exposures to MSG. Although the National Academy of Sciences, the WHO, and the FDA have not regulated MSG, I take precautionary measures. If you are interested in avoiding MSG, here are some tips.

01. MSG may be in hidden forms such as hydrolyzed vegetable protein, hydrolyzed yeast, autolyzed yeast, yeast extract, soy extracts, protein isolate, sodium and calcium caseinate, and various other forms of processed free glutamic acid.

02. Avoid foods containing hydrolyzed corn gluten and hydrolyzed wheat protein. Both are ingredients that may contain hidden MSG.

03. Request information from delis or restaurants about their use of MSG.

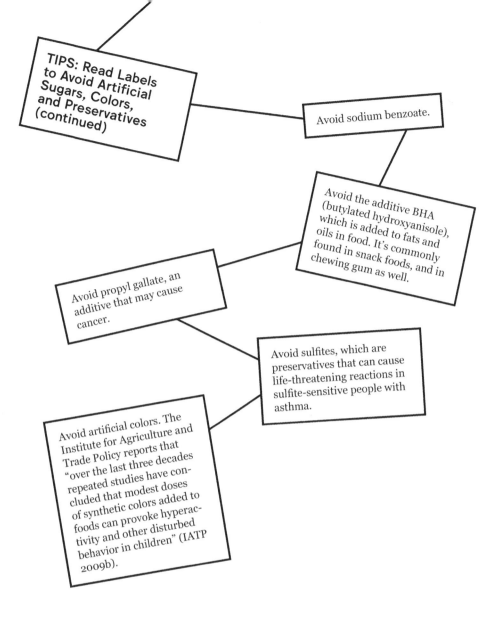

TIPS: Read Labels to Avoid Artificial Sugars, Colors, and Preservatives (continued)

Avoid sodium benzoate.

Avoid the additive BHA (butylated hydroxyanisole), which is added to fats and oils in food. It's commonly found in snack foods, and in chewing gum as well.

Avoid propyl gallate, an additive that may cause cancer.

Avoid sulfites, which are preservatives that can cause life-threatening reactions in sulfite-sensitive people with asthma.

Avoid artificial colors. The Institute for Agriculture and Trade Policy reports that "over the last three decades repeated studies have con-cluded that modest doses of synthetic colors added to foods can provoke hyperac-tivity and other disturbed behavior in children" (IATP 2009b).

Packaged and Processed Ingredients: Genetically Modified Ingredients

OVERVIEW

"Genetically modified foods" (GM foods), "genetically engineered foods" (GEs), or "genetically modified organisms" (GMOs) refer to plants or animals whose genetic material has been changed by adding DNA from other species, in ways that would not occur naturally or through traditional breeding. Genetic engineering can create desired traits, such as pest and disease resistance or cold tolerance. Available since the early 1990s, GMOs are now present in more than 60 percent of processed foods found in supermarkets in the US (Ackerman 2015). The US is among the largest producers and exporters of genetically modified crops (FAO 2012).

HOUSEHOLD REPEAT OFFENDERS

Toxicants

— Pesticides: GMOs require lots of pesticides (they even produce pesticides within their own cells); and they cross-contaminate other crops and harm wildlife (Koch 2011).

REPEAT ISSUES

— Lack of disclosure: The US does not require manufacturers to label products that contain GMO ingredients, even though 92 percent of Americans want GMO foods labeled and more than 40 countries have mandatory labeling of GMOs, according to the advocacy group Just Label It! Countries with such laws include the EU nations, Japan, China, Korea, Australia, and New Zealand.

ADDITIONAL ISSUES

— Unknown health risks: Because GMOs are a relatively new introduction into the food supply, their potential impact on our bodies isn't yet fully understood. Suspected health risks include allergies and increased cancer risk. In an animal study published in the *International Journal of Biological Sciences* in 2009, researchers found GM corn to be linked to impaired kidney and liver function. Adverse effects on the heart, adrenal glands, spleen, and blood cells were also reported (de Vendomois et al. 2009). Monsanto, a major producer of GMO seeds, attacked the study, saying "these claims are based on faulty analytical methods and reasoning and do not call into question the safety findings for these products" (Goldstein and Emami 2010).

— Trails of Contamination throughout our Homes

TIPS

Buy "Certified Organic." Seek foods with labels that state the product is either 95 or 100 percent organic.

Prioritize your budget for organic animal products— meat, dairy, and eggs. Conventional farms sometimes feed GMO corn to their animals.

The most common GMO crops grown in the US in 2014 were soy (94 percent of the total crop), cotton (91 percent), and corn (89 percent; USDA 2014). Many foods produced in the US with corn or high-fructose corn syrup, soybeans, and cottonseed or canola oils can contain genetically modified ingredients. Animal feed frequently contains these ingredients. Unless the label specifically says organic, it's likely that any food or product that contains soy, cotton, corn, or canola has been genetically changed. These products are wide ranging: tofu, tortilla chips, potato chips fried in cottonseed oil, diet sodas with aspartame (created by a fermentation process involving soy and corn), bed and bath linens, and clothing.

Avoid processed, packaged foods, many of which contain corn-based ingredients. As Michael Pollan (2007) stated in *The Omnivore's Dilemma*, "There are some 45,000 items in the average American supermarket and more than a quarter of them now contain corn."

Let your elected representatives know that you want mandatory GMO labeling laws. Learn more at JustLabelIt.org.

Use the Non-GMO Shopping Guide prepared by the Institute for Responsible Technology (nongmoshoppingguide.com).

Packaged and Processed Ingredients: Processed Sugars

HOUSEHOLD REPEAT OFFENDERS

Toxicants
— Arsenic
— Mercury

ADDITIONAL OFFENDERS

— Aspartame: Also sold as Nutra-Sweet and Equal, aspartame is a sugar substitute in many diet and sugar-free beverages and vitamins, including children's vitamins. A 2006 Italian study found that it was associated with unusually high rates of lymphoma, leukemia, and other cancers in rats (Soffritti et al. 2006).

— High-fructose corn syrup (HFCS): Because HFCS extends the shelf life of foods, and farm subsidies make it cheaper than other sugars, HFCS is used in a wide variety of processed foods, including breads, cereals, breakfast bars, crackers, baked goods, lunch meats, fruity yogurts, soups, condiments (salad dressings and ketchup), beverages, soft drinks, fruit juices, and many foods marketed to children.

For many, HFCS may be a significant additional source of elemental mercury. Daily per capita consumption of HFCS in the US averages about 50 grams, and daily mercury intake from HFCS ranges up to 28 micrograms (Wallinga et al. 2009). Teens and others with high intakes can ingest up to 80 percent more than the average amounts (IATP 2009a).

Currently, the EPA hasn't established a safe dose of elemental mercury, the kind found in corn syrup. The EPA has stated that "All forms of mercury are quite toxic, and each form exhibits different health effects" (EPA 2013b).

Mercury was detected in almost 50 percent of tested samples of commercial HFCS (Dufault et al. 2009). A separate study by the Institute for Agriculture and Trade Policy found that mercury was present in almost one-third of 55 prevalent, brand-name food and beverage items, which listed HFCS as either the first or second ingredient on their labels (Wallinga et al. 2009).

In addition, HFCS may increase the likelihood for obesity. Researchers at Princeton University found that when rats consumed HFCS at levels well below those in soda, they became obese (Bocarsly et al. 2010).

— Organic brown rice syrup: A common substitute for HFCS in organic products, brown rice syrup sometimes contains the type of arsenic that causes cancer, as part I explained. Products with organic brown rice syrup may introduce significant concentrations of arsenic into the diet.

TIPS: Navigating Sugar Options

Remember that too much of any kind of sugar isn't great for you. Below are popular ones among health foodies.

Coconut palm sugar is currently considered a healthier option.

Honey offers trace amounts of vitamins C and B-complex, amino acids, enzymes, and minerals. Raw honey is rich in antioxidants, enzymes, and various healing cofactors.

Raw agave nectar, once viewed as a healthy option, is no longer recommended, as it contains too much fructose.

Maple syrup and brown rice syrup have a fairly high glycemic index and can stress existing digestive issues. They are okay in moderation, if they are pure and high quality.

Organic raw cane sugar, organic Florida Crystals, and organic turbinado sugar are slightly better than refined sugar. They retain some nutrients and are better for the environment.

Opting for organic sugars reduces the Trails of Contamination of synthetic fertilizers and pesticides.

Packaged and Processed Ingredients: Soy

OVERVIEW

Soy became popular in the US soon after Americans started to associate it with the low rates of certain cancers and other Western diseases among people living in Asia, whose cultures have regarded soy as an important food crop for centuries. It became so popular that soy and soy-related products started to be incorporated into a wide range of innovative products in the form of substances called soy protein isolate, soy isoflavones, soy lecithin, and textured vegetable protein.

However, rather than eat it in its more natural forms of tofu and edamame, we eat it in processed foods: veggie burgers, tofu hot dogs, chicken-free nuggets and other imitation meats; soy ice creams, energy bars, tempeh, tofu yogurt, soy butter, soy nut butter, soy milk, soy cheese, bean curd, seitan, and soy noodles. Soybean flour is found in products such as chorizo, salchichón, mortadella, boiled ham, doughnuts, and soup stock cubes. As a result, Americans now eat more soy than the Japanese or Chinese do. Asians also eat soy after it has been fermented, which provides healthy bacteria for our guts. Asians have eaten whole soy foods for centuries, but in much smaller quantities and in more natural forms.

REPEAT ISSUE

— Endocrine disruption: Soy isoflavones, compounds found in soy products, resemble estrogen and bind to human estrogen receptors. Whether these compounds impair our health is unclear. However, studies show that in addition to its health benefits, soy may pose risks as well. For example, heavy intake of the estrogen-mimicking compounds in soy is linked to reduced fertility in women (Chan 2009), early puberty (Delclos et al. 2009), and the disruption of fetal and childhood development (Latendresse et al. 2009).

ADDITIONAL ISSUES

— Genetically modified organisms: It is estimated that 94 percent of soy crops are genetically modified (USDA 2014).
— Soy offers health benefits: Low in fat and cholesterol and high in protein and fiber.
— The long-term effects of eating GMOs and soy are unknown but being studied.

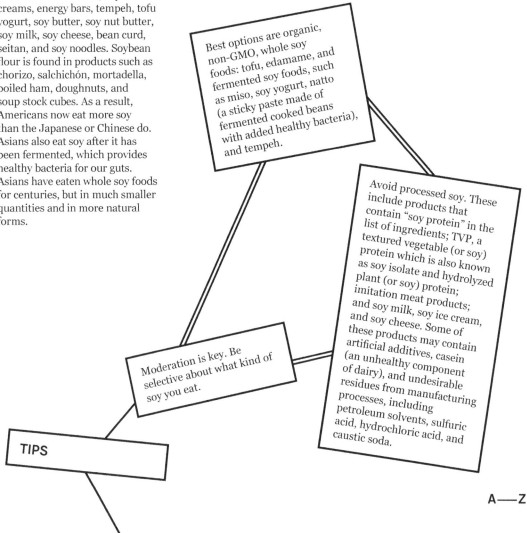

Best options are organic, non-GMO, whole soy foods: tofu, edamame, and fermented soy foods, such as miso, soy yogurt, natto (a sticky paste made of fermented cooked beans with added healthy bacteria), and tempeh.

Avoid processed soy. These include products that contain "soy protein" in the list of ingredients; TVP, a textured vegetable (or soy) protein which is also known as soy isolate and hydrolyzed plant (or soy) protein; imitation meat products; and soy milk, soy ice cream, and soy cheese. Some of these products may contain artificial additives, casein (an unhealthy component of dairy), and undesirable residues from manufacturing processes, including petroleum solvents, sulfuric acid, hydrochloric acid, and caustic soda.

Moderation is key. Be selective about what kind of soy you eat.

TIPS

Simple Strategies to Reduce Toxicants in Your Diet

Toxicants in your diet come from three main sources: the ingredients, what the food has touched, and sometimes how it was cooked or manufactured. Be curious about the four key tips below. Ultimately, you should increase your diet's portion of nourishing home-cooked meals.

01. Assess the ingredients

To reduce your chemical body burden, eat things that are lower on the food chain (they have fewer links in the food web). A diverse diet that contains lots of veggies, fruits, nuts, legumes, and whole grains will lower and diversify your exposure to toxicants. The nutrients in a plant-based diet not only boost your immunity but may also help counteract the negative effects of toxicants. Since animals and animal by-products can still be part of a healthy diet, consider those that are organic and grass-fed.

Choose organic ingredients as much as possible, but prioritize animals and their by-products. To learn which fruits and vegetables have the most and the fewest pesticides, see the EWG's "Dirty Dozen" and "Clean Fifteen" lists (ewg.org/foodnews/). Studies led by Chensheng Lu of Emory University and published in 2006 and 2008 found that pesticides in elementary school–age children peaked during the summer, when they ate the most fresh produce. After five days of being on an all-organic diet, participants became essentially pesticide-free (Lu et al. 2006; Lu et al. 2008). Eating organic will reduce exposures to pesticides, artificial growth hormones, artificial additives, and genetically modified ingredients. Regardless, eating even conventional fruits and vegetables is still healthier than eating none at all.

Minimize your diet's portion of processed and packaged foods. Not only will this reduce your exposure to chemicals from manufacturing and packaging, but it will also help you avoid concerning ingredients. The FDA's database "Everything Added to Food in the United States" lists nearly 4,000 chemicals (FDA 2013a), and the agency acknowledges that this is only a partial list (FDA 2014b). These ingredients help color, stabilize, emulsify, bleach, texturize, soften, sweeten, flavor, deodorize, and preserve the food products they are added to. Some are known carcinogens, and some may be linked to diabetes, obesity, and hyperactivity in children.

Seek simple, recognizable ingredients.

02. Consider what your food has come into contact with

Consider what your food ate before it reached your plate. Think about its possible body burden of toxicants and the environment in which it lived.

Minimize exposure to food packaging, including plastic containers, plastic wrap, styrofoam, takeout or delivery containers, and metal cans. Heat can encourage the leaching of toxicants from containers or plastic wrap into the food or drinks that touch them. So when you must use them (they are impossible to avoid completely), never heat them in the microwave and avoid washing them in the dishwasher.

Avoid using nonstick pots and pans, and choose cast iron or stainless steel instead. C8, a common ingredient in nonstick chemical formulas, was phased out due to health risks, but its replacement chemical may not be safer (EWG 2015s).

Cookware: Choose cast iron and stainless steel interiors.

When storing food and beverages, opt for stainless steel and glass containers and unbleached wax paper.

Avoid heating any kind of plastic, as it encourages leaching. Use glass.

When you can't avoid plastic, stick to safer reusable plastics like #2, #4, and #5.

Minimize consumption of foods that were stored in metal cans.

03. How was it cooked?

Avoid processed, packaged foods whenever possible. Sometimes support is available. For example, in New York City there are services that offer home-cooked meals made of nourishing ingredients.

Was part of the meal wrapped in plastic? Was it microwaved in plastic? Is it charred? Were delicate oils, like olive oil, cooked at temperatures that are beyond its safe heat threshold? Asking these questions can help reduce your exposure to toxicants. Since it is hard to get comfortable with meals that have been prepared outside your home, increasing your intake of wholesome, home-cooked foods is a good solution.

Oils with high heat thresholds that are good to cook with: coconut, grapeseed, and canola. Healthy oils with lower heat thresholds are great as a finishing touch, such as olive (fine if heated below 325 degrees Fahrenheit), sesame, and flaxseed.

Avoid overcooking, and do not eat any food that is charred.

04. Detox your beverages

Skip bottled water. Drink filtered tap water instead. Use a food-grade stainless steel bottle as a container for filtered tap water. And think critically about your local sources of water and potential nearby sources of pollution.

Choose organic beverages whenever you can. Pesticides and other synthetic chemicals are sometimes found in juice, soda, wine, beer, coffee, tea, milk, and yogurt drinks.

Beverage packaging: Avoid disposable packaging materials. Opt for reusable stainless steel bottles.

Water: Filtered is generally best, but it depends on the local tap water and the water filter.

Juice boxes: Avoid. Make your own juice out of organic ingredients, or from produce included on EWG's Clean 15 list.

Wine and beer: Choose certified organic beer and certified organic or biodynamic wine.

Coffee and tea: Certified organic helps minimize ingestion of pesticides. Beware of decaffeinated coffee.

Chapter III.3
Interior Furnishings

CONVENTIONAL INTERIOR FURNISHINGS: WHAT'S IN THEM?

Certain toxicants can be two to five times—and even *100 times* (EPA 2012a)—higher indoors than outdoors. Why is that so? A broad offender is the category of interior furnishings. Included in this category are furniture, carpets, mattresses, window treatments, paints, wallpaper, and building materials.

Most of us cannot change our building materials, but there are many interior furnishings that we can change, and that's what this section focuses on. Readers who are about to build a home, renovate, or prepare a room for a new baby may find this section of special interest.

IN THIS CHAPTER:

— Household Repeat Offenders in conventional interior furnishings
   — Blinds
   — Candles
   — Conventional carpets
   — Curtains
   — Floor materials
   — Furniture
   — In the Bathroom
   — In the Bedroom: Mattresses; headboards and bed frames; blankets, comforters, pillows, and sheets
   — Paints and finishes
   — Renovations, maintenance, and repairs
   — Wallpaper
   — Wallpaper adhesives
— Simple Strategies for healthier interior furnishings

HOUSEHOLD REPEAT OFFENDERS

Toxicants
— Benzene
— BPA
— Chlorine
— Formaldehyde
— Lead
— Methylene chloride
— PBDEs
— PFCs
— Phthalates
— Tris flame retardants
— Unintentionals

Ingredients
— Artificial colors and dyes
— Chemical flame retardants
— Inerts
— Nanoparticles
— Petroleum distillates
— Solvents

Materials
— Adhesives
— Conventional textiles
— Paints
— Plastics, including vinyl
— Polyurethane foam
— Wood

OTHER OFFENDERS
— Potentially toxic additives, HAPs, and VOCs such as toluene and xylene
— Preservatives, fungicides, and biocides, which may contain toxic chemicals such as copper, arsenic disulfide, phenol, styrene, and quaternary ammonium compounds

REPEAT ISSUES
— Hidden hazards
— Ingredients detected in humans
— Lack of disclosure of ingredients or of toxicity, or potential toxicity
— Lack of required safety testing by an objective third party
— Little or no regulation of validity of label claims
— No regulation of levels of toxic ingredients used in consumer products
— The necessity of ventilation and other precautionary measures because even the safest options may emit toxic chemicals
— Trails of Contamination throughout our Homes
— Unintentional Potential Effects

Blinds

OVERVIEW

In the mid-1990s, some children experienced significant lead exposure from their homes' PVC (or vinyl) mini-blinds. Lead had been used as a stabilizer in some blinds made in Indonesia, China, Taiwan, and Mexico, and the lead was being released into dust after exposure to light and heat.

The CPSC found that on certain blinds, lead levels were so high that if a child ingested the dust from less than a square inch of blinds each day for 15 to 30 days, his or her blood level of lead could exceed 10 micrograms per deciliter, the level that the CPSC considers dangerous (CPSC 1996). While most manufacturers agreed to reformulate their blinds to be lead-free, there is no premarket testing to determine whether current blinds are safe, even if they bear a "lead-free" label. Your best bet is to remove any blinds that were purchased before 1997 from your home and replace them with either curtains or non-PVC blinds.

HOUSEHOLD REPEAT OFFENDERS

Toxicants
— Lead
— Phthalates

Ingredients
— Adhesives
— Solvents

Materials
— Paints
— Vinyl
— Wood

REPEAT ISSUES
— Off-gassing and leaching of toxicants into indoor air and house dust

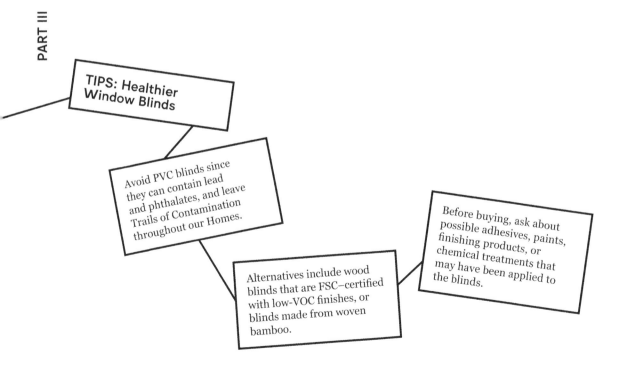

TIPS: Healthier Window Blinds

Avoid PVC blinds since they can contain lead and phthalates, and leave Trails of Contamination throughout our Homes.

Alternatives include wood blinds that are FSC–certified with low-VOC finishes, or blinds made from woven bamboo.

Before buying, ask about possible adhesives, paints, finishing products, or chemical treatments that may have been applied to the blinds.

A—Z

Candles

OVERVIEW

Burning anything usually releases by-products including nanoparticles and polycyclic aromatic hydrocarbons (PAHs), which are carcinogenic and have been linked to lower birth weights in babies of exposed mothers. PAHs have been found to reach "inordinately high levels in churches after candles or incense is burned" (*National Geographic* 2008). So think twice about what you burn at home.

Most household candles are made with paraffin wax, a petroleum-based product that releases toxic chemicals when heated or burned. Lead has been found in candle wicks. According to LEAD Group Inc. (2000), an organization that fights for global reduction of lead, "The characteristics observed in candle emissions match those of diesel emissions in the aspects considered to contribute to toxicity."

HOUSEHOLD REPEAT OFFENDERS

Toxicants
— Benzene
— Fragrance
— Lead
— Phthalates

Ingredients
— Nanoparticles: Can be created from a burning candle.
— Solvents

REPEAT ISSUES
— EDCs
— Likely carcinogens (like styrene)
— Petroleum-based ingredients
— Polluting indoor air with toxic chemicals like benzene, toluene, naphthalene, acetylaldehyde, ethanol, methyl ethyl ketone
— Trails of Contamination
— Unintentional Potential Effects
— Unique vulnerabilities
— VOCs

ADDITIONAL ISSUES
— Scented candles may emit soot, lead, and phthalates. In one study, 63 percent of scented candles and 45 percent of non-scented candles produced soot (LEAD Group Inc 2000).

TIPS: Healthier Candles

Burning anything pollutes the air, so be selective about what, when, and how often you burn.

Beeswax, which has been used for centuries in candles, is an excellent substitute for paraffin.

100 percent soy wax is better than petroleum-containing candles. It's created from hydrogenated soybean oil and has a texture that's slightly softer than beeswax. It's usually less expensive than beeswax. Non-GMO soy is ideal.

Gel candles are usually petroleum-derived.

Beware of added fragrances, since their chemical formulas are complex. Scents from 100 percent essential oils are a good choice if you must have fragrance.

Choose all-cotton cloth wicks. Conventional candle wicks may contain metals like zinc, tin, and even lead. As the candle burns, these toxins can contaminate your air and settle onto surfaces. Detecting lead in a candle wick can be confirmed only by laboratory testing. However, a wick with a metal core is more likely to contain some lead, even if a candle's packaging says the product is lead-free.

Imported candles may contain more hazardous ingredients than domestic ones, unless the country of manufacture has strong regulations. For example, while the US banned lead in candle wicks in 2003, lead is still found in them, possibly because of importation.

Conventional Carpets

OVERVIEW

After hundreds of people—including employees of the EPA—reported adverse health effects after 27,000 square yards of new carpet was installed in their offices in 1987, several teams investigated whether carpet emissions could be the culprit. No causal relationships were determined from these studies, but hundreds of toxicants were detected in carpet emissions.

— The EPA: A study for the EPA identified more than 200 compounds in carpet emissions (EPA 1994). The EPA (2014c) acknowledges that carpet materials can emit VOCs; however, the identities and quantities of VOC emissions are hard to predict based solely on the chemical composition of the materials in the carpet. Common ones include 4-PC, formaldehyde (a human carcinogen), and styrene (a possible human carcinogen).

— An independent laboratory: In 1992, an independent toxicology laboratory exposed mice to carpet fumes from at least 300 carpet samples and found neurotoxic reactions. Minor symptoms included irritation of the eyes, nose, and throat as well as labored breathing; more severe reactions included tremors, paralysis of the legs, convulsions, and death. And some carpet samples were 12 years old! (Bader 2009; Gram 1993). While the results of this study were not replicated by other scientists, I consider it as a cautionary tale.

Why Do Carpet Emissions Affect Some People?

— *The unknown cocktail effect.* Two or more of the many chemicals emitted from a carpet may interact to cause a greater impact than that of any one substance.

— *Carpet samples may vary widely in their emissions.* Even samples of the same carpet.

— *People have unique vulnerabilities.* While not entirely understood, some people have more vulnerable immune systems, and each person's unique body burden is at a different proximity to his or her tipping point. For some people the tipping point may be a new carpet; for others it may be the cumulative cocktail produced by a new or newly renovated home.

HOUSEHOLD REPEAT OFFENDERS

Toxicants
— Benzene
— Dioxins (and furans): Created at the end of a carpet's life cycle.
— Formaldehyde
— Unintentional Toxicants

Ingredients
— Adhesives
— Chemical flame retardants
— Nanoparticles
— Synthetic colors

Materials
— Conventional textiles
— Polyurethane foam
— Plastics, including vinyl

REPEAT ISSUES
— VOCs and HAPs off-gassing and leaching into indoor air and house dust
— The difference between "no proof of harm" and "proof of safety"
— Trails of Contamination

ADDITIONAL TOXICANTS
— Conventional carpeting has been found to off-gas chemicals such as acetonitrile, azulene, diphenyl ethers, dodecane, tetrachloroethylene, ethylbenzene, styrene, toluene, xylene, and 4-phenylcyclohexene (4-PC). The latter has been found to irritate the mucous membranes, eyes, skin, and respiratory system (Washington Toxics Coalition 2000).

TIPS: Buying for Cleanability

According to the late John W. Roberts, "Mr. Dust," the following four traits make carpets easier to clean (Roberts et al. 2009):

01. Short-fiber impermeable carpets can reduce exposures to allergens and pollutants.

04. "Deep plush and shag carpets are the most difficult to clean."

02. "Flat and level loop carpets, often found in office buildings, are easiest to clean."

03. "Short plush carpets are the next easiest to clean."

Outdoor contaminants: These may be tracked in on the bottom of shoes. Soil, additional pesticides, and coal tar have been found in carpet studies.

TIPS: Area Rugs and Carpets

The healthiest choice is to have NO carpets or area rugs, since carpets trap contaminants. Indoors, contaminants cannot be broken down by sunlight and removed by wind, so they accumulate in carpets. Frequent vacuuming cannot remove everything. Bare floors, on the other hand, can be easily and thoroughly cleaned and dried.

Indoor contaminants: These include pet dander, fungal spores, bacteria, and dust mites and their droppings. One study found an average of 67 grams of dust per square meter of carpet (Roberts et al. 1999).

If you must purchase carpet, then the following tips will help you make healthier choices. Remember that in general, the main sources of carpet fumes are the backing, adhesives, seam sealants, and cushion or pad.

Avoid wall-to-wall carpeting: It is usually of synthetic components, installed with potentially toxic glues, and pretreated with a toxic stain guard.

Check labels to find options with the low toxic emissions.

Select a carpet with a lower pile.

Consider natural fibers.

Consider modular carpet tiles, which don't require glues. Individual tiles may be recycled and replaced as necessary.

Look for small, washable rugs that are stitched, not glued, to backing or that use low- to no-VOC glues.

Opt for area rugs.

Choose carpets that are made of untreated natural fibers such as 100 percent wool, sisal, hemp, silk, cotton, or sea grass. Great options are unbacked, organic cotton area rugs that can be laundered. Wool fibers are absorbent, so they may be more likely than synthetic fibers to trap contaminants such as formaldehyde and nitrogen oxides.

TIPS: Carpet Fibers

TIPS: Carpet Treatments

Carpet sealant
Specify low-VOC seam sealant. Seam sealants may emit significantly more pollutants than the other carpet components, especially during the first few weeks after installation.

Carpet dyes
Traditionally, carpet dyeing is a very polluting stage in the carpet manufacturing process. Dyes (as well as insecticides, pesticides, and fungicides) may contaminate your indoor air and dust.

Carpet treatments
Avoid stain- and water-repellents. Also investigate whether the carpet has antistatic, antimicrobial, or mothproofing treatments.

Another popular backing is vinyl or PVC. If unavoidable, try to find PVC that's woven on, not glued. Good alternatives to PVC as backing material: natural rubber, jute, or other natural plant fibers. Felt or recycled-rag pads are also better than PVC.

Styrene-butadiene rubber (SB latex) is commonly glued to the backs of carpets (rather than sewn on). SB latex may emit styrene and 4-PC (4-phenylcyclohexene). Styrene is a known toxin and suspected carcinogen. While there isn't proof of harm from 4-PC, this is the chemical most responsible for the distinctive smell associated with new carpets. It continues to be emitted at measurable levels for longer periods than other carpet chemicals.

Limit carpets that use polyurethane foam, another standard backing. It leaves a Trails of Contamination that may include flame retardants, isocyanates, toluene, diamines, and the ozone-depleting gases methylene chloride and chlorofluorocarbons.

Woven carpets, because they are inherently more stable than tufted carpets, require much less adhesive backing.

Backing materials can be a main source of toxic carpet emissions. Because they may off-gas chemicals, try to avoid synthetic backings.

TIPS: Carpet Backing

The Carpet Profile: The Devil Is in the Details

Understanding carpet components (such as their materials and ingredients) and their method of manufacturing can help you make more informed purchasing and editing decisions. Generally, common carpet components include textile, backing material, cushioning, adhesives, and other chemicals. Each of these may pollute the indoor environment. Furthermore, because carpets are thick, tightly woven, and insulating, contaminants accumulate in carpets and are hard to remove, even with regular vacuuming.

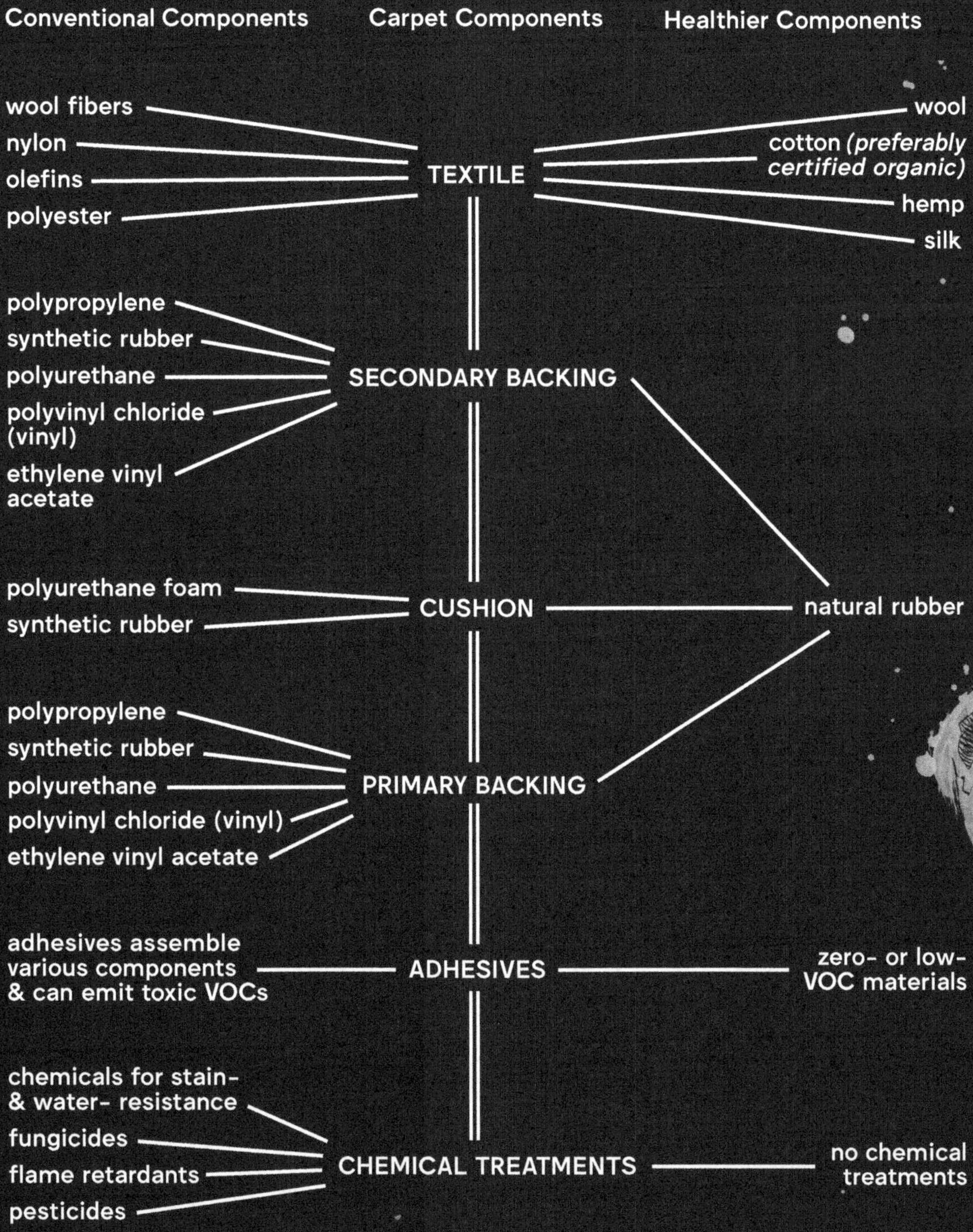

Conventional Components	Carpet Components	Healthier Components

TEXTILE

Conventional: wool fibers, nylon, olefins, polyester

Healthier: wool, cotton *(preferably certified organic)*, hemp, silk

SECONDARY BACKING

Conventional: polypropylene, synthetic rubber, polyurethane, polyvinyl chloride (vinyl), ethylene vinyl acetate

Healthier: natural rubber

CUSHION

Conventional: polyurethane foam, synthetic rubber

Healthier: natural rubber

PRIMARY BACKING

Conventional: polypropylene, synthetic rubber, polyurethane, polyvinyl chloride (vinyl), ethylene vinyl acetate

Healthier: natural rubber

ADHESIVES

Conventional: adhesives assemble various components & can emit toxic VOCs

Healthier: zero- or low-VOC materials

CHEMICAL TREATMENTS

Conventional: chemicals for stain- & water- resistance, fungicides, flame retardants, pesticides

Healthier: no chemical treatments

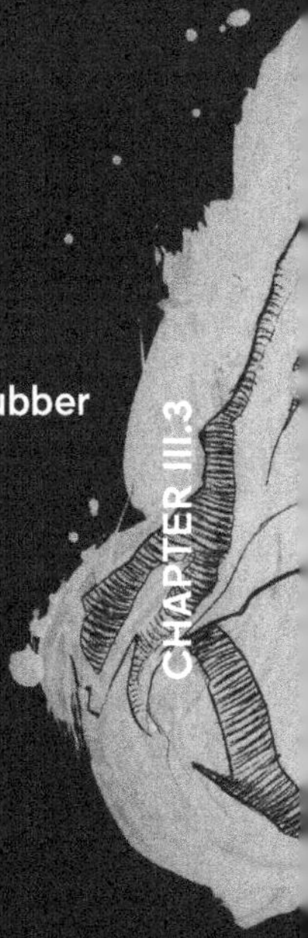

FIGURE #11　　　　　　　　　　　　　　　　　　　　　245

TIPS: Carpet Adhesives

Avoid adhesives if possible.

When adhesives are unavoidable, seek solvent-free, low-VOC varieties (check out "solvent-free" or water-based formulations or other "green" alternatives). Be aware that these products could be more vulnerable to temperature and humidity, so be sure to consult the manufacturer's directions to get directions on care. Nowadays, a number of manufacturers offer low-VOC products, defined as less than 50 grams per liter.

Alternative carpet-fastening methods include:
— Tackless strips, which are typically used for residential jobs.
— Hook-and-loop tape systems (such as Velcro®), which allow removing, adjusting, and reattachment of carpet as needed.
— Peel-and-stick adhesive systems, which are considered a safer option, and are often used on modular carpet tiles (Wilson and Piepkorn 2008).

Look for certifications. For instance, look for the Carpet and Rug Institute's Green Label Plus, which is given to carpet products, including adhesives, that are low in VOC emissions.

TIPS: Warranties of Safety

If your remodeling work is significant enough to get a manufacturer's attention, ask for more information. Some indoor air quality consultants recommend seeking products that emit VOCs below 100 micrograms per square meter per hour, when tested after 24 hours. Ask the manufacturer for information on any adhesives used, and for a warranty of VOC emissions as a result of installation (Building Green 2015).

Opt for rugs and padding that have a Green Label Plus designation from the Carpet and Rug Institute. This means that the product meets or exceed California's indoor environmental standards for low-emission products in commercial settings (National Geographic 2008). Be aware that this does not guarantee a safe carpet, only that a minimum standard has been met. Green Label tests for a short list of chemicals, and only a few carpet samples are assessed (Washington Toxics Coalition 2000). Learn more at carpet-rug.org.

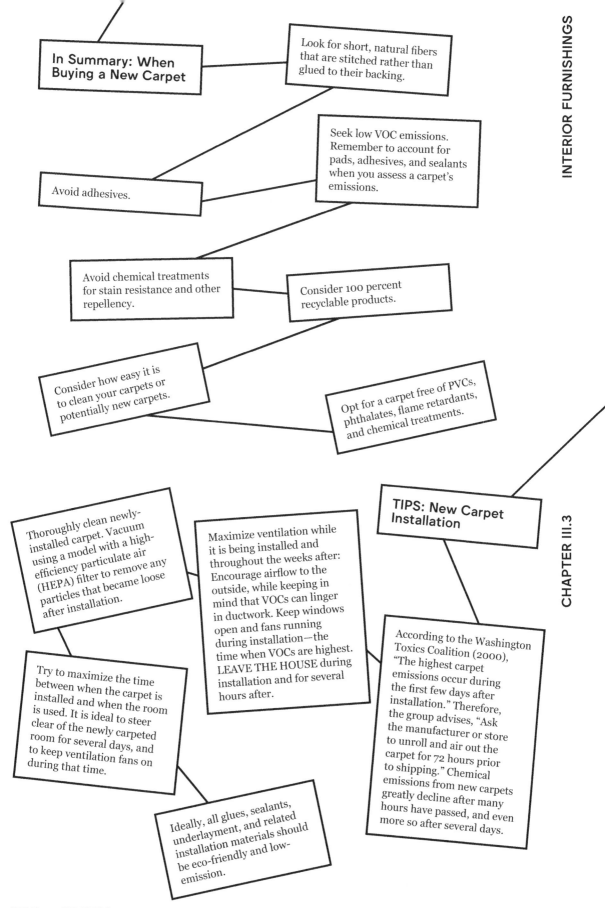

In Summary: When Buying a New Carpet

Look for short, natural fibers that are stitched rather than glued to their backing.

Seek low VOC emissions. Remember to account for pads, adhesives, and sealants when you assess a carpet's emissions.

Avoid adhesives.

Avoid chemical treatments for stain resistance and other repellency.

Consider 100 percent recyclable products.

Consider how easy it is to clean your carpets or potentially new carpets.

Opt for a carpet free of PVCs, phthalates, flame retardants, and chemical treatments.

TIPS: New Carpet Installation

Thoroughly clean newly-installed carpet. Vacuum using a model with a high-efficiency particulate air (HEPA) filter to remove any particles that became loose after installation.

Maximize ventilation while it is being installed and throughout the weeks after: Encourage airflow to the outside, while keeping in mind that VOCs can linger in ductwork. Keep windows open and fans running during installation—the time when VOCs are highest. LEAVE THE HOUSE during installation and for several hours after.

Try to maximize the time between when the carpet is installed and when the room is used. It is ideal to steer clear of the newly carpeted room for several days, and to keep ventilation fans on during that time.

Ideally, all glues, sealants, underlayment, and related installation materials should be eco-friendly and low-emission.

According to the Washington Toxics Coalition (2000), "The highest carpet emissions occur during the first few days after installation." Therefore, the group advises, "Ask the manufacturer or store to unroll and air out the carpet for 72 hours prior to shipping." Chemical emissions from new carpets greatly decline after many hours have passed, and even more so after several days.

TIPS: Old Carpet Removal

Clean old carpet before removal
Carpets filter and collect all varieties of dust and dirt. During removal, much of this can be released, circulating into the air and HVAC systems.

Remove old carpet with care
Do your best to isolate your work space from other areas of your home.

Take special care to clean
After removing old carpet, thoroughly clean the area to eliminate pollutants and dirt that have lingered underneath the carpet.

TIPS: Maintenance and Treatment of Carpets

Wipe your shoes or remove them before you come indoors!

Vacuum frequently with a vacuum that uses a HEPA filter. Vacuuming is especially crucial if your home has wall-to-wall carpeting. Regular vacuums can recirculate dust into the air, whereas HEPA filters are capable of removing finer particles, as small as 0.3 microns.

For deep cleaning, consider hiring a technician to perform hot water extraction. Steam cleaning can result in mold, so avoid it for wall-to-wall carpets, which can't ventilate well. If you do steam clean, don't let the carpet get overly wet.

Throw away wet carpet. Mold and mildew growth is likely to occur in carpets that have been significantly wet for more than one day, which is notoriously hard to remedy. Cleaning is often done with harsh chemicals, which may leave behind toxic residues and lead to human exposure. To avoid the health repercussions of these pollutants, experts often suggest replacing the carpet.

Properly ventilate to minimize concentrations of indoor toxicants. Ventilation should be continuous and well distributed throughout the space. The carpet industry claims that carpets only off-gas during their initial installation. But older carpets may be just as, or worse than, new ones. (Bader 2011)

A—Z

Curtains

HOUSEHOLD REPEAT OFFENDERS

Toxicants
— Chlorine
— Dioxins
— Formaldehyde
— Heavy metals
— Pesticides
— PFCs

Ingredients
— Artificial dyes
— Chemical flame retardants
— Nanoparticles

Materials
— Conventional cotton
— Synthetic fibers

ADDITIONAL OFFENDERS
— Perc, if curtains are dry cleaned

REPEAT ISSUES
— Fabric treatments
— Off-gassing VOCs
— Petroleum-based ingredients
— Trails of Contamination
— Unintentional Potential Effects

TIPS

To minimize your curtains' contribution to indoor air and dust contamination, select curtains made of natural fabrics, such as 100 percent organic cotton, canvas, linen, or hemp. Consider other options for window treatments too, since fabric can absorb VOCs and release them later under certain conditions.

Avoid chemical treatments that impart resistance to water, stains, or fire. If you're concerned about the fire risk posed by untreated fabrics, consider wool, which is naturally fire-resistant and doesn't stain as easily as other fabrics.

If adhesives are used to adhere curtain materials to each other or to hang from a wall, then refer to chapter II.3 for healthier adhesives.

Window treatments can harbor dust, so washable ones are best. Maintain your drapes properly, as the layers of fabric can collect indoor air pollutants such as dust, mold, and airborne chemicals, all of which can lead to respiratory problems.

Vacuum curtains weekly using a model with a HEPA filter to remove loose particles.

If buying blackout curtains, try to avoid PVC.

Dirty drapes made of cotton, linen, and wool can often be hand-laundered and hung to dry. Even delicate fabrics like silk can sometimes be washed at home. Check the label to be sure.

Avoid dry-cleaning your drapes, since they can off-gas perchloroethylene, a toxic solvent used by most dry cleaners. Refer to chapter III.1 for tips on dry cleaning.

Floor Materials

HOUSEHOLD REPEAT OFFENDERS

Toxicants
— Chlorine
— Formaldehyde

Ingredients
— Adhesives
— Nanoparticles
— Solvents

Materials
— Paints and stains
— Vinyl
— Wood

REPEAT ISSUES
— Off-gassing and leaching of toxicants into indoor air and house dust
— Trails of Contamination

TIPS: Floors

Consider the preexisting floor material you will be disturbing before you install new flooring. Concerns include vinyl/PVC and wall-to-wall carpeting.

Oil-based polyurethane sealants are often used for hardwood, like oak, and are known respiratory irritants. For a better option, look for water-based sealants, which emit fewer VOCs. Water-based finishing products dry quickly and therefore several coats can be applied in a single workday, and are comparable to solvent-based products in terms of durability.

Have wood pre-finished before delivery, which eliminates the need to seal it at home. Try to let the wood ventilate at the factory for a while after it has been treated.

Ventilate as much as possible after your new floor is installed.

Buy from companies that use no- or low-VOC adhesives, stains, paints, sealers, etc.

TIPS: Healthier Floor Materials

Some flooring materials, including "green" options, can contaminate your indoor environment. For example, polyvinyl chloride (PVC) flooring and laminates may emit harmful chemicals. What follows are tips for selecting healthier floor materials.

Consider refinishing your existing floors

Sanding down your existing wood floor (and then coating it with a water-based sealant) can sometimes be easier and more eco-friendly than completely replacing floor materials.

Wood laminate

Investigate adhesives that are used in the lamination process. Seek options that are low-VOC, and have a retailer lend you sample boards to ensure that the smell does not bother you. If so, consider other brands.

Hardwood

Avoid composite woods, such as particleboards or fiberboards, and laminated woods. The most eco-friendly options are FSC–certified. The FSC is a nonprofit organization established in 1993 to encourage responsible, sustainable forest management. It provides certifications for hardwood flooring that was made from sustainably managed forests. Learn more at us.fsc.org.

Eco–flooring options

Renewable options include cork, bamboo, coconut and sugar palm, and sisal, which are usually finished with a nontoxic surface coating. Also consider sustainably grown or certified hardwood, natural linoleum (made with cork and linseed oil), tile, and even "green" wall-to-wall carpets. Not all eco-friendly options are healthy, though: Bamboo is frequently produced with adhesives containing formaldehyde. Ask the manufacturers if they have third-party certifications, if they have set reduction goals to diminish their carbon footprint, and if they are tracking and reporting their waste and emissions.

Reclaimed wood

It is eco-friendly, and sometimes of higher quality than brand-new wood flooring. If you are replacing flooring that is in fair condition, research (start by asking your contractor) vendors that may be interested in reusing your materials.

Stone and tile

Though not renewable, stone and tile absorb heat and release it back into the home, making them popular choices for floors that often come into contact with the sun. They also wear more slowly than wood, carpets, and cork.

Rubber

If considering rubber flooring, natural rubber is better than synthetic varieties. Confirm that it is free of contaminants and chlorine. Recycled rubber flooring helps the planet but has a strong odor.

Furniture

OVERVIEW

Furniture usually consists of composite woods, like particleboards and medium-density fiberboards, held together by formaldehyde-containing glues. This material costs significantly less than furniture made of solid wood, which is increasingly hard to find. Although its lower price makes composite-wood furniture tempting, minimize how much of it you have at home, especially in bedrooms, because formaldehyde and other harmful chemicals can off-gas.

Focusing on eco-friendly furniture is a good start, but be aware of potential greenwashing. Assess whether materials may contain Household Repeat Offenders.

HOUSEHOLD REPEAT OFFENDERS

Toxicants
— Formaldehyde
— Heavy metals
— PBDEs
— PFCs
— Tris flame retardants

Ingredients
— Artificial dyes
— Chemical flame retardants
— Nanoparticles
— Solvents: Used in adhesives, paints, and wood stains.

Materials
— Paints
— Plastics
— Polyurethane foam
— Synthetic textiles
— Wood

REPEAT ISSUES
— Petroleum ingredients
— Toxicants release into indoor air and house dust
— Trails of Contamination
— Unintentional Potential Effects

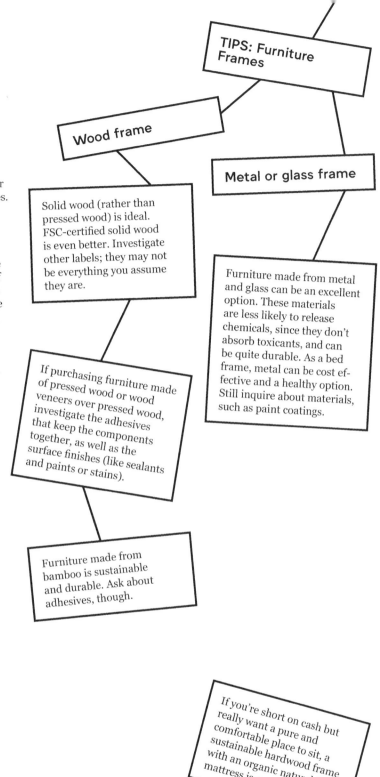

TIPS: Furniture Frames

Wood frame

Metal or glass frame

Solid wood (rather than pressed wood) is ideal. FSC-certified solid wood is even better. Investigate other labels; they may not be everything you assume they are.

Furniture made from metal and glass can be an excellent option. These materials are less likely to release chemicals, since they don't absorb toxicants, and can be quite durable. As a bed frame, metal can be cost effective and a healthy option. Still inquire about materials, such as paint coatings.

If purchasing furniture made of pressed wood or wood veneers over pressed wood, investigate the adhesives that keep the components together, as well as the surface finishes (like sealants and paints or stains).

Furniture made from bamboo is sustainable and durable. Ask about adhesives, though.

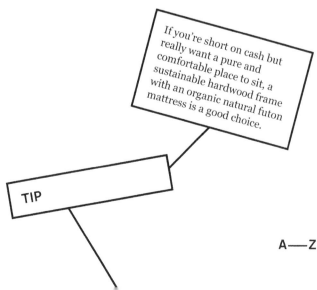

If you're short on cash but really want a pure and comfortable place to sit, a sustainable hardwood frame with an organic natural futon mattress is a good choice.

TIP

TIPS: Wood Finishes

The purest furniture is made of unfinished hardwood, which allows you to apply a finish of your choice.

If you want to buy your wood furniture finished, then investigate with the manufacturer about the finishes.

If you desire a polyurethane coating—which is often touted as a nontoxic sealant that may be applied to furniture to reduce the amount of VOCs—then seek a water-based one.

Natural finishes include linseed oil or beeswax. Other healthier finishes include zero- or low-VOC paints and stains (water-based as opposed to oil-based stains and urethane finishes).

Even if furniture is upholstered in chemical-free fabric, there may be chemicals used on its wood frame, in the cushions, and in the dyes. Inquire with the manufacturer.

TIPS: Furniture Covers

Wool and linen may be the most convenient choices, as many mainstream retailers sell couches, love seats, and other furniture upholstered in a variety of these fabrics.

Opt for furniture upholstered with natural fabrics like wool, hemp, or linen, which typically use few (if any) pesticides in processing, and that are either undyed or dyed using plant-based pigments. Hemp-covered furniture is rare, but it exists. Research online.

Consider materials inside your upholstered furniture and mattresses. Natural materials include cotton batting, wool fill, water-based glues, natural latex, natural twine and webbing, recycled-content metal springs, and free-range down and feathers. Their purity also depends on how these are grown, extracted, processed, and manufactured. See tips on Healthier Cushioning in this chapter.

TIPS: Interior Materials

Consider Greenguard Gold Certification and other certifications based on the California Department of Public Health standard method (also known as CA Section 01350), which outlines environmental and public health considerations for building projects.

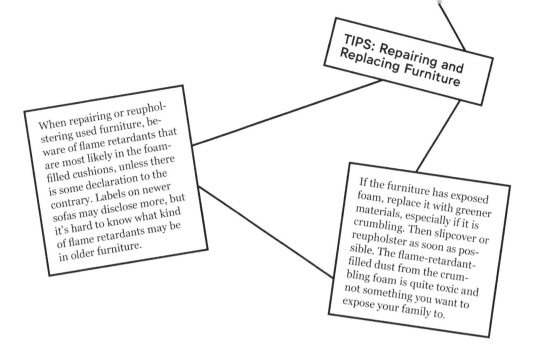

TIPS: Repairing and Replacing Furniture

When repairing or reupholstering used furniture, beware of flame retardants that are most likely in the foam-filled cushions, unless there is some declaration to the contrary. Labels on newer sofas may disclose more, but it's hard to know what kind of flame retardants may be in older furniture.

If the furniture has exposed foam, replace it with greener materials, especially if it is crumbling. Then slipcover or reupholster as soon as possible. The flame-retardant-filled dust from the crumbling foam is quite toxic and not something you want to expose your family to.

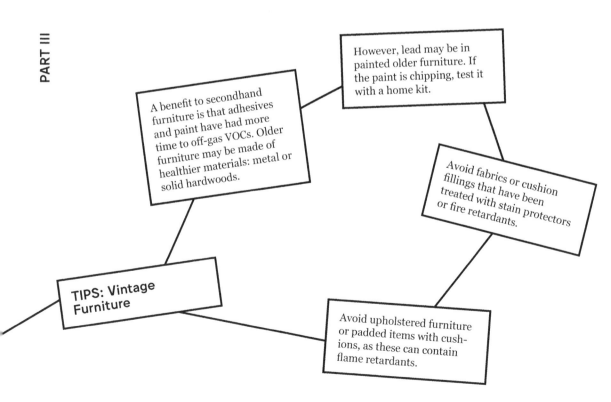

However, lead may be in painted older furniture. If the paint is chipping, test it with a home kit.

A benefit to secondhand furniture is that adhesives and paint have had more time to off-gas VOCs. Older furniture may be made of healthier materials: metal or solid hardwoods.

Avoid fabrics or cushion fillings that have been treated with stain protectors or fire retardants.

TIPS: Vintage Furniture

Avoid upholstered furniture or padded items with cushions, as these can contain flame retardants.

Furniture: Cushions and Cushioning

OVERVIEW

Cushions are generally made of polyurethane foam, which is a Household Material of Concern. While phased out since the mid-2000s, PBDEs, a popular class of flame retardants, may be in your cushioning if it was made before their phase-out. Since PBDEs are easily released into the air and inhaled, your house dust is probably contaminated with them.

Arlene Blum PhD, chemist at the University of California, Berkeley, conducted research in the 1970s that resulted in the removal of chlorinated Tris, a flame retardant, from children's pajamas (Blum and Ames 1977). She was concerned about pregnant women's exposure because the flame retardants can cross the placenta and alter brain development in the fetus. (In one study of fetal tissues, PBDEs were found at levels equalling those in the mother's body [Mazdai et al. 2003]). Oddly, many couches and nursing pillows still contain chlorinated Tris, and may not include warning labels (Kristof 2012).

HOUSEHOLD REPEAT OFFENDERS

Toxicants
— Benzene
— Chlorine
— Formaldehyde
— Methylene chloride
— PBDEs
— PFOS
— Tris flame retardants: Banned from children's pajamas in the late 1970s due to their mutagenic and carcinogenic effects. Tris retardants were selected to replace PBDEs in cushions and other products as PBDEs were phased out in the 2000s. Tris flame retardants have been detected in house dust, indoor air, breast milk, urine, food, and drinking water.

Ingredients
— Chemical flame retardants
— Fabric treatments
— Nanoparticles
— Solvents

Materials
— Polyurethane foam
— Synthetic textiles

REPEAT ISSUES
— Polluting indoor air and house dust with toxicants
— EDCs, VOCs, and HAPs
— Petroleum-based ingredients
— Contribution to body burdens
— Trails of Contamination

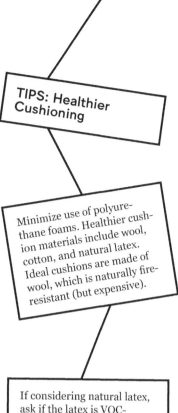

TIPS: Healthier Cushioning

Minimize use of polyurethane foams. Healthier cushion materials include wool, cotton, and natural latex. Ideal cushions are made of wool, which is naturally fire-resistant (but expensive).

If considering natural latex, ask if the latex is VOC-free. "Natural" latex foam may also contain flame retardants.

When using foam (because it's unavoidable):
— Replace pieces that have ripped covers or crumbling foam. If you can't replace them, then keep the foam in a protective cover.
— If reupholstering foam furniture, hire a professional to do it, since the process increases exposure to fire retardants.
— If selecting foam material, try to find foam that's untreated with flame retardants and antimicrobial chemicals.
— If foam has flame retardants, then learn more. New foam won't contain PBDEs, but may have other brominated fire retardants.

In the Bathroom

TIPS: Healthier Bathroom

HOUSEHOLD REPEAT OFFENDERS

Toxicants
— Chlorine
— Dioxins
— Formaldehyde
— Unintentional Toxicants

Ingredients
— Adhesives
— Artificial dyes
— Chemical flame retardants
— Inerts
— Nanoparticles
— Polyurethane foam for backing in bath mats
— Solvents

Materials
— Conventional textiles

REPEAT ISSUES
— Contamination of indoor air and dust with VOCs, HAPs, carcinogens, neurotoxins, and other toxicants
— Trails of Contamination throughout our Homes
— Unintentional Potential Effects

PRODUCTS OF CONCERN
— Cleaning products, interior furnishings, and personal care products

---

01. Avoid potentially dangerous products
Read product labels, and avoid those that contain words such as "caution," "hazardous," or "dangerous," as well as those that don't list their ingredients.

02. Ventilate often
To avoid mildew and mold in the bathroom, open a window or use a fan to ventilate. Never clean any surface of the bathroom without ventilation.

03. Should you incorporate water filters?
Check your local water supply to see if you may be experiencing repeated exposure to unwanted contaminants, like chlorine. If so, then consider a water filter for your shower head.

04. Use healthier towels
The best ones for our Homes are the ones that we already own. But if you're buying new towels, then consider fabrics that are 100 percent certified organic cotton, hemp, or linen. Bamboo is very energy-intensive to turn into fabric. However, it's naturally anti-bacterial, which is helpful in a damp bathroom. Buy towels made from fibers that are grown without chemicals and dye-free or eco-dyed since dyes and chemical treatments can produce VOCs that can be absorbed by your skin. One source recommended washing them at least five times before using.

05. Evaluate your bath mats
Bath mats are often made with plastics that leave Trails of Contamination. They may also contain antimicrobial chemicals. Opt for mats made of organic cotton or those without backing. Seek materials that are free of antibacterial chemicals and PVC.

06. Assess your shower curtain

01. Avoid vinyl.

02. If you do stick with vinyl, leave new items outside to off-gas for a few days before using.

03. If you see mold on a fabric shower curtain, spray it with a peroxide cleaner or put it in the washing machine, adding half a cup of hydrogen peroxide along with your detergent. As for drying, hanging it outside is best. Otherwise, line-dry in a well-ventilated room or tumble-dry in the dryer. A glass shower door is a great alternative.

04. Healthier fabrics include certified organic cotton or hemp. Cotton curtains are mold-prone, though, and you may need two (one as a liner and one as a decorative curtain). Other alternatives include polyethylene vinyl acetate (PEVA), ethylene vinyl acetate (EVA), and nylon (Liu, Schade, and Simpson 2008).

05. Polyester is less toxic than vinyl.

In the Bedroom:
Blankets, Comforters, Pillows, and Sheets

HOUSEHOLD REPEAT OFFENDERS

Toxicants
— Chlorine
— Formaldehyde
— Heavy metals
— PBDEs
— Pesticides, such as herbicides, boric acid, and fungicides
— PFCs

Ingredients
— Chemical flame retardants
— Nanoparticles
— Polyurethane foam, such as in pillows
— Synthetic colors (dyes)

Materials
— Conventional textiles

ADDITIONAL OFFENDERS
— Other chemical treatments, to impart qualities like wrinkle resistance

REPEAT ISSUES
— Contamination of indoor air and dust with VOCs, HAPs, carcinogens, neurotoxins, and other toxicants
— Trails of Contamination throughout our Homes

TIPS: Healthier Bedding

01. Sheets, blankets, and pillows are all capable of emitting VOCs. They're made with petroleum-based fibers and cotton grown with pesticides, herbicides, and defoliants. The yarns are treated with chemicals for fire and wrinkle resistance, and these chemicals are incorporated directly into the yarns to ensure that the treatment will survive many washings.

The greenest sheets are the ones you already have. If you're buying new, then the tips below will help you choose healthier materials.

02. Choose natural fibers. (Bamboo sheets can be made of mainly rayon, which would make them not as eco-friendly as 100 percent bamboo products.)

03. Avoid buying sheets that have been dyed. Dyes can rub off on skin. The dyeing process also pollutes our Homes. Even "low-impact" dyes use chemicals in their processes.

04. Cotton can be tricky.

"Green" cotton doesn't necessarily mean that it's organic. It could be conventional cotton that hasn't been bleached with chlorine or treated with formaldehyde.

Be aware that these claims may not be true: "100 percent natural cotton," "undyed and unbleached cotton," or "green cotton." These marketing expressions all describe cotton grown with pesticides, and the product may still be treated with chemicals.

Exposure to toxicants from contact with cotton while sleeping is minimal, so choosing organic is more about reducing the Trail of Contamination throughout our Homes.

05. While fabric treatments add convenience, they may also add risks. While sleeping on cotton may not pose a significant health issue, fabrics with various treatments may come with added risks. Avoid permanent-press, crease-resistant, shrinkproof, stain-resistant, and water-repellent fabrics. They are probably treated with chemicals and may release formaldehyde, PFCs, and PBDEs, which you may inhale or absorb through your skin while you sleep. Wash all new bedding in hot water at least once before use. A 1999 study showed that a single washing of permanent-press fabrics could reduce formaldehyde emissions by 60 percent (Kelly, Smith, and Satola 1999).

Organic cotton fabric tends to be softer and more comfortable. However, it also rips more easily so it tends to be less durable than conventional textiles.

TIPS: Blankets and Comforters

For blankets, organic cotton for summer and organic wool for winter are good options. Wool comforters offer lightweight comfort plus insulating qualities. Other low-toxin options include linen and hemp.

Organic wool is not moth-resistant, so it's usually treated with mothproofing insecticides. And, depending on how the sheep were raised, wool may also contain other insecticide residues from chemical baths to rid the sheep of parasites. To avoid these, look for certified organic wool or California "Pure Grow" wool, which comes from ranches that do not treat their sheep with chemicals.

Think twice about electric blankets, especially if you are pregnant. Some worry that overheating can increase the risk of miscarriage and birth defects. Further, there's concern that metal can create an electromagnetic field that's stressful to our bodies. If you have one and would like to use it, turn it on to warm the bed before you climb in, and turn it off when sleeping.

TIPS: Label Insight

"Hypoallergenic" means that the bedding is less likely to trigger allergic reactions. However, it has no medical definition, and there is no certification process or organization that reviews the accuracy of a "hypoallergenic" claim.

TIPS: Organic Pillows

Polyfill pillows may be inexpensive and hypoallergenic, but they are made of synthetic chemical fibers or foams that have been disinfected with undisclosed chemicals (like flame retardants). As environmental advocate Annie Leonard says in the Story of Stuff (storyofstuff.org), "We take our pillows, we douse them in a neurotoxin, then we bring them home and put our heads on them for eight hours a night to sleep" (Leonard 2015). Check with the manufacturer to find out what's in your pillow.

Organic pillows are made with the same materials used in organic mattresses: wool, cotton, natural rubber latex, kapok (silky fibers from the ceiba tree), buckwheat, or even down. Consider using an organic cotton pillow protector to make it last longer.

Use an under-bed pad for wood-slat platform beds

Today many mattresses are used without a traditional box-spring foundation, the mattress instead being placed directly upon a wood-slat platform. This raises several dust concerns. Use an under-bed pad to protect the bottom of the mattress—not just from dust—but also from abrasive damage caused by the mattress rubbing against the wood surface of the platform bed.

Vacuum

Thoroughly vacuum the surface of a flipped mattress before sleeping on it. When people dust or vacuum under their beds, or when air currents disturb the area under a bed, the dust rises, and contaminants adhere to the fabric on the bottom of the mattress. When the mattress is flipped, the dust layer is then positioned next to the sleeper's face.

TIPS: Minimize the Effects of Under-Bed Dust

In the Bedroom: Headboards and Bed Frames

HOUSEHOLD REPEAT OFFENDERS

Toxicants
— Formaldehyde
— Heavy metals
— Pesticides, such as herbicides, boric acid, and fungicides
— Unintentional Toxicants

Ingredients
— Adhesives
— Chemical flame retardants
— Inerts
— Nanoparticles
— Paints, wood stains, and other wood treatments
— Solvents

Materials
— Polyurethane foam
— Synthetic textiles
— Woods

REPEAT ISSUES
— Contamination of indoor air and dust with VOCs, HAPs, carcinogens, neurotoxins, and other toxicants
— Potential to create EMFs
— Unintentional Potential Effects

TIPS: Headboards, Frames, and Cribs

Opt for hardwood or metal frames, though the effects of metal amid EMFs are unknown.
— Seek out local hardwood and a frame that's made locally, with minimal or no particleboard or composite wood.
— Look for the few furniture brands that have received third-party certifications for their cribs from the FSC or Greenguard.
— If you must use a composite wood, remember that plywood off-gasses less than particleboard or fiberboard. Choose formaldehyde-free plywood or plywood made with phenol-formaldehyde (PF) resin. Plywood can still emit formaldehyde, though, when urea-formaldehyde (UF) is used as the adhesive.

Avoid upholstered headboards or footboards, which are havens for dust mites and might contain foam.

Choose low-VOC stains, paints, and finishes. Water-based versions are best.

Consider options that eliminate the need to buy a box spring. Instead, wooden slats may exist to support the mattress and facilitate air exchange.

TIPS: Healthier Box Springs

To avoid any chemicals in your box springs, look for the simplest one you can find: solid, untreated wood (preferably sourced from an FSC-certified forest) covered in untreated cotton, preferably organic.

Hardwood platforms are another good choice since they don't require a box spring. Do not place mattresses directly on the floor; air needs to circulate around them. Check the materials of your platform for the presence of toxicants, such as formaldehyde glues in pressed wood.

Avoid products coated with high-VOC finishes.

Also known as foundations, box springs support the mattress. Traditional box springs pose health concerns similar to those of conventional mattresses because they are constructed of similar materials. They can be created from combinations of composite wood, steel springs, rigid polyurethane, high-density polypropylene, covering fabrics, synthetic paddings, nails, staples, and adhesives.

The labels on foundations suffer from the same scarcity of information as do those on mattresses, so consumers are not always able to thoroughly evaluate the health and environmental hazards associated with these products.

In the Bedroom: Mattresses

OVERVIEW

Since most of us spend one-third of our lives sleeping, the bedroom is a high-impact area on which to focus. Generally, bedrooms contain several sources of toxicants, and a major one can be your mattress.

Toxicants can be emitted from toxic mattress components, such as polyurethane foam or vinyl. However, unintentional contamination can also occur in their production environments. In the simplest scenario, the manufacturer is a "true manufacturer;" one that completes the entire manufacturing process—including quilting, cutting, and sewing—on its own premises. There are only a few that produce organic mattresses and bedding.

More common is an "assembler," a manufacturer that purchases mattress components from various sources, and then assembles them into the final product. With more parties and environments involved in this process, it's harder to determine the purity of the mattress components because environments and standards vary.

Moreover, toxicants can contaminate otherwise "pure" mattresses through cross-contamination: Some makers of organic mattresses also produce conventional or "chemical" products in the same facility, which creates the risk of chemical cross-contamination from nonorganic materials or products. This can be even more of a concern for assembler environments, where components from a number of outside sources converge.

In this section, I share key information that led me to purchase safer mattresses for my household. When I was evaluating crib mattresses, prices ranged from $59.99 to $550. With health claims including neurotoxicity and SIDs, I was willing to invest in the purest mattress for my children. However, I wanted to understand the benefits at different price points.

On the following pages, you will learn about toxic fumes that have been detected from mattresses, and key components of mattresses. Understanding the components—including conventional materials and their healthier alternatives—will help you identify and explore answers to strategic questions to make a purchasing decision that suits your budget.

Since salespeople may not fully understand these details, do your own research and check with the manufacturer.

HOUSEHOLD REPEAT OFFENDERS

Toxicants

— Chlorine
— Dioxins
— Formaldehyde
— Heavy metals
— Pesticides, such as herbicides, boric acid, and fungicides
— Phthalates
— Unintentional Toxicants
— VOCs

Ingredients

— Adhesives
— Chemical flame retardants
— Inerts
— Nanoparticles
— Solvents
— Synthetic colors

Materials

— Conventional textiles:
Vinyl: Common in mattresses. Generally, the cheaper the mattress, the more likely it is that vinyl is a component.
Polyester: A common synthetic fiber used in conventional mattresses. It is polyethylene in fabric form. While it is less toxic than other plastics, it may contain hidden additives and contaminants, such as antimony.
Conventional cotton: Grown with environmentally toxic pesticides, fungicides, herbicides, and defoliants. It may also be treated with chemicals for waterproofing and antibacterial properties.
— Polyurethane foam
— Latex mattresses: Can be a hybrid of natural (more expensive) and synthetic latex (cheaper). Both natural and synthetic latex use chemical additives, such as natural soaps, zinc, sulfur, fatty acids, antioxidants, and accelerators. While this is not ideal, latex (whether 100 percent pure, synthetic, or a hybrid) is considered preferable to polyurethane foam.
— Synthetic latex: Manufactured from styrene (a potential carcinogen that may affect liver function, irritate the eyes, and impair motor skills) and butadiene (which can cause cancer, harm the nervous system, and irritate eyes and skin). Other chemicals and VOCs are used as well. For some people, however, synthetic latex is good because it is not allergenic.

(Bader 2011)

It is easiest to assess the purity of a mattress's components when a manufacturer completes the entire manufacturing process on their own premises. This is referred to as a "true manufacturer." There are only a handful that produce organic mattresses and bedding.

More common is an "assembler," a manufacturer that purchases mattress components from various sources, and then assembles them into the final product. With more parties and environments involved in this process, it's harder to determine the purity of the mattress components.

TIPS: Are You Buying From a True Manufacturer or an Assembler?

How serious are the potential adverse health effects from mattresses?

Methylene Chlorine
A suspected carcinogen.

Styrene
Toxic to the lungs, liver, and brain and a possible carcinogen.

2,4- AND 2,6 TOLUENE DIISOCYANATE
Possible human carcinogens, causes irritation and sensitization of the respiratory tract, typical emissions from polyurethane foam.

Dichlorobenzene
Carcinogen.

Ethylbenzene
Toxic to the liver, kidneys, and brain.

FORMALDEHYDE
Human carcinogen, most likely emitted from mattress textiles.

SOLVENTS & ADHESIVES

CONVENTIONAL MEMORY FOAM MATTRESS

Organic mattress maker Walter Bader sent a popular memory foam mattress to a lab for analysis. Sixty-one different VOCs were identified, with the mattress emitting 7,958 micrograms per unit-hour in the first four hours. Meanwhile, an organic natural rubber mattress sent for testing released 95 percent fewer VOC emissions during that same time period. After 48 hours, total emissions were 127 micrograms per unit-hour (Bader 2011).

CONVENTIONAL INNERSPRING MATTRESS

Some 39 VOCs were identified in a typical innerspring/pillow-top mattress, giving off 4,002 micrograms per unit-hour over a 24-hour period. The organic alternative gave off 97.5 percent fewer VOC emissions during the same period (Bader 2011).

Boric Acid
Added to interior fabric. It can irritate eyes and the respiratory tract (Clean and Healthy New York 2011).

CHEMICAL FLAME RETARDANTS

Halogenated Flame Retardants
Linked to endocrine and thyroid disruption, immuno-toxicity, reproductive toxicity, cancer, and harm to fetal and child development (Shaw et al. 2010).

Tris Flame Retardants
May alter DNA, contribute to cancer, harm sperm even across two generations, and harm brain and nerve function (Clean and Healthy New York 2011).

PBDEs
Some are possible human carcinogens. The broader group of PBDEs may delay puberty and reproductive development, disrupt thyroid hormones, and cause neurobehavioral changes (Clean and Healthy New York 2011).

Antimony
A toxic heavy metal that can impact the lungs, heart, and eyes (Clean and Healthy New York 2011).

FIGURE #12

The Mattress Profile: the devil is in the details

Conventional Components	Mattress Components	Healthier Components
Synthetic fibers (nylon, polyester, polypropylene, acrylic, vinyl), conventional cotton, or a blend of the aforementioned.	**FABRIC COVERING**	Organic natural fibers: wool, cotton, hemp, or silk.
Padding layers insulate the mattresses' core and add structure and support. Conventional materials include polyurethane or other petroleum-based foam, synthetic-fiber pads, polyester, and conventional cotton. When layers of padding are manufactured, adhesives and other chemical treatments can be used to bond and maintain the fibers.	**PADDING**	Organic natural fibers, such as wool and cotton.

Organic 100 percent natural rubber, 100 percent natural latex foam, innerspring, certified organic cotton, and wool. Fibers from coconut husks are also available; if you have a latex allergy, then investigate whether these fibers, called coir, are bonded by latex, which may not be listed on the label. |
| Polyurethane foam, memory foam, synthetic rubber/latex, and innerspring. Pressed wood for a frame or support. | **SUPPORTING CORE** | — Natural rubber latex: Made from the sap of rubber trees and has many practical strengths for a mattress core. It is naturally antibacterial, has high flexibility in both hot and cold temperatures, and has long-term resilience. The proteins in natural latex can trigger rare but serious allergic reactions, so beware. How latex is covered in mattresses may affect those who are allergic. Ask for "VOC-free" latex since VOCs may be added during processing.
— Natural latex foam: A good option if you want a foam core.
— Hardwood
— Innerspring: Investigate the padding of innerspring mattresses. Ideal padding is of organic cotton or wool. |
| Toxic fumes (such as styrene and benzene) may off-gas from the solvents of conventional adhesives. | **ADHESIVES** | Zero- or low- VOC adhesives, or none (components sewed together). |
| The materials, especially the fabrics, may receive chemical applications such as toxic dyes; chemicals designed to create resistance to stains, water, wrinkles, microbes, and flames; and fungicides and pesticides. | **CHEMICAL TREATMENTS** | Organic mattresses use wool beneath the exterior cover fabric to meet flammability standards so no chemical flame retardants are needed. Wool is naturally water-repellent too. However, some people are allergic to lanolin, a waxy substance on wool fibers. Interior wool is unlikely to cause skin irritation, however. |

TIPS: For Any Type of Mattress

Vacuum frequently

Even after a mattress has off-gassed considerably, its synthetic and chemically-based construction becomes an environment for dust and dust mites, whose excrement is the leading trigger for asthma attacks.

Ventilate

Regardless of whether you have a conventional or organic natural rubber mattress, open your bedroom windows to let your bedroom breathe. When purchasing a new mattress, let it off-gas outside the bedroom for as long as possible. While the volume of new mattress off-gassing lessens over time (most emissions occur in the first 60 days), it never really stops (Bader 2009).

TIPS: Conventional Mattress

There are probably no consumer products that are completely free of chemicals. Consider that when you read a "nontoxic" claim.

If you have a crib mattress from an older sibling that you want to reuse, it may be preferable to replace it. Consider whether it contains toxic flame retardants, accumulated dust, or Household Repeat Offenders. Read about crib mattresses in chapter III.5, Children's Stuff.

Precautionary measures can reduce your toxic exposures from a new conventional mattress.

If you do use a secondhand mattress, consider encasing it to minimize exposure to chemical dust.

In a crib, an untreated cotton mattress cover provides a barrier between a sleeping baby and off-gassing chemicals while also absorbing accidental leaks. Cotton won't seal fumes and odors entirely, but it will provide a partial barrier.

TIPS: Mattress Protectors

Avoid polyethylene, surgical rubber, and PVC mattress covers, which do not allow the mattress to breathe and create a breeding ground for bacteria and mold. PVC covers themselves also release VOCs.

Consider adding a naturally water-resistant wool pad between the organic cotton mattress cover and the crib sheet. It is a good barrier.

TIPS: Buying a Healthier Mattress

Healthy mattresses are expensive purchases. To understand the value you get for your money, it is important to know the components of a mattress, how it is manufactured, and the materials that go into it. Six questions to investigate: What fabrics cover the mattress? What is the padding made of? What composes the supporting core? What adhesives are used? What chemical treatments have been applied? Are there unbiased certifications for components of the mattress?

01. Consider organic cotton

It is great for mattress padding and cover fabrics. Certified organic is most reliable. Other claims—green cotton, unbleached and undyed cotton, or 100 percent natural cotton—may be used to describe cotton grown with pesticides and other chemicals.

02. Consider organic wool

It is also great for mattress padding. Wool is a safe, natural, mildew-resistant fiber that is breathable, versatile, and fire resistant. Its insulating properties keep us cooler in summer and warmer in winter. Organic wool is an ideal material for beds and bedding.

03. Consider 100 percent natural rubber or natural latex

It is excellent as a supporting core material. It's durable and helps regulate heat and moisture. It is also free of innersprings so those concerned about metal innersprings creating EMFs should rest better with a metal-free mattress. Among organic mattresses, natural latex is very often used.
— Find latex that's VOC-free.
— Some people have allergic reactions to natural latex.
— Mattresses can be promoted as "natural latex," or "natural rubber" and still be primarily synthetic. Labeling laws don't require a manufacturer to disclose what portion of the latex is natural. Therefore, a mattress label can say "Made from Natural Rubber" and contain only 10 percent natural versus 90 percent synthetic. Verify that a mattress is made completely from 100 percent natural, organic material derived from the milk of the rubber tree.

04. Beware of polyurethane memory foams

05. Avoid adhesives or seek options that used low- or zero-VOC adhesives.

Some mattresses avoid adhesives by having components sewn together.

06. Research certifications

These are meaningful when they are conducted by an organization that has no financial or other ties to the industry or company. According to Walter Bader (2009), the founder of two organic mattress companies, ideally, you'll be able to find third-party verification that each roll of fabric or bale of cotton is organic; that the mattress is made in a factory that conforms to organic standards; and that the organic components have met a certifying organization's published standards for toxic emissions.

08. Avoid chemical treatments

They are used to create resistance to stains-, water-, wrinkles-, and flames. Ask whether other additives, such as fungicides, antibacterial chemicals, and pesticides, were used. Were toxic dyes used in any components of the mattress? Ask how the mattress meets federal flammability requirements. There are concerns with most flame retardants, such as Tris. Boric acid is used sometimes. It has risks but is preferable to antimony, which is preferable to brominated flame retardants. If you want to avoid chemical flame retardants altogether, then you can.

07. Does your mattress contain metal?

Some are concerned that metal contributes to electromagnetic fields. This has not been proven true or false.

Paints and Finishes

OVERVIEW

Paints and other paint-like finishes contain chemicals that serve important roles: VOCs help paints and finishes dry; pigments add color; fungicides and biocides guard against mildew and prolong a product's shelf life; additives act as dryers, hardeners, surfactants, anti-foaming agents, or emulsifiers; and solvents suspend ingredients and allow them to be spready easily.

Unfortunately, even years after application, these ingredients may evaporate toxicants into your indoor air or settle into your household dust to be inhaled and ingested.

Fortunately, manufacturers disclose enough information on labels, material safety data sheets, and on their websites for consumers to select healthier options. One key thing to look for on labels is what type of solvent was used: natural- or oil-based. Oil-based, or alkyd, paints are made with petroleum-based ingredients. According to the EPA (Chang 2001), oil-based coatings can contain as many as 100 different VOCs. Natural-based paints are healthier.

The second key thing to decide on is low- or zero-VOC products. However, remember that when the EPA set VOC standards, the intention was to address outdoor air quality issues, mainly smog, and not indoor air quality. Therefore, the criteria for earning the label "zero-VOC" does not consider the indoor environment. In fact, "zero-VOC," "green," or "environmentally friendly" products may still contain toxicants that can contaminate your indoor environment.

The EPA has a category of "exempt compounds" that includes VOCs that do not significantly pollute outdoor air but may be unhealthy for the indoor environment. For example, ammonia is a common VOC in paint. However, since it does not promote smog, the EPA does not classify it as a VOC, and it is not required to appear on paint labels even though it is unhealthy for us to inhale and its use indoors should be avoided.

The tips on the next page offer guidance on selecting and using paints, followed by tips to follow when painting.

HOUSEHOLD REPEAT OFFENDERS

Toxicants
— Benzene
— Formaldehyde
— Lead: While lead was banned from paint, toys, and furniture in 1977, it's still found in paint. According to the CPSC (2015b), "lead-free" paint does not contain lead concentrations greater than 0.0009 percent.
— Methylene chloride
— Unintentional Toxicants

Ingredients
— Adhesives
— Inerts
— Nanoparticles
— Petroleum distillates
— Preservatives
— Solvents
— VOCs

OTHER OFFENDERS
— Fungicides and biocides, which may contain toxic chemicals like copper, arsenic disulfide, phenol, formaldehyde and quaternary ammonium compounds
— Some hazardous air pollutants may be allowed in products that bear a "zero-VOC" label, such as ammonia, toluene, and xylene.

REPEAT ISSUES
— Petroleum-based ingredients
— Trails of Contamination
— Unknown Potential Effects
— Unique vulnerabilities

TIPS: Selecting and Using Healthier Paints and Finishes

01. Seek "natural" paints

They are made from natural ingredients like water, plant dyes, oils and resins, essential oils, clay, chalk, talcum, milk casein, natural latex, beeswax, and mineral dyes.

Water-based (latex) paints and finishes are nearly odorless and generally emit far fewer chemicals and chemical vapors than oil-based paints (EPA 2000b).

02. Read labels for VOC information

According to the EPA (2011), approximately 40 to 65 percent of a paint or coating is made up of VOCs. The EPA (2010) has shown that formulations with formaldehyde can off-gas, despite manufacturer claims (EWG 2011). By selecting zero- or low-VOC paints, VOC air emissions are reduced.

02A. Find good options

Products that use water-based solvents, like low-VOC paints, stains, and varnishes. Certified low-VOC products should contain much lower amounts of heavy metals and formaldehyde; note that levels of VOCs in these products will vary, so check the container or the material safety data sheet for more information.

02B. Consider better options

Zero-VOC paints have fewer harmful VOCs like benzene, methylene chloride, and formaldehyde, which are known or suspected carcinogens and may trigger allergies, asthma, or chemical sensitivities.

01. The EPA's federal VOC limits are 250 g/l for flat paints and coatings and 380 g/l for non-flat varieties (EPA 2015a). Some states and regions have more stringent regulations for VOC levels in paints. (*Consumer Reports* 2009).

02. Paints that are certified with the Green Seal Standard (GS-11) have a VOC level lower than 50 g/l for flat sheen, or 150 g/l for non-flat sheen. Generally, low-VOC products from reputable manufacturers meet the 50 g/l threshold, which is lower than the strictest VOC regulations in California (Wilson and Piepkorn 2008).

03. Be aware that "certain paints marketed as 'low-VOC' may still emit significant quantities of air pollutants including HAPs," according to the EPA (Chang 2001). These fumes are more threatening when they are confined indoors. So ventilate! If you are sensitive, get paint that contains less than 25 g/l of VOCs.

05. Consider buying paints that have certifications. According to the Better Business Bureau, a major paint manufacturer was claiming its paint to be nontoxic while using colorants full of toxic VOCs (Hirshberg 2015). Certifications that help identify safer paints include Green Seal certification, as well as a high Pharos User Toxicity score. Pharos is an organization working to create more transparency in the components of building materials.

01. Zero-VOC products may contain up to 5 g/l of VOCs.

02. Zero-VOC paints may also contain colorants, biocides, and fungicides along with various VOCs.

03. Color/color tints typically increase the amount of VOC's up to 10 g/l, which is still considered a low level.

04. Ask manufacturers if their zero-VOC designation takes into account compounds or hazardous air pollutants considered "exempt" by the EPA because they either do not create smog or have negligible "photochemical reactivity."

TIPS: Selecting and Using Healthier Paints and Finishes (continued)

03. Take precautionary measures with water-based products too

Remember that while water reducible paints and finishes do not have volatile thinners, they may still contain VOCs, petroleum distillates, and other potentially harmful additives. These may introduce more VOCs into the air, especially on a short-term basis.

06. Use healthier oil-based products

If you use oil-based products, then look for ones that have a VOC no higher than 380 g/l. Varnishes cannot have VOC levels that exceed 300 g/l.

04. Aesthetic results can vary

When selecting paint, remember that each type of paint has different performances and aesthetics. For example, milk-based paints have an old-fashioned, country aesthetic.

05. Don't use exterior products indoors

Do not use exterior paints indoors.

07. Minimize leftovers

If you have leftover paint and finishing products that you intend to keep, be sure to close containers tightly. Try not to store paint or similar products in your home, because even in closed containers they may release VOCs.

Buy only what you need; dispose of any unused paint.

Material Safety Data Sheets (MSDS)

Some products (like paints) have a material safety data sheet that you can obtain. Because these sheets are designed for workers who handle the profiled products, they will not tell consumers everything they should know about the potential health risks, but they do provide useful information. The MSDS should list "known hazards" and provide information on how to deal with them. I have used MSDS information to help me choose paint and wooden stain products.

A few weaknesses of the MSDS to keep in mind:
— Information is voluntary, with no government oversight or third-party verification.
— Most chemicals have never been tested on humans.
— Some 17,000 chemicals are classified as trade secrets (EWG 2013a), making it difficult to identify all the compounds in a product if the manufacturer chooses not to disclose the information.

Proposition 65

Beware of Prop 65 labels when shopping. A result of California law, the state is mandated by Proposition 65 to release a comprehensive list of chemicals that cause cancer, birth defects or reproductive harm. The list is updated annually, and has expanded to about 800 chemicals since it was established in 1987. Some businesses have added Prop 65 warning labels to their products, but not all products with harmful ingredients will have a warning label. When in doubt, compare the product's ingredients to the Current Proposition 65 List.

TIPS: For Savvy Consumers

TIPS: When Painting

01. Try to schedule painting for a time when you can open all windows.

02. Create conditions inside your home that encourage rapid drying, and ventilate odors out of the house as rapidly as possible. To encourage vapors to dissipate, place window-mounted box fans near the work area. If fans cannot be used, ensure adequate cross-ventilation in rooms being painted. Indoor VOC levels can become over 1,000 times higher than outdoor levels after installing a high-VOC-emitting product (NRDC 2015).

03. Minimize time spent in newly-painted areas for several weeks. If possible, keep your children out of the house during painting and for two or three days afterward.

04. If you are pregnant, then let someone else do the painting.

05. Continue to keep the room well ventilated after the paint job is completed. While wet-applied items, like paint, release the highest amount of VOCs right after curing, off-gassing can occur long after the job has been finished.
From the EPA (2012e): "Under normal temperature and humidity, most emissions occur during drying, in the first few days after painting." Generally, no-VOC paint takes longer to dry. Remember that even no-VOC paint can contain toxicants.

06. Apartment dweller? Vapors can pass through shared walls, space that surround pipes, as well as electrical outlets. Consider asking your apartment manager to give you advance notice when a unit will be painted. Ask management to optimize the units' ventilation capabilities during paint jobs and for at least two to three days afterward. Box fans are a good answer to poor ventilation, which can help move VOCs outside when apartments (and neighboring units) are being painted.

07. In a home built or renovated pre-1978, don't attempt to sand or strip old paint. Even if the top few coats of paint are lead-free, underlying layers may contain lead that you shouldn't disturb. Clean up and repair peeling or chipping paint.

08. Be aware that fibers absorb and retain chemicals emitted from paint, releasing them long after the paint has dried. Clear the space to be painted of its contents during painting and drying. Cover all soft surfaces while painting and provide direct ventilation until the paint is dry. Wool fibers seem to be especially efficient at trapping VOCs in comparison to synthetic fibers.

09. Read the labels on all products and follow directions. They will advise you about the working conditions needed to reduce exposure to VOCs.

10. For more information, check out the EPA and CPSC's online brochure for healthy indoor painting habits (cpsc.gov/PageFiles/121965/456.pdf).

Renovations, Maintenance, and Repairs

HOUSEHOLD REPEAT OFFENDERS

Toxicants
— Triclosan

Ingredients
— Adhesives
— Chemical flame retardants
— Inerts
— Nanoparticles
— Solvents
— Unintentional Toxicants

Materials
— Conventional Textiles
— Paints
— Plastics
— Wood

REPEAT ISSUES
— Dust
— HAPs
— Trails of Contamination
— Unintentional Toxicants
— Unintentional Potential Effects
— VOCs

TIPS: Building Materials

Renovations
Renovation releases an unknown cocktail of dust. When renovating, consider using the healthier materials identified in Simple Strategies in chapter III.3. Try to vacate your home during the process. If you're freshening up a room with a coat of paint, investigate the materials underneath to make sure there is no lead paint—especially around windows and door frames. If there is, research your safest options for either removing it or sealing it in.

Adhesives
Construction materials can contain chemicals that off-gas toxicants into your home. For glues, putties, grouts, and more, look for no- or low-VOC formulations. Avoid mildewcides or antibacterial agents in these products, if you can. The best options may be to find a retailer who specializes in eco-friendly building materials. Look for labels that disclose all ingredients or manufacturers that make their material safety data sheets easy to access on the Web.

Piping
Forgo PVC pipes as material to transport drinking water, and other materials in your home. Better alternatives include HDPE (high-density polyethylene), iron, steel, concrete vitrified clay, and copper (Liu, Schade, and Simpson 2008).

Insulation
If you're dealing with insulation choices during a building or renovation project, remember that plastic or polyurethane foam insulation contains petrochemicals and chemical flame retardants. Options that may be better for our Homes include insulation using cotton denim, mineral wool, and cellulose. Better options should become available with increased consumer demand.

Roofing
Try to keep roofing PVC-free, by choosing thermoplastic polyolefin (TPO), ethylene propylene diene monomer (EPDM), nitrile butadiene polymer (NBP), and low-slope metal roofing (Liu, Schade, and Simpson 2008).

Shutters
Safe shutter choices are wood, aluminum, or plastic that does not contain PVC (Liu, Schade, and Simpson 2008).

Siding
Healthy choices include fiber-cement board, stucco, oriented strand board (OSB), brick, polypropylene (PP) siding, and recycled, reclaimed, or FSC-certified wood (Liu, Schade, and Simpson 2008).

Windows and doors
Avoid vinyl, which can contain harmful phthalates. For windows, look to wood, metal, or fiberglass, with blinds made of metal or wood. Good choices for drapes and window treatments include fabric, wood, and bamboo (Liu, Schade, and Simpson 2008).

Wallpaper

HOUSEHOLD REPEAT OFFENDERS

Toxicants
— Dioxins
— Phthalates

Ingredients
— Adhesives
— Nanoparticles

Materials
— Vinyl

REPEAT ISSUES
— EDCs
— HAPs
— Petroleum-based ingredients
— Trails of Contamination
— VOCs

TIPS

Vinyl is a popular material for wallpaper. Not only does this leave a Trail of Contamination throughout our Homes, but it's also more likely to promote mold growth because it can trap moisture behind the wall coverings, creating a mold-friendly environment. Therefore, in kitchens, bathrooms, and any other rooms where moisture is present, low-VOC paint is safer than vinyl wallpaper. In the event of a house fire, incinerated vinyl can release high amounts of dioxin into the air. However, once installed, vinyl wallpaper generally off-gasses fewer chemicals than most types of commercial wall paint.

Choose wallpaper made of paper, linen, grass cloth, or other plant materials. And avoid pre-applied adhesives.

Alternatives include paint, wood paneling, and vintage wallpapers. Vinyl wallpaper wasn't introduced until 1947, so papers made before that date are a good bet.

Call the manufacturer whose wallpapers you like and ask which of its products are free of vinyl and adhesives. Doing so will also let the company know that its customers are interested in green products.

Wallpaper Adhesives

HOUSEHOLD REPEAT OFFENDERS

Ingredients
— Adhesives
— Preservatives
— Solvents

REPEAT ISSUES
— Unique vulnerabilities
— Unintentional Potential Effects
— VOCs

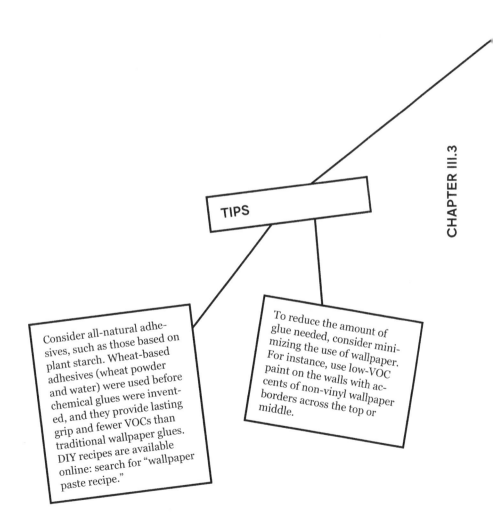

TIPS

Consider all-natural adhesives, such as those based on plant starch. Wheat-based adhesives (wheat powder and water) were used before chemical glues were invented, and they provide lasting grip and fewer VOCs than traditional wallpaper glues. DIY recipes are available online: search for "wallpaper paste recipe."

To reduce the amount of glue needed, consider minimizing the use of wallpaper. For instance, use low-VOC paint on the walls with accents of non-vinyl wallpaper borders across the top or middle.

Simple Strategies: Healthier Interior Furnishings

Area of Concern	Conventional Options	Healthier Options
Adhesives, caulks, sealants	These can be significant sources of short-term VOCs. Avoid conventional adhesives whose solvents are petroleum-based.	Healthier adhesives are water-based and low-toxic or nontoxic (<10g/l). They contain no formaldehyde.
Carpets and area rugs	Carpet components can off-gas toxic fumes. Key offenders include adhesives, synthetic fibers, and cushioning. Chemical treatments are also of concern.	Avoid wall-to-wall carpeting. Minimize area rugs too since they collect contaminants. Select healthier textiles, zero-VOC adhesives, 100 percent natural rubber backing material, and no chemical treatments. Vacuum frequently.
Dyes	Manufacturing dyes can involve heavy metals that are toxic to the environment and present risks to plant workers and consumers.	Labels with "low-impact" dyes indicate that the dye meets requirements set by Oeko-Tex Standard 100. There is no policing of the term's use, however, and some "low-impact" dyes contain many of the same petrochemicals and heavy metals as conventional dyes.
Flooring materials	Contaminants may be released from floor materials, such as composite woods, vinyl, paints, stains, adhesives, and sealants.	Healthier floor materials include hardwood, preferably FSC-certified. Bamboo is eco-friendly, but it is often made with adhesives that contain formaldehyde. Safer pressed woods exist. Stone and tile are good options too.
Furniture	Furniture components can release toxicants; key components include conventional textiles, wood, polyurethane foam in cushions, and chemical treatments (for resistance to fire, stains, and water).	Healthier furniture frame materials are made of solid wood, metal, or glass. They are filled with healthier cushion materials and wrapped with healthier textiles (both are explained in chapter II.3).
Mattresses	Mattress components may release contaminants; key components include conventional textiles, interior components (polyurethane/memory foam), composite woods, adhesives, flame- and water-retardants.	Healthier mattress components include organic cotton, wool, natural rubber latex, and solid wood; and they have no fire retardants, harmful adhesives, or toxic dyes.
Mattress foundations	Components of mattress foundations can release contaminants; key components include composite woods, adhesives, plastics, conventional textiles, and other chemical treatments	Heathier mattress foundations are made of untreated solid wood, healthier textiles, low VOC adhesives, and do not have chemical treatments.

Area of Concern	Conventional Options	Healthier Options
On the walls	Contaminants such as VOCs and HAPs may be released from paints and wallpaper materials, including wallpaper adhesives.	Use zero- or low-VOC paints. Avoid vinyl wallpaper and choose the lowest-VOC adhesive you can find.
Stains/paints	These are petroleum-based products that can off-gas significant levels of VOCs for years.	Healthier paints and stains do not contain mostly petroleum-based ingredients; products from Europe must meet stricter standards.
Textiles	Conventional textiles are generally associated with petroleum, pesticides, bleaching, and synthetic dyes. Beware of labels that state 'Permanent Press," "No Iron," 'Water Repellent," Antimicrobial," and "Flame Retardants."	Healthier textiles include organic cotton, wool, linen, and hemp. Bamboo is eco-friendly, but some bamboo textiles may contain formaldehyde. Avoid fabric treatments when possible.
Underneath the fabric	Cushion stuffing may pose risks. Popular ones include polyurethane foam and synthetic latex.	100 percent natural rubber or wool.
Wood products	Composite woods are of concern because of off-gassing from their adhesives and glues, sealants and sealers, and paints and stains.	Solid wood (investigate "solid wood" with veneers), reclaimed wood, and FSC-certified wood. If using composite wood, investigate adhesives (avoid formaldehyde). Vintage may be a good option, but avoid leaded paint.

Chapter III.4
Personal Care Products

CONVENTIONAL PERSONAL CARE PRODUCTS: WHAT'S IN THEM?

Of the 82,000+ chemicals that are registered with the EPA, one out of seven are used in personal care products (Houlihan 2015). And, as with other products, federal laws protect proprietary information, so manufacturers don't need to disclose all product ingredients, and product labels don't inform us of possible health effects (EWG 2013a).

Further, there is no unbiased oversight for product safety. The EWG estimates that 89 percent of the 10,500 chemicals used in personal care products have not been assessed by the FDA (EWG 2007a). Many ingredients are petroleum-based. Some threaten our health and exacerbate environmental issues. Worse, unlike chemicals in food and water that are found at low levels (parts per million or even parts per billion), these petroleum-based ingredients are staple components of personal care products, like flour's importance in a bread recipe.

Historically, tests of personal care product safety, including those conducted by the industry-funded Cosmetic Ingredient Review (CIR) safety panel, examined exposure to one chemical at a time (EWG 2015i). However, our typical morning routine exposes us to toxicants from a variety of products. For men, it may include toothpaste, soap, shampoo, hair conditioner, deodorant, body lotion, sunscreen, cologne/fragrance, and shaving products. For women, add cosmetics and other hair products. Each product can contain a dozen or more chemicals, of which the cumulative, long-term effects are unknown. According to the EWG (2015q), the average person applies 126 unique ingredients onto the skin per day.

I keep my beauty cabinet simple, as you can see in the Simple Strategies at the end of this chapter. These strategies most efficiently help me avoid the long list of Repeat Offenders you will see on the next page. If you do buy off-the-shelf products, read labels to avoid the Repeat Offenders. In general, though, the best approach is to eliminate or reduce unnecessary products.

IN THIS CHAPTER:

— Household Repeat Offenders in conventional personal care products
— Tips for buying healthier off-the-shelf products
　— Acne products
　— Antiperspirants and deodorants
　— Cleansers and soaps
　— Cosmetics
　— Dental products
　— Feminine care products
　— Fragrance
　— Hair dyes
　— Insect repellents
　— Moisturizers
　— Over-the-counter drugs
　— Shampoos and other hair products
　— Shaving cream and aftershave
　— Sun protection
— Simple Strategies: Simplify your personal care

A—Z

HOUSEHOLD REPEAT OFFENDERS

Toxicants

— Formaldehyde
— Heavy metals, such as lead and mercury
— Methylene chloride
— Phthalates
— Triclosan
— Unintentional Toxicants: Dioxane, a human carcinogen, has been found to unintentionally contaminate personal care products.

Ingredients

— Coal tar
— Fragrance: Federal laws allow companies to keep ingredients of fragrance confidential.
— Inerts
— Microbeads
— Nanoparticles
— Preservatives like parabens
— Surfactants: Can dry skin and hair by removing oils that protect them. Skin and hair then become prone to irritation, dryness, and damage.

OTHER OFFENDERS

Preservatives and solvents

— Acetone: Found in cologne and nail polish remover.
— Formaldehyde, toluene, and phthalates: Can be found in nail polish.
— Mercury: Found in some personal care products as a preservative. According to the FDA, "mercury compounds are readily absorbed through the skin on topical application and tend to accumulate in the body." The FDA has banned mercury from all cosmetics except those used around the eyes, where levels may not exceed 65 parts per million (ppm) (FDA 2015). In 2007, the state of Minnesota banned all uses of mercury in cosmetics.

Anti-aging Ingredients

— Alpha hydroxy acids (AHAs): Found in products that claim to enhance the appearance of skin, it may double users' vulnerability to skin damage caused by UV rays (EWG 2015r).
— Hydroquinone: Used to reduce age spots and to lighten skin, it's found in skin creams and undereye treatments. It is neurotoxic and allergenic; limited evidence suggests it may cause cancer in lab animals.
— Retinyl palmitate and retinol (vitamin A): Popular ingredients for improving the appearance of aging skin. Retinyl palmitate can expedite the growth of skin tumors and lesions when treated skin is exposed to sunlight (Lunder 2011). Pregnant women should also be aware that excessive exposure during pregnancy can cause severe birth defects.

Other Concerns

— PTFE or perfluoro in the ingredients
— Talc: A naturally occurring mineral that may pose health risks. While science hasn't proven harm, it has suggested possible links to ovarian cancer in women who use it in the genital area (Epstein 2015). There are also unknown risks from inhaling it, which can occur more easily as talc is used in powder form.

REPEAT ISSUES

— Ingredients from personal care products have been detected in our environment and in humans.
— Lack of disclosure of toxicity, and potential toxicity
— Lack of regulation of validity of label claims and of levels of toxic ingredients used in consumer products
— No required safety testing by an objective third party
— Unintentional By-products
— Unintentional Potential Effects
— Unintentional Toxicants

ADDITIONAL ISSUES

— We can inhale toxic chemicals in our personal care products through powders and sprays that we use, such as hair sprays, cologne/perfume, spray antiperspirants, or spray sunscreens. We can ingest lead or other toxic chemicals that may be in lipstick. We can also absorb chemicals from the moisturizers, sun blocks, or makeup that we put on our skin.
— Designed to penetrate, some cosmetic ingredients have been detected in both wildlife and humans. Some ingredients have been found to cross the placenta.

TIPS: Buying Off-the-Shelf Personal Care Products

Review your products at the EWG's Skin Deep Cosmetic Database (ewg.org/skindeep/). EWG publishes ratings for over 68,000 products by comparing ingredients to the information found in 60 definitive toxicity and regulatory databases. Products receive a score between 1 and 10 based on the group's standards of safety.

Visit Campaign for Safe Cosmetics (SafeCosmetics.org) to see which companies have signed the group's compact. Members' products must meet the criteria of the EU's Cosmetics Directive 76/768/EEC. The voluntary group of companies pledge to meet (or exceed) EU standards and to avoid using ingredients that are known to be, or suspected of being, hazardous to human health.

Check out The Good Guide (GoodGuide.com), which has a database of over 250,000 product reviews based on scientific ratings.

As you familiarize yourself with the toxic ingredients commonly found in personal care products, start reading the fine print on their labels. Don't feel you have to know every ingredient on the list; just get used to thinking about what you put on your body. If you gravitate toward products whose ingredients you recognize (sunflower seed oil, cocoa butter, aloe vera, rosemary essential oil), you are more likely to use products that are better for you.

Shop at drugstores, natural foods stores, and beauty boutiques that have flexible return policies so you can easily return or exchange the product if you find out that your new shampoo or lotion contains chemicals of concern.

Third-party certifications may help identify safer products. Certifying organizations include the USDA (USDA Organics, ams.usda.gov/nop), NSF (nsf.org), the Soil Association (soilassociation.org), BDIH (kontrollierte-naturkosmetik.de), Eco-Cert (ecocert.com), and the National Products Association (npainfo.org). Some standards are stricter than others. Regardless, it's still important to read the labels!

Acne Products

HOUSEHOLD REPEAT OFFENDERS

Toxicants
— Parabens

Ingredients
— Nanoparticles
— Triclosan

Materials
— Plastics

ADDITIONAL OFFENDERS
— Benzoyl peroxide
— Ceteareth
— PEG
— Polyethylene
— Salicylic acid

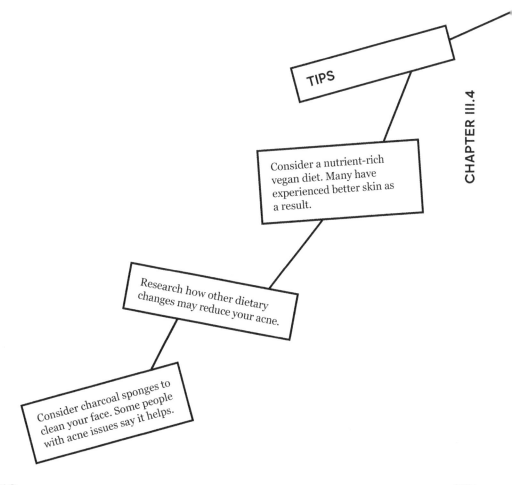

TIPS

Consider a nutrient-rich vegan diet. Many have experienced better skin as a result.

Research how other dietary changes may reduce your acne.

Consider charcoal sponges to clean your face. Some people with acne issues say it helps.

Antiperspirants and Deodorants

HOUSEHOLD REPEAT OFFENDERS

Toxicants
— Parabens
— Phthalates

Ingredients
— Fragrance
— Nanoparticles
— Triclosan or other antibacterial agents

Materials
— Plastics

ADDITIONAL OFFENDERS
— Antiperspirants: Compounds like aluminum, zinc, and zirconium salts that are used to keep your underarms dry (by blocking pores and reducing sweat production) can cause skin irritation and asthma.
— Deodorizing ingredients: Perfumes that mask odors may contain phthalates and trigger allergies, and antibacterial agents that prevent sweat from combining with surface bacteria may promote antibiotic-resistant bacteria.

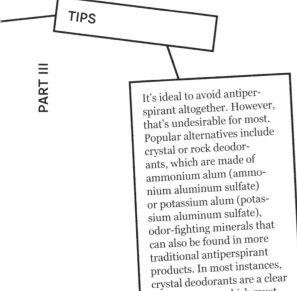

TIPS

It's ideal to avoid antiperspirant altogether. However, that's undesirable for most. Popular alternatives include crystal or rock deodorants, which are made of ammonium alum (ammonium aluminum sulfate) or potassium alum (potassium aluminum sulfate), odor-fighting minerals that can also be found in more traditional antiperspirant products. In most instances, crystal deodorants are a clear or white stone, which must be moistened with water before use (*National Geographic* 2008). They need to be applied more often than conventional products.

Natural herbal extracts like lavender, rosemary, sage, and mint produce odor-neutralizing scents. These plants serve as antiseptics and their odors are natural, so they are good choices for use in deodorant and antiperspirant products, which can be found at natural food stores as well as online (*National Geographic* 2008).

Cleansers and Soaps

HOUSEHOLD REPEAT OFFENDERS

Toxicants
— Formaldehyde
— Phthalates

Ingredients
— Fragrance
— Glycols
— Parabens
— Microbeads
— Nanoparticles
— Sulfates, a group of surfactants
— Synthetic colors
— Unintentionals, such as formaldehyde-releasing ingredients

Materials
— Plastics

ADDITIONAL OFFENDERS
— Petroleum ingredients
— Triclocarbon

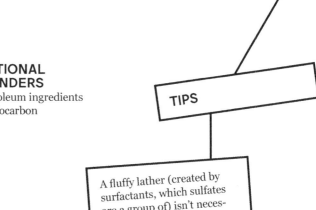

TIPS

A fluffy lather (created by surfactants, which sulfates are a group of) isn't necessary to remove dirt and oil. Consider cleansers with low-sudsing formulas that are free of sulfates, DEA, TEA, and MEA. Gentler cleansers can include milder surfactants like cocamidopropyl betaine, sorbitan laurate, sorbitan palmitate, and sorbitan stearate.

Choose soap that is color-free and fragrance-free (or uses essential oil fragrances exclusively).

Choose vegetable-based soaps such as castile soap. Although true castile soap is an olive oil–based formula historically crafted in the Castile region of Spain, today the term is loosely applied to other vegetable-based formulas. I used organic castile soap to wash my face, body, and hair throughout my pregnancies and periods of nursing.

Cosmetics

HOUSEHOLD REPEAT OFFENDERS

Toxicants
— Formaldehyde
— Heavy metals, like lead and mercury
— Phthalates

Ingredients
— Artificial coloring
— Fragrance
— Glycols
— Microbeads
— Nanoparticles
— Preservatives, such as parabens and formaldehyde-based

Materials
— Plastics

ADDITIONAL OFFENDERS
— Irritants
— Nanoparticles in powders
— Talc
— Vitamin A: May appear as retinol, retinyl palmitate, and retinyl acetate (EWG 2015r).

REPEAT ISSUES
— Petroleum-based ingredients
— Unintentional Potential Effects
— Unique vulnerabilities
— Unknown risks from chronic exposure

TIPS

Reduce how often and how much you use cosmetics. For example, limiting use of mascara to special occasions may reduce exposure to mercury, which is found in the preservative thimerosal. It is more commonly used in "lash-building" mascaras. Also, lead is sometimes added as an ingredient in cosmetics, or is present as an impurity.

Many cosmetics brands have signed the Campaign for Safe Cosmetics, pledging to replace toxic compounds with safer ingredients in their products. These brands are safer bets in general, though you should always read labels to see what your products contain. Visit the organization's website (SafeCosmetics.org) for a current list of participating companies.

E-retailers often list products' ingredients, which you can compare against the EWG's list of Dirty Dozen ingredients before you buy.

Increasingly, less-toxic products may be found among national retailers. Natural foods stores frequently stock cosmetics that contain fewer toxins. Read labels to avoid Household Repeat Offenders and ingredients on the EWG's Dirty Dozen list.

Beware of nanoparticles. When buying mineral-based foundations and powdered cosmetics, choose products made without them. The primary minerals used in foundations are zinc oxide and titanium dioxide, along with mica and iron oxides (for pigment and iridescence). The particles are often fragmented down to nanometers in order to increase the products' blendability and texture, but it's unclear whether this increases their absorption, or whether there are health consequences if the particles are absorbed. Their affect on the environment and wildlife are also unknown.

Read ingredient lists carefully to see what else the formulas contain. Some manufacturers coat mineral particles with petroleum-based silicone oils, including dimethicone, to help foundation spread more evenly. A better alternative is lauryl lysine, a combination of the amino acid lysine and coconut oil–derived lauric acid.

Cosmetics: Anti-Aging Products

HOUSEHOLD REPEAT OFFENDERS

Ingredients
— Fragrance
— Glycols
— Nanoparticles
— Preservatives, like parabens

Materials
— Plastics

ADDITIONAL OFFENDERS
— Alpha hydroxy acids (AHAs)
— Hydroquinone: Sometimes found in skin-lightening products, hydroquinone can harm the skin and cause permanent damage.
— Mercury: Has been found in illegally imported skin lighteners. Pregnant women should be extra mindful. Always avoid products with mercury, calomel, mercurio or mercurio chloride on the label (EWG 2015r).
— Retinyl palmitate and retinol (vitamin A)

TIPS: Healthier Ways to Delay Wrinkles and Other Signs of Aging

Eat a nourishing diet. Lycopene from cooked tomatoes, paired with olive oil or avocado, and vitamins C and E from blueberries, kiwi, and sweet potatoes can help protect your skin from sun damage. Antioxidant-rich foods include artichokes, beans, berries, russet potatoes, some spices, and nuts. Also, omega 3s in salmon, cod, and walnuts can improve the appearance of wrinkles.

Sleep!

Consider alternative therapies for acne, eczema, or itchy skin but consult your physician first. Together, you may be able to identify an underlying issue.

Drink lots of water. Limit dehydrating beverages such as coffee and wine. Get a healthy amount of sleep. Protect your skin from the sun. Be extra careful of the sun if you use products with alpha hydroxy or beta hydroxy acids, lactic acid, and glycolic acid.

Conventional skin lighteners may contain potentially unsafe ingredients like phenacetin, which is a probable human carcinogen, or hydroquinone, according to the US government (EPA 2015b).

Taken orally or applied topically, the antioxidant vitamins A, C, and E may help fight off damage to healthy cells and lessen wrinkles and other signs of aging.

Boost collagen formation. Some peptides boost the skin's production of collagen when applied topically. The "plumping" effect may reduce the appearance of wrinkles and sagging skin. Zinc, which is necessary for collagen development, may be found in high doses in foods such as yogurt, red meat, white kidney beans, and oysters.

Cosmetics: Lip Color

OVERVIEW

Lip color can contain toxic ingredients too. For example, in February 2012, the FDA conducted a study of lead in lipstick. Lead was detected in most of the 400 lipsticks assessed in that study (Hepp 2012). The FDA said there was no cause for alarm because the levels detected were "within the limits recommended by global public health authorities for cosmetics, including lipstick" (Lipka 2012).

Just be careful of whom you kiss or share drinks with: The EPA has said that there is no known safe level of lead, especially for children (EPA 2014b).

HOUSEHOLD REPEAT OFFENDERS

Toxicants
— Heavy metals like lead and mercury
— Nanoparticles

Ingredients
— Petroleum distillates
— Preservatives
— Synthetic colors

Materials
— Plastics

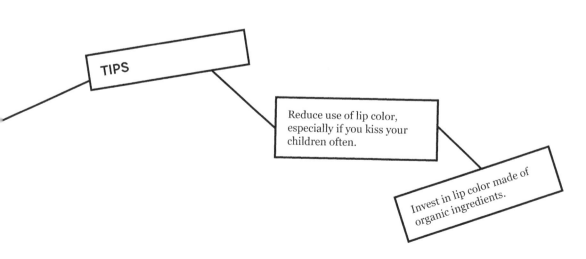

TIPS

Reduce use of lip color, especially if you kiss your children often.

Invest in lip color made of organic ingredients.

Cosmetics:
Nail Polish

HOUSEHOLD REPEAT OFFENDERS

Toxicants
— Formaldehyde: Used as a preservative in nail products. One study found a three-inch-square coating of wet nail polishes to emit significantly more formaldehyde than an equal area of particleboard (Kelly, Smith, and Satola 1999).
— Nanoparticles
— Phthalates

Ingredients
— Solvents
— Synthetic colors
— Triclosan
— VOCs

Materials
— Plastics

ADDITIONAL OFFENDERS
— Acetone: A neurotoxin that may also harm the liver, kidneys, and a developing fetus (EHANS 2015).
— Toluene: A common nail polish solvent that's also used as a paint thinner. A volatile petrochemical, it is a potent neurotoxicant and may also contribute to immune system damage, malignant lymphoma (EWG 2015r), and adverse respiratory effects including the onset of asthma and asthma attacks (*National Geographic* 2008). In utero exposure may impair fetal development (EWG 2015r).

REPEAT ISSUE
— The unknown safety of these chemical ingredients established on your nails for days.
— While nail polish without the most notorious trio of toxic ingredients (dibutyl phthalate, toluene, and formaldehyde) now exist, substitute chemicals may not be safer.

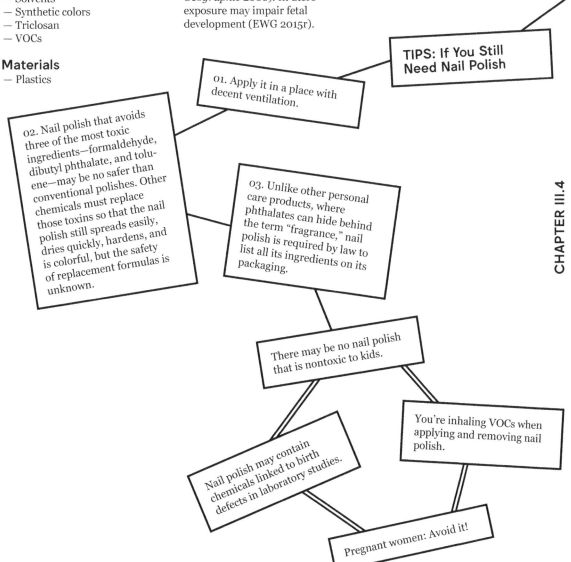

TIPS: If You Still Need Nail Polish

01. Apply it in a place with decent ventilation.

02. Nail polish that avoids three of the most toxic ingredients—formaldehyde, dibutyl phthalate, and toluene—may be no safer than conventional polishes. Other chemicals must replace those toxins so that the nail polish still spreads easily, dries quickly, hardens, and is colorful, but the safety of replacement formulas is unknown.

03. Unlike other personal care products, where phthalates can hide behind the term "fragrance," nail polish is required by law to list all its ingredients on its packaging.

There may be no nail polish that is nontoxic to kids.

You're inhaling VOCs when applying and removing nail polish.

Nail polish may contain chemicals linked to birth defects in laboratory studies.

Pregnant women: Avoid it!

Dental Products: Dental Floss

HOUSEHOLD REPEAT OFFENDERS

Toxicants
— PFCs: Some flosses may contain perfluorochemicals.

Ingredients
— Synthetic fragrance

Materials
— Conventional textiles, such as nylon, silk, and rubber
— Plastics

ADDITIONAL OFFENDERS
— Petroleum-based ingredients, such as polytetrafluoroethylene (PTFE), also known as Teflon

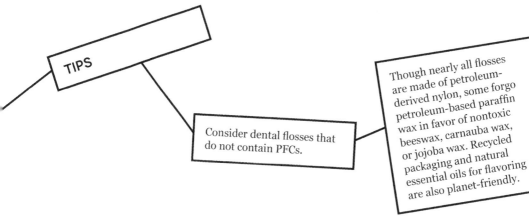

TIPS

Consider dental flosses that do not contain PFCs.

Though nearly all flosses are made of petroleum-derived nylon, some forgo petroleum-based paraffin wax in favor of nontoxic beeswax, carnauba wax, or jojoba wax. Recycled packaging and natural essential oils for flavoring are also planet-friendly.

Dental Products: Fluoride

OVERVIEW

According to the American Dental Association (ADA 2015b), fluoride helps reduce decay in baby and adult teeth. However, there has been debate about children's chronic exposures to fluoride since fluoride is also a developmental neurotoxin.

While fluoride is naturally occurring, it is also added to tap water, toothpaste, mouth rinses, soda, juices, baby food, and other processed products that are manufactured in a fluoridated community.

The EPA has set a legal limit on fluoride in drinking water of four parts per million (EPA 2013a). But studies have found up to an average IQ loss of seven points in children exposed to fluoride at less than four ppm, according to an article published by Philippe Grandjean MD DMSc, Harvard School of Public Health, and Philip Landrigan MD MSc, Icahn School of Medicine, in the March 2014 issue of *Lancet Neurology*.

Since fluoride protects against tooth decay, the key is getting the proper amount. The American Dental Association advises that for children under three, parents should begin brushing when children start growing teeth, and that a small amount (about the size of a grain of rice) of fluorinated toothpaste is appropriate (ADA 2015b). Too much fluoride can also cause opaque white patches or permanent brown discoloraton on teeth.

TIPS: Fluoride in Water

There seems to be no consensus on what fluoride levels are safe. Below is a collection of notes from my research, meant to help jump-start your own inquiry.

Learn what the fluoride levels are in your tap water from your local water company or department of public health. Each year, companies are required to provide their customers with water quality reports, known as a Consumer Confidence Report. This report highlights what chemicals and other substances there are in the water, including fluoride (EPA 2013e). Check out the EPA's Safe Drinking Water Hotline at water.epa.gov/drink/hotline/ for more general information about the safety of drinking water.

If you drink water from a private source, such as a well, you can have fluoride levels tested by a reputable laboratory. Keep in mind that even without fluoridation, some areas may have natural amounts of fluoride in water that exceed four mg/l. While public water systems in such areas are required to lower the fluoride level to the acceptable standard, private water sources may still be higher.

If your tap water is fluoridated, you may want to use nonfluoridated spring water to reduce your exposure to fluoride.

Water filters, including a reverse-osmosis or water-distillation unit, can help reduce fluoride levels that exceed 1.2 ppm (*National Geographic* 2008).

Dental Products: Mouthwash

HOUSEHOLD REPEAT OFFENDERS

Ingredients
— Glycols
— Nanoparticles
— Preservatives, such as sodium benzoate
— Sulfates, such as sodium lauryl sulfate (SLS)
— Synthetic colors, such as those made from coal tar. The common colorants FD&C Blue 1, Green 3, Yellow 5, and Yellow 6 may be harmful to human health.

Materials
— Plastics

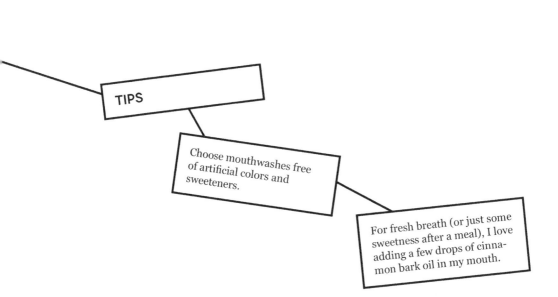

TIPS

Choose mouthwashes free of artificial colors and sweeteners.

For fresh breath (or just some sweetness after a meal), I love adding a few drops of cinnamon bark oil in my mouth.

Dental Products: Toothpaste

HOUSEHOLD REPEAT OFFENDERS

Toxicants
— Lead

Ingredients
— Microbeads
— Nanoparticles
— Preservatives, like parabens
— Surfactants, like sodium lauryl and laureth sulfates
— Synthetic colors
— Triclosan

Materials
— Plastics

ADDITIONAL OFFENDERS
— Artificial sweeteners
— Cleansing agents
— Synthetic flavors

ON PROBATION
— Fluoride

TIPS

Look for the American Dental Association seal of approval.

Look for a product that's free of artificial colors, sugars, and microbeads. Download the app, "Beat the Microbeads," for help (BeatTheMicrobead.org).

Note that fluoride-free toothpastes may not provide the same level of cavity protection as fluoride-containing varieties.

Avoid the common ingredient, hydrated silica, which may lead to the unintentional presence of lead.

Children under 6 should not use fluoridated mouth rinses, because they may swallow them.

Parents with concerns should use a pea-size amount of toothpaste for their children's brushing and try to prevent their children from swallowing toothpaste.

The American Dental Association recommends that children over the age of three brush at least twice a day with a fluoridated toothpaste and that adults help them floss once daily (ADA 2014; ADA 2015a).

Feminine Care Products

OVERVIEW

A female's most private areas are among the most delicate and absorbent ones of her body. Therefore, careful consideration should be given to which toxicants these areas may be exposed. For example, dioxins, a potential unintentional contaminant in the cotton and rayon used in tampons and menstrual pads, may be absorbed.

While the long-term health effects are not known, Philip Tierno MS PhD, director of clinical microbiology and diagnostic immunology at the New York University Medical Center and expert on the risks associated with tampon use, is among those that believe that even trace levels of dioxin can be harmful (Dudley, Nassar, and Hartman 2009). In animals, dioxins cause cancer, and one type (TCDD) is known to cause cancer in people (WHO 2014). Other potential health effects in humans from exposure to dioxins include damage to the reproductive system (higher likelihood of pelvic inflammatory disease, endometriosis, reduced fertility, lowered sperm count and birth defects), nervous system, immune system, endocrine system, and development (Hollender and Zissu 2010; Rier and Foster 2002; EPA 2014a; EPA 2015e; EWG 2015k; WHO 2014).

If you use tampons regularly, then consider the unknown effects from chronic exposure. In "A Question for Women's Health: Chemicals in Feminine Hygiene Products and Personal Lubricants," an article in *Environmental Health Perspectives*, Dr. Tierno observes, "A woman uses approximately 11,400 tampons in her menstrual life . . . . That's exposure to dioxins 11,400 times" (Nicole 2014).

HOUSEHOLD REPEAT OFFENDERS

Toxicants
— Chlorine: Often used to bleach materials.
— Dioxins: Created in the process of bleaching the cotton and rayon used in feminine products. Because they pervade our environment, they are suspected of also being in the cotton and rayon even before bleaching.
— Parabens: Various feminine products and personal lubricants use parabens as preservatives.
— Pesticides: According to *Planet Home*, "If every woman of menstruating age replaced one 16-count package of regular absorbency conventional cotton tampons with organic cotton ones, we could prevent 17,000 pounds of pesticides from polluting our rivers, lakes, and streams. For super absorbency, that number is 21,000 pounds of pesticides, and for super-plus, it goes up to 24,000 pounds" (Hollender and Zissu 2010).

Ingredients
— Fragrance

Materials
— Plastics
— Synthetic fibers: Absorb more moisture than cotton does, creating an environment that may foster more toxins (Hollender and Zissu 2010).

REPEAT ISSUES
— Allergens
— Carcinogens
— Endocrine disrupting chemicals
— Trails of Contamination throughout our Homes
— Unintentional By-Products
— Unintentional Potential Effects
— Unique vulnerabilities

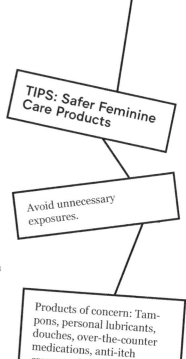

TIPS: Safer Feminine Care Products

Avoid unnecessary exposures.

Products of concern: Tampons, personal lubricants, douches, over-the-counter medications, anti-itch creams, wipes, yeast infection treatments, deodorizing sprays/powders/washes, and various homeopathic remedies.

Seek materials that are unbleached (or bleached with hydrogen peroxide), made of certified organic cotton, and free of dyes and fragrance.

Fragrance

OVERVIEW

There are over two dozen types of phthalates, which part II details. In cosmetics, the most common phthalate used is DEP (diethyl phthalate). Also used in personal care products, and among the most toxic, is DBP (dibutyl phthalate).

Due to loopholes in federal law, the cosmetics industry is not required to test or monitor phthalates for adverse effects. DBP is undergoing scientific scrutiny because of high levels found in women of reproductive age.

Phthalates (and other endocrine disruptors) can accumulate in the body, and even very small amounts can interact with other compounds to create adverse cocktail effects. It's a good idea to reduce unnecessary exposure. The European Parliaments prohibited the use of the phthalates DEHP (di-[2-ethylhexyl] phthalate) and DBP in cosmetics.

— A CDC study found seven types of phthalates in the bodies of 289 average Americans. Every person tested had DBP in his or her body (Blount et al. 2000).

— In one study, men who used cologne or aftershave had more than twice as much DEP in their urine samples as non-users did. Levels increased by 33 percent for each additional type of personal care product used (Duty et al. 2005).

— CDC researchers reported that women ages 20 to 40 appear to have the highest amounts of DBP in their bodies (Blount et al. 2000).

— Research conducted by the Harvard School of Public Health found that high amounts of DBP in men was correlated with lower sperm quality and motility (Hauser et al. 2006). Harvard researchers also found links between DEP and DNA damage in sperm, which can contribute to infertility and miscarriage (Hauser et al. 2007).

HOUSEHOLD REPEAT OFFENDERS

Toxicants
— Phthalates

Ingredients
— Preservatives
— Solvents
— Nanoparticles

Materials
— Plastics

ADDITIONAL OFFENDERS
— Petroleum-based ingredients

TIPS

Think twice about using perfume/cologne, especially if you will be around children. The profile about synthetic fragrance in chapter II.2, Ingredients of Concern, examines this in more depth. As perfumes/cologne sit on your skin, you and others can inhale or absorb toxicants. Even reducing your frequency of use is helpful.

For the special occasions that you would like to wear fragrance, healthier options exist. They are generally made of 100 percent pure essential oils.

Read labels of other products to avoid fragrance. They are in unexpected products such as garbage bags and dolls.

Examples of the wide variety of personal care products that may contain phthalates include cosmetics, skin-care products, nail polish, perfume, cologne, aftershave, hair spray, hair growth products, shampoo, conditioner, deodorant, and plastic packaging.

Hair Dyes

HOUSEHOLD REPEAT OFFENDERS

Toxicants
— Lead: Lead acetate is a color additive in some hair dyes.

Ingredients
— Coal tar: Used in some hair dyes, coal tar may penetrate the skin, enter the body, and break down into cancer-causing compounds (EWG 2015r).
— Nanoparticles
— Solvents

Materials
— Plastics

ADDITIONAL OFFENDERS
— Alkylphenyl ethoxylates (APEs): Synthetic surfactants used in some hair dyes, detergents, and cleaning products. APEs don't biodegrade easily and can create Unintentional By-products such as alkylphenols (some of which are potential endocrine disruptors) and nonylphenol. In one study, exposed wild salmon and other fish were found to have altered reproductive systems, feminization, hermaphrodism, and lower survival rates (Healthy Child Healthy World 2013).
— Nonylphenol: Regulated in the EU, but found in US products.
— Phenylenediamine (PPD): Commonly found in hair dyes, it can damage the nervous system and irritate lungs, severe allergic reactions, and blindness. It's also listed as 1,4-benzenediamine, p-aminoaniline, and 1,4-diaminobenzene.

TIPS

There are no truly nontoxic hair dyes, so avoid or minimize hair coloring. When you can't resist, then consider the following tips.

01. Avoid permanent, dark dyes
— While not all scientists are in agreement over the relationship between hair dye and cancer, a study published in the *International Journal of Cancer* found that women who colored their hair with permanent dyes every month were "twice as likely to get bladder cancer as women who don't dye their hair at all" (Gago-Dominguez et al. 2001).
— Some dyes contain ingredients, like coal tar, that increase the risk of cancer. Darker colors seem to contain more harmful chemicals, and prolonged exposure to permanent, dark hair dyes is correlated with a greater likelihood of developing non-Hodgkin's lymphoma and multiple myeloma (*National Geographic* 2008). Coal tar may be listed as aminophenol, diaminobenzene, or phenylenediamine.
— Pregnant women should be extra cautious, especially during the first trimester. While skin absorption of treatments is minimal, it's hard to know which levels pose risk to a fetus. Try to avoid ammonia, which can be in permanent hair dyes; inhaling fumes may harm the fetus.

02. Choose highlights
Highlights painted onto sections of hair instead of dyes that are applied all over can reduce your toxic exposures.

03. Choose dyes with plant-based ingredients
Less toxic options exist. While performance is different, safer hair dyes contain no petrochemicals. Remember that "natural" and "herbal" hair dyes can contain toxic chemicals too. But they'll most likely contain lower concentrations of them than standard dyes if they're made of mostly plant-based ingredients. They may be better for subtle color changes.

04. Be wary of straightening products
They may release toxic fumes.

05. Semipermanent dyes and light-colored permanent dyes are usually safer
Generally, the less drastic the color change, the less toxic.

Insect Repellents

ADDITIONAL OFFENDER
— N,N-diethyl-m-toluamide (DEET): Widely used since the late 1950s, it protects against insects, especially mosquitoes. However, DEET has been associated with eye and skin irritation (like blisters and rashes), adverse neurological symptoms (including lethargy, confusion, disorientation, and mood swings), seizures, and death.

REPEAT ISSUES
— Unintentional Potential Effects
— Unique vulnerabilities

Keep it external. Do not apply DEET-containing products to children's hands or faces, as it may enter eyes or be ingested. Keep it away from cuts, wounds, or sunburned skin.

Avoid sprays, since the chance of inhaling the chemicals will be higher.

When possible, use precautionary measures as your first line of defense rather than using sprays and lotions. For example, cover yourself with light colored clothing to help block ticks and mosquitoes and to make them easily visible. Wear shoes and socks. Learn which nearby wooded areas are hotbeds for ticks. Avoid being in those areas during high-risk seasons. Be sure to check bodies and scalps after spending time there.

Avoid formulas that combine sunscreen with DEET. While sunscreen should be reapplied frequently throughout the day, one application of DEET could suffice, and multiple reapplications increase your chances of being exposed to unsafe levels.

Use as little insect repellent as possible while maintaining the product's effectiveness, and apply it only to exposed skin.

Cleanse DEET-sprayed skin thoroughly with soap and water as soon as you come indoors.

01. While insect bites pose health risks, insect repellents may as well. Get to know what you're using, and think twice about the risk/reward profile. The consequences of insect bites from ticks and mosquitoes can be serious. For example, Lyme disease is common in parts of the northeastern US. In the trop-ics, mosquitoes may carry malaria or dengue fever.

Go for lower concentrations. A formula with 10 percent DEET will keep mosquitoes at bay for two hours. The effectiveness plateaus at 30 percent.

03. For those who wish to avoid DEET, herbal insect repellents that rely on botanical oils—citronella, lemongrass, lemon eucalyptus, pennyroyal, and others—can discourage insects, but are generally not as effective (and are more expensive) than DEET, providing protection for less than 20 minutes. Mesh clothing can protect some parts of your body. Check the EWG database for the safest off-the-shelf options.

02. When insect-borne disease is of concern, the risks of DEET use may be outweighed by its repellent reliability. If you decide that a DEET-containing repellent is necessary, take these precautions.

TIPS

Moisturizers

OVERVIEW

Toxicants in moisturizers can enter your body. If you are pregnant or nursing, then carefully evaluate what you put on your skin. In a study of 163 infants, the more phthalate-containing lotions, powders, and shampoos a mother reported using, the higher her infant's phthalate level. Over 80 percent of the infants had detectable phthalate levels, including monoethyl phthalate (MEP), monomethyl phthalate (MMP), and monoisobutyl phthalate (MiBP; Sathyanarayana et al. 2008).

Shanna Swan PhD, who coauthored the study and is an expert on the health effects of phthalate exposures on animals and humans, says that exposure to very low levels can add up to create a substantial effect (Smith and Lourie 2009).

HOUSEHOLD REPEAT OFFENDERS

Toxicants
— Phthalates

Ingredients
— Fragrance
— Glycols
— Microbeads
— Nanoparticles
— Preservatives, like parabens and formaldehyde-releasing ingredients
— Synthetic colors

Materials
— Plastics

REPEAT ISSUES
— Petroleum-based ingredients

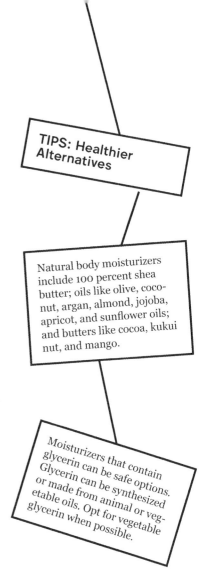

TIPS: Healthier Alternatives

Natural body moisturizers include 100 percent shea butter; oils like olive, coconut, argan, almond, jojoba, apricot, and sunflower oils; and butters like cocoa, kukui nut, and mango.

Moisturizers that contain glycerin can be safe options. Glycerin can be synthesized or made from animal or vegetable oils. Opt for vegetable glycerin when possible.

Over-the-Counter Drugs

REPEAT OFFENDERS

Toxicants
— Parabens
— Phthalates

Ingredients
— Preservatives
— Synthetic colors

Materials
— Plastics

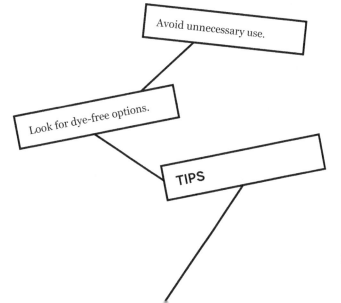

Avoid unnecessary use.

Look for dye-free options.

TIPS

Shampoos and Other Hair Products

HOUSEHOLD REPEAT OFFENDERS

Toxicants
— Coal tar
— Formaldehyde
— Lead
— Parabens
— Unintentional Toxicants

Ingredients
— Glycols
— Inerts
— Nanoparticles
— Surfactants
— Synthetic colors
— Synthetic fragrance

Materials
— Plastics

ADDITIONAL PRODUCTS OF CONCERN
— Aerosols
— Dandruff shampoos: There are FDA-approved active ingredients in dandruff shampoos that pose risks. Selenium sulfide, coal tar, and other common ingredients appear on the European or California lists of carcinogens and reproductive toxicants (ECHA 2015; CA EPA 2015). These compounds can also cause skin irritation, inflammation, and photosensitivity. Avoid unnecessary use, especially on children.
— Hair sprays and cosmetics: PVP/VA copolymer is commonly found in hair sprays and gels, as well as cosmetics, and is a harmful, petroleum-based chemical that may contaminate the lungs.
— Shampoos and texturizing products: May contain phenolphthalein, a probable human carcinogen.

REPEAT ISSUES
— Lack of unbiased safety review: In a study of shampoos published in 2004, every product contained ingredients that had not been assessed for safety by either the Cosmetic Ingredient Review panel or the FDA (*National Geographic* 2008).
— Petroleum-based ingredients
— Unknown ingredients
— Unintentional Potential Effects

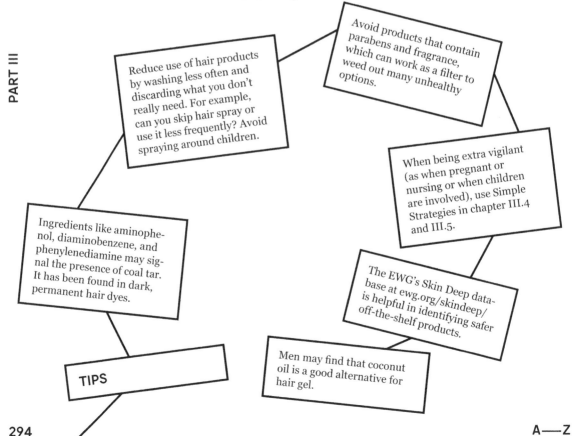

Reduce use of hair products by washing less often and discarding what you don't really need. For example, can you skip hair spray or use it less frequently? Avoid spraying around children.

Avoid products that contain parabens and fragrance, which can work as a filter to weed out many unhealthy options.

When being extra vigilant (as when pregnant or nursing or when children are involved), use Simple Strategies in chapter III.4 and III.5.

Ingredients like aminophenol, diaminobenzene, and phenylenediamine may signal the presence of coal tar. It has been found in dark, permanent hair dyes.

The EWG's Skin Deep database at ewg.org/skindeep/ is helpful in identifying safer off-the-shelf products.

TIPS

Men may find that coconut oil is a good alternative for hair gel.

Shaving Cream and Aftershave

HOUSEHOLD REPEAT OFFENDERS

Toxicants
— Phthalates
— Unintentional Toxicants

Ingredients
— Glycols
— Nanoparticles
— Preservatives
— Solvents
— Surfactants
— Synthetic colors
— Synthetic fragrance

Materials
— Plastics

ADDITIONAL OFFENDERS
— Isobutane: An extremely flammable ingredient
— Petroleum-based ingredients
— Triethanolamine (TEA): A skin irritant that may be related to an unintentional toxicant, nitrosamines, which are linked to cancer

TIPS

Beware that shaving cream containers can contain foam-producing propellants such as propane or isobutane. These chemicals are extremely flammable.

Use bar soap (such as castile) as shaving soap, working it into a lather with a shaving brush.

Use EWG's Safe Cosmetics database to find safer shaving creams (probably lower-foaming, but equally effective).

Sun Protection

OVERVIEW

Conventional Chemical Sunscreens

Most conventional sunscreens allow the sun's rays to reach the skin and rely on synthetic chemicals to protect against damage. While these chemicals are effective at preventing sunburn and reducing your risk of skin cancer, they can penetrate the skin and may pose health risks. For example, oxybenzone, the popular ingredient in chemical sunscreens profiled as an Additional Offender, has been detected in nearly every American and in breast milk (EWG 2015t).

Mineral-based Sunblocks

Mineral-based sunscreens work by creating a physical barrier that deflects both UVA and UVB rays. Currently, this is considered a safer choice than chemical formulations.

Titanium dioxide and zinc oxide are the most commonly used minerals. In the past, zinc-based sunscreens were distinguishable by the white streaks they left on users' skin. These days, mineral sunscreens are more transparent and blend better due to nanotechnology, which significantly reduces the size of the mineral particles used. Nanotechnology is not without health concerns, as is explained earlier in this chapter.

HOUSEHOLD REPEAT OFFENDERS

Ingredients
— Glycols
— Nanoparticles: In sunscreen creams available in the US, zinc oxide and titanium dioxide nanoparticles are considered the safer and more effective active ingredients. They appear to not penetrate the skin. However, avoid nanoparticles in powder and spray products as inhaling them is dangerous (EWG 2015m).
— Preservatives
— Synthetic colors
— Synthetic fragrance

Materials
— Plastics

ADDITIONAL OFFENDERS
— Benzophenone-3 (or oxybenzone): A common active ingredient in sunscreen. It raises concern due to its developmental and reproductive toxicity, its immunotoxicity, and its ability to cause biochemical or cellular-level changes as well as endocrine disruption. It is also linked to allergies. Its persistence and bioaccumulation is also cause for concern (EWG 2015n).
— Petroleum-based ingredients

ON PROBATION
— Paraffins
— Silicons

ISSUES
— The higher the SPF, the more chemicals are used.
— Some sunscreen ingredients may contribute to skin cancer.
— Prolonged sun exposure causes some of these toxins to mutate into more harmful compounds. Titanium dioxide and zinc oxide nanoparticles don't appear to break down in the sun (EWG 2015m).
— The CDC estimates that certain sunscreen ingredients (such as oxybenzone) are present in nearly all Americans (EWG 2008a).

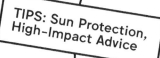

TIPS: Sun Protection, High-Impact Advice

Sunscreen should not be your primary defense against skin cancer (IARC 2001). The FDA says that relevant studies "do not demonstrate that even [broad-spectrum products with SPF greater than 15] alone reduce the risk of skin cancer and early skin aging" (FDA 2011). In fact, studies have found that sunscreen users have a heightened risk of melanoma. Scientists suggest several possible explanations: Sunscreen users are typically in the sun for long durations of time and are therefore exposed to more radiation, Unintentional Toxicants (such as breakdown products from sunlight) may have negative health effects, and low-quality sunscreens with inadequate UVA protection are very prevalent in the market.

01. The first line of defense
Use hats, shade, UVA-blocking sunglasses, protective clothing, and avoid the sun when its rays are strongest (generally, 10 a.m. to 4 p.m.). Not all brands of sun-protective clothing will offer equal protection. Look for brands that have been specifically recommended by dermatologists and skin cancer groups.

TIPS: Sun Protection, High-Impact Advice (continued)

Opt for a lotion, not a spray or powder. Inhalation of powders and sprays is a concern.

02. When choosing a sunscreen

Pick SPF 30 to 50. Anything over SPF 50 provides a false sense of security under the sun, as the extra protection from SPF concentrations over 50 are negligible (EWG 2015u) and users may not reapply as often as is needed.

Look for these on the labels:
— Broad-spectrum, which will guard against both UVA and UVB rays
— Water-resistant
— Safer key ingredients include zinc oxide and titanium dioxide, preferably without nanoparticles. If they are not available, then select avobenzone at 3 percent.

Use the Safe Cosmetics database to identify products that have a low hazard assessment.

Avoid products that contain these ingredients:
— Oxybenzone, popular among SPF products
— Vitamin A (retinyl palmitate): When applied in sunlight, vitamin A may promote the formation of skin tumors and lesions (EWG 2015o; NTP 2012).
— Insect repellent: If you need it, then buy it separately and apply it first.

03. Apply generously and frequently
Most people use just 25 to 50 percent of the recommended amount of sunscreen, says the Skin Cancer Foundation (2015). Follow the application instructions precisely.

04. Avoid applying over open wounds
When applied topically, chemicals may enter the body through open wounds.

05. The EWG
Check its annual review of the best and worst sun protection. The EWG reviews hundreds of studies and gives safety and effectiveness ratings for more than 700 products (EWG 2015h).

Simple Strategies:
Simplify Your Personal Care

The ideal solution is to buy less stuff, use less stuff, and reallocate your budget toward a few healthy products and a healthier diet. A nutrient-dense diet will improve your skin, your energy, and your glow. For the personal care products that you do use, here is a simple guide to follow until you identify the healthier products that meet your preferences.

01 . Remember that less is best
Eliminate or reduce the use of unnecessary products. Save more toxic ones, like perfume and hair spray, for special occasions.

02. Prioritize your budget
Prioritize your budget to focus on products that sit on your skin for long periods of time: lotions, creams, sunscreens and cosmetics. Good resources include ewg.org/skindeep/ from the EWG and SafeCosmetics.org from the Campaign for Safe Cosmetics.

03. Invest in your diet
Research which dietary changes may improve your skin, energy, and glow.

04. Use organic castille soap
Use organic castille soap to replace cleansers for body, face, and hair. I did that when pregnant and nursing. After I was no longer pregnant or nursing, I started incorporating more off-the-shelf shampoos and conditioners.

05. Replace moisturizers
Replace moisturizers with organic olive oil, coconut oil, or 100 percent pure shea butter. Organic oils are effective too, like argan oil.

06. Avoid powders and sprays
They are quickly inhaled into the body.

07. Avoid artificial colors and flavors in things that you may ingest
Avoid artificial colors and flavors in things that you may ingest: toothpaste, mouthwash, and pharmaceuticals.

08. Use pharmaceuticals conservatively

09. Minimize use of nail polish
This is especially important when pregnant. Also minimize visits to the nail salon.

10. Avoid bleached products, especially for private areas
Choose nonchlorine-bleached (or, ideally, unbleached) feminine products and diapers.

11. Avoid darkening your hair
It is best to avoid all hair coloring, but if you cannot, then choose semipermanent hair dye in lighter shades. Limiting yourself to highlights is even better.

12. Strategies for sun exposure
— Minimize your exposure during the sun's strongest hours (generally 10 a.m. to 4 p.m.).
— Wear clothing that guards from the sun, like hats and light, long-sleeved shirts.
— When buying sunscreen, pick a broad-spectrum formula with SPF 30 to 50 in a lotion form (not spray or powder). Also look for zinc oxide, titanium dioxide, and water resistance. Avoid oxybenzone, vitamin A (retinyl palmitate), and added insect repellent. Apply lotion liberally and reapply often.

13. Invest in your inner peace
Yoga and meditation can transform your inner and outer beauty.

Chapter III.5
Children's Stuff

CONVENTIONAL PRODUCTS: WHAT'S IN THEM?

In many instances, Household Repeat Offenders are even more common in children's things because they tend to be made of relatively inexpensive materials, like vinyl.

In this section, I highlight the key products of concern and their Household Repeat Offenders. This should help you edit your possessions and purchases more critically.

IN THIS CHAPTER:

— Household Repeat Offenders in conventional children's products
— Baby bottles
— Baby bottle nipples, pacifiers, and teethers
— Baby formula
— Baby and children's gear
— Children's apparel
— Food and beverage containers
— Children's personal care products
— Healthier bedrooms
— Toys
— Simple Strategies to reduce your children's exposures

HOUSEHOLD REPEAT OFFENDERS

Toxicants
— BPA
— Cadmium
— Chlorine
— Heavy metals, including lead
— Phthalates: The prevalence of phthalates in products used by children increases the likelihood of exposure. According to the EPA (2007b), key sources of daily exposure for children include breast milk, cow's milk, infant formulas, plastic-packaged foods, plastic toys, cups and bowls used for feeding; and indoor air.
— Unintentional Toxicants

Ingredients
— Chemical flame retardants
— Glycols
— Preservatives
— Solvents
— Surfactants/Sulfates
— Synthetic colors
— Synthetic fragrance
— Triclosan

Materials
— Adhesives
— Conventional textiles
— Paints
— Plastics, especially vinyl
— Polyurethane foam
— Woods

REPEAT ISSUES
— Accidental poisonings
— Children's unique vulnerability
— Hidden hazards: VOCs, HAPs, EDCs, respiratory irritants, carcinogens, and neurotoxins
— Ingredients detected in humans
— Lack of disclosure of ingredients and potential toxicity. These ingredients are part of proprietary formulas that manufacturers aren't required to divulge.
— Lack of required safety testing by an objective third party
— Manipulative Business Strategies
— Misleading and confusing label claims; and difficulty of determining safe products
— No regulation of levels of toxic ingredients used in consumer products
— Our choices contribute to Trails of Contamination
— Spray products, which are a common exposure route
— Unintentional By-products
— Unintentional Potential Effects in children's bodies

Baby Bottles

HOUSEHOLD REPEAT OFFENDERS

Toxicants
— BPA
— Phthalates

Materials
— Plastics: Plastic bottles can leach chemicals, like BPA, into formula and stored breast milk.

According to the *Green Guide*, breast milk stored in plastic may lose a high percentage of its antibodies for *E. coli* bacteria and much of its fat content, since fat tends to adhere to the plastic and may be left in the bottle (*National Geographic* 2008).

TIPS: Healthier Baby Bottles

01. Freezing and warming plastic bottles promotes leaching of chemicals.

Glass is a safe and durable option. If glass is not an option, then consider stainless steel or safer plastic bottles. Polyethylene (#2, #4, or #5) has not been found to leach potential hormone disruptors; many mainstream companies manufacture baby bottles using these types of plastic.

02. Discard scratched baby bottles, since scratched plastics (especially polycarbonate #7) are more likely to leach toxic chemicals.

Wide-mouth glass canning jars are a decent choice for storage, as they won't crack when heated or chilled. Just be sure to leave room at the top of the jar, as liquid expands as it freezes.

03. Follow the maintenance and care instructions for your bottles.

TIPS: Bottle Feeding

Plastic bottle liners: Forgo these, as chemicals can leach from the plastic liners, and enter into formula and breast milk. This is especially true when the liners are heated.

Heating: Avoid microwaving baby bottles. Warm them in a pan of hot water on the stovetop.

Baby Bottle Nipples, Pacifiers, and Teethers

HOUSEHOLD REPEAT OFFENDERS

Toxicants
— Phthalates: Beginning in 1986, manufacturers voluntarily discontinued the use of phthalates in bottle nipples and pacifiers. However, the safety of substitutes is not fully understood.

Materials
— Latex: This can cause allergic reactions and, according to the EWG (2008c), can contain impurities linked to cancer.
— Vinyl

TIPS: Healthier Baby Bottle Nipples, Pacifiers, and Teethers

01. Avoid PVC (vinyl) in nipples and in anything else going into the mouth.

02. Materials for baby bottle nipples include rubber, latex, and silicone. Silicone, which is nitrosamine-free, is the safest option. Opt for medical-grade of clear silicone if you can find it. They last longer and are safer than the amber-colored rubber ones, which can contain low levels of nitrosamines. These substances have been found to cause cancer in lab animals, but it's unknown whether exposure via bottle nipples increases cancer risk in humans. The FDA has established limits for nitrosamines in rubber nipples, but low levels are permissible.

03. Inspect all bottle nipples regularly. Discard any with cracks or tears, which can encourage bacteria growth and pose a choking hazard. Throw away thinning or discolored nipples as well.

04. Pacifiers should be entirely silicone. Avoid ones made of hard plastic unless you can easily find out what the plastic is (this isn't always obvious). There are also one-piece natural rubber pacifiers on the market. This rubber isn't synthetic; it's harvested from rubber trees.

05. Give your baby a frozen washcloth rather than vinyl teethers.

Baby Formula

HOUSEHOLD REPEAT OFFENDERS

Toxicants
— Arsenic: This may come from brown rice syrup, which is frequently used in organic foods.
— BPA
— Lead
— Phthalates

Ingredients
— Contaminants in water
— Heavy metals

Materials
— Plastics: Plastic containers and metal cans can leach BPA and phthalates into breast milk and infant formula.

OTHER OFFENDERS
— Metal cans
— Offenders from dairy or soy
— Perc: This dry cleaning toxin has been detected in formula.

TIPS: Infant Formula

01. Despite the potential risks of contamination, the benefits from infant formula outweigh the potential risk of BPA exposure. Consider the following tips for selecting healthier formula, from the perspective of minimizing environmental toxins.

02. Powdered, iron-fortified infant formula is the safest choice, as well as being the most nutritious alternative to breast milk.

03. Avoid ready-to-eat or liquid formula sold in metal cans. Recent tests by the EWG (2007c) and the Canadian government (Cao et al. 2008), and a 1990s test by the FDA (1996), found BPA leaching from metal cans into all brands of liquid formula. Powdered formula appears to be BPA-free.

04. When powdered formula is not available or if your pediatrician suggests a liquid formula, choose one sold in glass or plastic containers.

05. Soy formula: The American Association of Pediatricians suggests that only infants with particular medical conditions be given soy formula. Some studies suggest that natural plant estrogens in soy formula may hinder development in infants. While these results have raised concern, current research is inconclusive (Bhatia and Greer 2008).

06. Check the water section in chapter III.2 for tips on healthier water. The American Dental Association states that making formula with fluoridated water may increase the risk for enamel fluorosis, but urges parents to consult their dentist (ADA 2015a). Some experts believe that fluoridated water can cause damage to babies' developing teeth.

07. Review guidelines from physicians and the American Academy of Pediatrics, and discuss any changes to your baby's diet with your pediatrician.

Baby and Children's Gear

REPEAT OFFENDERS

Toxicants
— PBDEs
— Phthalates
— Tris flame retardants

Ingredients
— Adhesives
— Chemical flame retardants
— Solvents

Materials
— Conventional textiles
— Plastics, especially PVC
— Polyurethane foam

REPEAT ISSUES
— Contamination of air and dust and onto hands

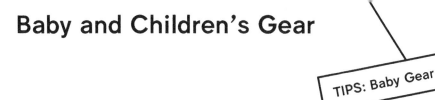

TIPS: Baby Gear

01. Buy just what you really need. Conventional textiles and polyurethane foam are common components of children's gear: car seats, baby carriers, rocking chairs, high chairs, strollers, sleep positioners, crib mattresses, nursing pillows, changing table pads, and much more. This means that those products will also tend to have toxic flame retardants. In one study of 101 baby products that contained polyurethane foam, 80 percent were found to have chemical flame retardants: 36 percent had TDCPP (listed as a carcinogen under Proposition 65 in California and a suspected developmental neurotoxin), 17 percent had Firemaster 550, and others had TCEP (considered a carcinogen by California) and PBDEs (banned in many countries).

07. If purchasing a changing pad cover, then consider a cloth one that you can remove and launder. Unbleached, undyed organic cotton is best.

02. Purchase baby items early so they can off-gas in a well-ventilated, infrequently used place. (But don't expose yourself to VOCs while you're pregnant.)

06. Consider skipping a changing pad altogether. Instead, cushion the changing table with a folded wool or organic cotton blanket.

03. Wash what you can, as frequently as you can, to remove residual chemicals on textiles. Check Simple Strategies in chapter III.1 for tips on healthier detergents.

05. Vinyl often covers polyurethane foam in high chairs, changing pads, and playpens. It may also be used in rain covers for strollers, and in toys. Try to avoid it. More detail is provided later in this chapter under the Toys section.

04. Investigate the cushioning materials found in diaper changing pads, high chairs, car seats, nursing pillows, playpens, play mats, and more. Polyurethane foam may release small amounts of toxic chemicals.

Children's Apparel

HOUSEHOLD REPEAT OFFENDERS

Toxicants
— Formaldehyde
— Pesticides

Ingredients
— Chemical flame retardants
— Synthetic colors

Materials
— Conventional textiles
— Plastics, especially vinyl

REPEAT ISSUES
— Skin absorption of residual toxicants on textiles
— Trails of Contamination throughout our Homes
— VOCs

TIPS: Children's Apparel

Try to find PVC-free materials for rainwear products (e.g., rain boots and raincoats), prints on clothing, and accessories. Inspect the product packaging and labeling, and on the underside of the item, look for a "3" inside a triangular recycling symbol, with the letter "V" or word "vinyl" written underneath the triangle. This label isn't used for all vinyl products, but a significant number of items carry it. A flexible, rubbery consistency and a distinct smell can indicate that the product contains vinyl ingredients. The CHEJ offers a guide to PVC-free products, called *Pass Up the Poison Plastic*, which can be found online.

Safer rain jackets are made with fabrics coated in polyurethane. Although it is still a synthetic plastic polymer, it is significantly less hazardous than vinyl. Nylon and polyester are also better choices than vinyl.

Natural rubber or EVA (a safer alternative for PVC) is a better material choice for rain boots than vinyl.

Choose organic, natural fabrics for children's products:

Snug-fitting pajamas that avoid flame retardants are good options for the kids. Conventional pajamas and nightgowns generally contain fire retardants that may penetrate their skin.

Healthier textiles, discussed in chapter II.3, also apply to children's clothes and bedding. Organic cotton is good for underwear, and Pure Grow wool is free of pesticides.

Check out the Organic Consumers Association website for help locating manufacturers and retailers of safer, organic clothing.

Secondhand clothes and what you already own are the best options.

Try to avoid clothes that need to be dry cleaned.

If you don't buy organic clothes, then wash the clothes before having your children wear them (the more washings the better).

Children's Personal Care Products

OVERVIEW
Generally, children's personal care products contain the same Household Repeat Offenders that adults' personal care products have. For my children, I keep it really simple. Especially when they were really young, I tried to use products that were safe enough to eat.

HOUSEHOLD REPEAT OFFENDERS

Toxicants
— Chlorine
— Dioxins from bleaching fibers for diapers or baby wipes
— Formaldehyde
— Phthalates
— Triclosan
— Unintentional Toxicants, like 1,4 dioxane. 1,4 dioxane was detected in an iconic baby shampoo in 2009. In 2012, the manufacturer announced that it would reformulate its product to make it safer.

Ingredients
— Fragrance
— Petroleum distillates
— Preservatives
— Solvents: May be found in children's nail polishes, baby wipes, and hand sanitizers.
— Synthetic colors

Materials
— Conventional textiles: Used in diapers.

ON PROBATION
— Fluoride

ADDITIONAL OFFENDERS
— Alcohol
— Other petroleum-based ingredients
— Talc

REPEAT ISSUES
— Inhaling toxicants from powder and spray products

SPECIAL CONCERN
— Babies can absorb chemicals more easily due to their thinner skin.

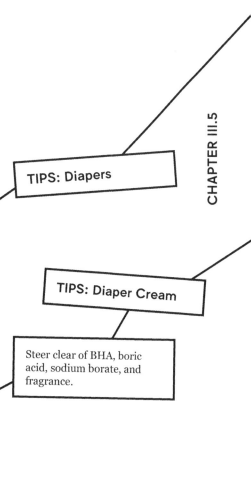

TIPS: Diapers

Look for unbleached, unscented diapers. Conventional disposables may emit VOCs and hormone disrupting fragrance, and their manufacture releases dioxins.

EWG (2015p) says to avoid 2-bromo-2-nitropropane-1,3-diol (bronopol), DMDM hydantoin, and fragrance.

TIPS: Diaper Cream

Steer clear of BHA, boric acid, sodium borate, and fragrance.

Try 100 percent pure, organic shea butter (if there's no allergy to it) or organic coconut oil.

TIPS: Children's Personal Care Products

Use just what is really needed. On average, children are exposed to 61 unique ingredients every day (EWG 2010). These ingredients are found in products such as lotions, shampoos, conditioners, diaper cream, and baby powder. While these products serve useful roles, the safety of these exposures is not fully understood. In fact, the EWG found that 77 percent of the ingredients in 1,700 children's products have not been tested for safety (EWG 2007b).

Moisturizers:
— Olive oil (organic, cold-pressed, light, not treated with chemicals)
— Coconut oil (raw, organic)
— Plant oils such as argan, jojoba, apricot seed, sunflower, and almond
— For very dry skin or to prevent diaper rash, organic plant butters such as cocoa and shea. I rely on organic shea butter in the winter.

Use pure castile soap to wash your infant's skin and hair. I used it on myself when pregnant and nursing.

Avoid fragrance.

When it comes to what products to use, less is more. When you cannot avoid them, remember that a little goes a long way. Use only small amounts of safer, off-the-shelf products on children—and not every day.

Use baking soda in the nursery to control odors, by adding some to your diaper pail after tossing disposable diapers.

Research fluoride in water and toothpaste to decide what you are comfortable giving your children.

Avoid powder and spray forms of sunscreen and insect repellent. Inhaling toxicants is a fast track to the bloodstream. If you really need baby powder, then use pure, organic cornstarch, which can be found in your grocery store's baking aisle.

Interpret marketing claims critically. Companies are rarely required to substantiate them, and claims like "hypoallergenic" and "natural" don't necessarily mean what you may think they mean. EWG's (2010) investigation of children's body care products found that 81 percent of items labeled "gentle" or "hypoallergenic" contained allergens or skin and eye irritants. According to the EWG (2015l), 35 percent of children's products that claimed to be "natural" had artificial preservatives. While the FDA attempted to officially define the term "natural," their efforts were overturned in court (Lewis 1998).

In choosing an off-the-shelf product at either a retail store or online, use the EWG's Skin Deep database at ewg.org/skindeep/ to find the safest products. USDA-certified organic or third-party-certified natural baby products are ideal.

TIPS: Baby Wipes

Minimize use of conventional baby wipes since many contain alcohol, perfumes, and preservatives like quaternium-15 and parabens. The wipes themselves, which are usually made of cotton or wood pulp, are also typically bleached using chlorine, which contaminates our Homes with dioxin.

For infants, healthy options include reusable cloths or a little water on paper towels, toilet paper, or organic cotton balls.

Choose wipes that are unbleached and free of chlorine, alcohol, fragrance, and parabens. Buying biodegradable ones is ideal.

Choose organic cotton in wipes (and other products, such as cotton balls and swabs, diapers, clothing, and bedding) to reduce pesticide used in farming cotton crops.

TIPS: Baby Powder

Fine powder can be a lung irritant. If you must use it, then organic cornstarch is a healthier substitute.

Avoid talc in baby powders. Talc is a natural mineral that can be contaminated with asbestiform fibers. If you need a store-bought product, then look for fragrance-free, cornstarch-based baby powders, which provide ample protection against diaper rash.

TIPS: Dental Care

Try to avoid the synthetic colors and sugars often found in children's mouthwashes and fluoride rinses.

Use small amounts (about the size of a grain of rice) of fluoride toothpaste for children under three, as recommended by the American Dental Association (ADA 2015b). See the general toothpaste guidelines in chapter III.4 for more information.

Refer to the sunscreen section in chapter III.4 for sun protection strategies, including tips on selecting healthier sunscreens.

Babies under six months shouldn't wear sunscreen and should be kept out of direct sunlight.

TIPS: Children's Medications

Consider whether natural remedies may be appropriate to try first.

Read product labels on cold, allergy, and other medicines to avoid parabens and artificial colors when possible.

TIPS: Sun Protection

Invest in a diet that boosts immunity.

Healthier Bedrooms

OVERVIEW

This section reviews the key concerns that have already been covered in the other chapters of part III. It is hard to believe that health risks found in consumer products for adults also exist in children's products. But they do.

The point of reiterating information in this section is to underscore that children's products are not safer; too often, they are even more toxic. For example, crib mattresses are often made of several Materials of Concern. An investigation by Clean and Healthy NY (2011) of 190 crib mattress models, made by 28 manufacturers for the US market, found the following:

— 72 percent used at least one chemical of concern (such as antimony, vinyl, polyurethane, and other VOCs).

— 40 percent used vinyl coverings.

— 22 percent used proprietary formulas for waterproofing, flame retardancy, and antibacterials. This keeps potential adverse health impacts unknown.

— 20 percent used "green" components but did not guarantee that their products were free of toxicants.

— Most crib manufacturers did not fully disclose all the materials that they used. Twenty-six of the 28 mattress manufacturers surveyed required one to five direct requests for more information. The information most often withheld was the type of flame retardant used.

On the next page, you can read about the theory that crib mattresses may contribute to SIDs.

HOUSEHOLD REPEAT OFFENDERS

Toxicants
— Chlorine
— Formaldehyde
— Phthalates
— Unintentional Toxicants

Ingredients
— Adhesives
— Chemical flame retardants
— Inerts
— Solvents
— Synthetic fragrance

Materials
— Conventional textiles
— Paints
— Plastics, like vinyl
— Polyurethane foam

REPEAT ISSUES
— Contamination of air and dust
— Manipulative Business Strategies
— Unintentional Potential Effects
— VOCs

PRODUCTS OF CONCERN
— Products in part III to consider: Cleaning products, personal care products, toys, interior furnishings (paints/wallpaper, conventional textiles, mattresses, bedding, and carpets), and products that create electromagnetic fields

TIPS: Healthier Crib

An organic solid-wood crib is the safest choice. If you can't get certified organic, then choose solid wood (preferably other than pine) rather than pressed-wood products.

Seek out furniture that has been finished with water-based solvents. Look for no- or low-VOC paints or lacquers.

You could buy an unfinished crib that you can finish yourself. Consider VOC-free beeswax. Read product labels, as not all store-bought beeswax is VOC-free; some formulations even have danger, flammable, or poison warnings. Seal all composite wood parts with a product proven to reduce formaldehyde emissions, such as AFM Safecoat Safe Seal (AFMSafeCoat.com).

If using an older crib, test the paint for lead. The EPA's National Lead Information Center can help you identify potential lead-based paint in used furniture. Also, check that it has not been recalled by the US CPSC (cpsc.gov), and make sure it meets the latest federal safety standards.

Remember that even "green" cribs may be finished with petrochemicals and constructed with formaldehyde-emitting woods.

Crib Mattresses and Bedding Materials

AN OVERLOOKED RISK?

Sudden infant death syndrome (SIDS) is a leading cause of death in infants up to 12 months of age. Yet, even after more than 50 years of research, the causes of SIDS are still not fully understood.

Risk factors have been identified, such as physical and environmental conditions. However, explanations remain mysterious; hence, contributing factors remain unidentified. The toxic gas theory proposes that toxic nerve gases result from the mixture of common household microorganisms and toxicants in mattresses, such as flame retardants (Richardson 1994). Believers in the theory allege that, when inhaled, toxic gases can cause inflammatory responses or lead to the cessation of heart functioning and breathing.

Barry Richardson, a British chemist who specialized in the deterioration and preservation of materials, published research starting in the late 1980s that supported this theory. Jim Sprott MSc PhD, a New Zealand scientist and chemist who also believed the theory, led a crib mattress wrapping campaign in New Zealand.

Before this campaign, New Zealand suffered from the world's highest rate of SIDS with 2.1 deaths per 1,000 live births (Sheppard 2015). Since this campaign began in 1995, the rate of SIDS in New Zealand has dropped 80 percent, according to CotLife2000.co.nz, an arguably unbiased source since the site also sells crib mattress covers that were used in this campaign. As of 2013, there had been no reported SIDS cases among the more than 235,000 babies who slept on a properly wrapped mattress. Among babies not involved in the study during that same time, 1,020 experienced SIDS (CotLife2000 2015).

While scientists have studied the toxic gas theory, there is still no consensus on the hypothesis. In 1998, a well known report among those who follow the issue, the UK Limerick Report, published its findings. The report claims that its investigation disproved the toxic gas theory. However, some scientists attacked the report's scientific analysis in detail, asserting that the investigations did not disprove the theory.

Searching for facts was challenging: The contents of referenced articles were missing more often than usual. The controversies and debates that I read about reminded me of patterns similar to the Manipulative Business Strategies discussed in chapter I.12. For parents who are inclined to take precautionary measures, I was struck by the following two reports:

— Hannes Kapuste MD, a German environmental medicine practitioner, conducted a statistical analysis on the data related to the crib mattress-wrapping campaign. The results were published in the German peer-reviewed journal *Zeitschrift fuer Umweltmedizin (Journal of Environmental Medicine 2002; 44:18-22)*, which is noted online but which I could not find. Dr. Kapuste determined that the statistical proof that mattress-wrapping prevents SIDS is "one billion billion times the level of proof which medical researchers generally regard as constituting certain proof of a scientific proposition," according to Stop Sids Now (2015), also an arguably unbiased source. According to the website StopSidsNow.com, "Dr. Kapuste described the toxic gas theory for crib death and mattress-wrapping for crib death prevention as having 'overwhelming reliability.'"

— Separately, a study was conducted on the influences of certain bedding materials (like vinyl, polyurethane foam, and organic cotton, materials often used in conventional crib mattresses) on the respiration of mice. The synthetic materials were found to impair breathing: Polyurethane foam covered with vinyl caused the largest air flow decrease, affecting 26 percent of mouse breaths. Organic cotton padding caused very different results: After mice were exposed to this bedding, their respiratory rate and volume of air increased. In other words, organic cotton bedding improved respiration (Anderson and Anderson 2000).

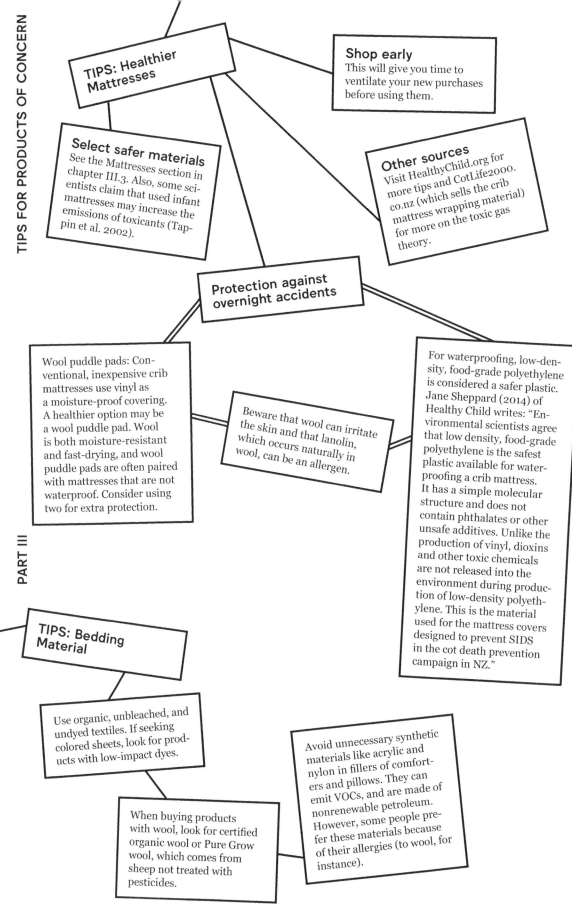

TIPS: Healthier Mattresses

Shop early
This will give you time to ventilate your new purchases before using them.

Select safer materials
See the Mattresses section in chapter III.3. Also, some scientists claim that used infant mattresses may increase the emissions of toxicants (Tappin et al. 2002).

Other sources
Visit HealthyChild.org for more tips and CotLife2000.co.nz (which sells the crib mattress wrapping material) for more on the toxic gas theory.

Protection against overnight accidents

Wool puddle pads: Conventional, inexpensive crib mattresses use vinyl as a moisture-proof covering. A healthier option may be a wool puddle pad. Wool is both moisture-resistant and fast-drying, and wool puddle pads are often paired with mattresses that are not waterproof. Consider using two for extra protection.

Beware that wool can irritate the skin and that lanolin, which occurs naturally in wool, can be an allergen.

For waterproofing, low-density, food-grade polyethylene is considered a safer plastic. Jane Sheppard (2014) of Healthy Child writes: "Environmental scientists agree that low density, food-grade polyethylene is the safest plastic available for waterproofing a crib mattress. It has a simple molecular structure and does not contain phthalates or other unsafe additives. Unlike the production of vinyl, dioxins and other toxic chemicals are not released into the environment during production of low-density polyethylene. This is the material used for the mattress covers designed to prevent SIDS in the cot death prevention campaign in NZ."

TIPS: Bedding Material

Use organic, unbleached, and undyed textiles. If seeking colored sheets, look for products with low-impact dyes.

When buying products with wool, look for certified organic wool or Pure Grow wool, which comes from sheep not treated with pesticides.

Avoid unnecessary synthetic materials like acrylic and nylon in fillers of comforters and pillows. They can emit VOCs, and are made of nonrenewable petroleum. However, some people prefer these materials because of their allergies (to wool, for instance).

Toys

TIPS: Guidelines for Safer Toys

HOUSEHOLD REPEAT OFFENDERS

Toxicants
— BPA
— Cadmium
— Lead
— Phthalates

Ingredients
— Chemical flame retardants
— Heavy metals
— Synthetic colors
— Synthetic fragrance

Materials
— Conventional textiles
— Plastics, like vinyl
— Polyurethane foam

02. If your child's painted toys show signs of wear, such as scratches or flaking, then dispose of them. It's safer to skip toys coated with any kind of paint unless labels or manufacturers' statements specifically indicate that they're free of lead, cadmium, and so on.

01. Review the website of the US CPSC to see if products in your home have been the subject of safety warnings. Don't assume that everything on store shelves is safe. While retailers are required to comply with all major recalls, the logistics of removing millions of recalled products is difficult, and some will continue to be sold.

03. If you suspect a toy might contain lead, test it with a home kit. When it comes to lead, no amount is safe.

04. Reduce the number of toys that are made of plastic, especially for infants and toddlers.

05. Wash toys and stuffed animals regularly to reduce dust accumulation.

07. Online shopping and research is an efficient way to find healthier toys. Healthy-Stuff.org is a great resource.

06. No matter what material your tub toys are made of, they should be towel-dried post-bath or lined up on the side of the tub until they're good and dry, then stored in a well-ventilated area so mold won't grow. Clean toys with soap and water or soak them in vinegar and water. If you have a toy that seems a little grimy, scrub with a little peroxide, then rinse. It will kill bacteria and mold, but not mold spores. However, spores won't multiply on dry surfaces, so make sure the toys are thoroughly dried.

09. The Simple Strategies at the end of this chapter highlight five key questions you can investigate to rule out most toys that pose a toxicant risk.

08. Although toys made in China have been implicated in many safety recalls, don't assume that toys made elsewhere are safe. One of the highest lead levels detected (190,943 ppm) in one study was on a Halloween Pumpkin Pin made in the US. HealthyStuff.org reports that it has found no correlation between the presence of toxicants and the country of origin (Healthy Stuff 2015).

TIPS: Accessories

01. Seek materials besides plastic when purchasing accessories like purses and jewelry, like jacquard, velvet, crinkled crepe, satin, wood, and metal.

02. Beware of cheap jewelry. Costume jewelry regularly tests positive for high levels of lead and cadmium, and there have been a number of recalls by the CPSC because of it. As lead has become a significant consumer concern, cadmium has increasingly been used as a substitute in paint, toys, and children's jewelry. Children can become exposed to cadmium (which is a neurotoxin and carcinogen) when they touch, chew, or swallow a product. Hazards as a result of lead or cadmium exposure include permanent brain damage, and children are the most vulnerable to these health risks.

Instead, have children make their own jewelry out of safer materials, like wood beads and dried pasta. Recently, my daughter thoroughly enjoyed drawing her own jewelry on paper and then cutting it out and taping it on.

Avoid jewelry that has plastic cords, dull metallic components, or artificial pearls, as these pieces may can contain lead.

In March 2012, HealthyStuff.org announced the results of a study in which researchers studied low-cost children's and adult jewelry for chemicals, including lead, cadmium, arsenic, mercury, bromine, and chlorine (in PVC). Over half (57 percent) of the tested products were of high concern because they contained high levels of one or more dangerous chemicals. Four products contained more than 10 percent cadmium. Lead was found in fifty percent of the products, half of which contained amounts higher than 100 ppm in one more components, which exceeds the CPSC's limit of lead in children's products (Ecology Center 2012a).

03. Forgo shiny and colorful plastic umbrellas, as they are commonly produced with PVC. Instead, choose products made from nylon or other materials.

04. Read more about costumes in chapter III.6.

TIPS: Helpful
Resources

01. CPSC (cspc.gov)
maintains a list of toy recalls.

02. GoodGuide.com ranks
products (including toys),
based on criteria like
environmental hazards and
health effects.

03. HealthyStuff.org, run
by the Ecology Center, a
nonprofit organization based
in Ann Arbor, Michigan,
tests a range of consumer
products for toxicants. Since
2007, Healthystuff.org has
screened more than 5,000
toys and ranks product items
by their level of concern,
based on roughly 10 priority
chemicals. While it uses an
X-ray technology to detect
harmful substances, the
technology cannot detect all
chemicals.

04. When shopping for
older children interested
in electronics, consult
Greenpeace's Guide to
Greener Electronics
(greenpeace.org) before
purchasing.

TIPS: Children's
Beauty Products

Avoid children's makeup,
temporary tattoos, and
nail polish, even when
labeled nontoxic. This is
not a regulated claim, and
they rarely are nontoxic.
They probably contain
solvents, artificial colors,
preservatives, and heavy
metals. Some temporary
tattoos and costume makeup
have been found with lead
and cadmium.

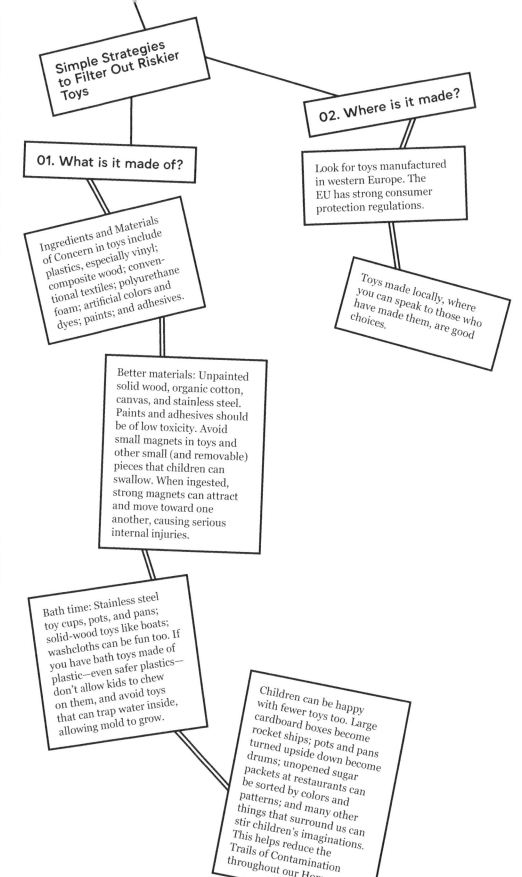

Simple Strategies to Filter Out Riskier Toys

01. What is it made of?

Ingredients and Materials of Concern in toys include plastics, especially vinyl; composite wood; conventional textiles; polyurethane foam; artificial colors and dyes; paints; and adhesives.

Better materials: Unpainted solid wood, organic cotton, canvas, and stainless steel. Paints and adhesives should be of low toxicity. Avoid small magnets in toys and other small (and removable) pieces that children can swallow. When ingested, strong magnets can attract and move toward one another, causing serious internal injuries.

Bath time: Stainless steel toy cups, pots, and pans; solid-wood toys like boats; washcloths can be fun too. If you have bath toys made of plastic—even safer plastics—don't allow kids to chew on them, and avoid toys that can trap water inside, allowing mold to grow.

Children can be happy with fewer toys too. Large cardboard boxes become rocket ships; pots and pans turned upside down become drums; unopened sugar packets at restaurants can be sorted by colors and patterns; and many other things that surround us can stir children's imaginations. This helps reduce the Trails of Contamination throughout our Homes.

02. Where is it made?

Look for toys manufactured in western Europe. The EU has strong consumer protection regulations.

Toys made locally, where you can speak to those who have made them, are good choices.

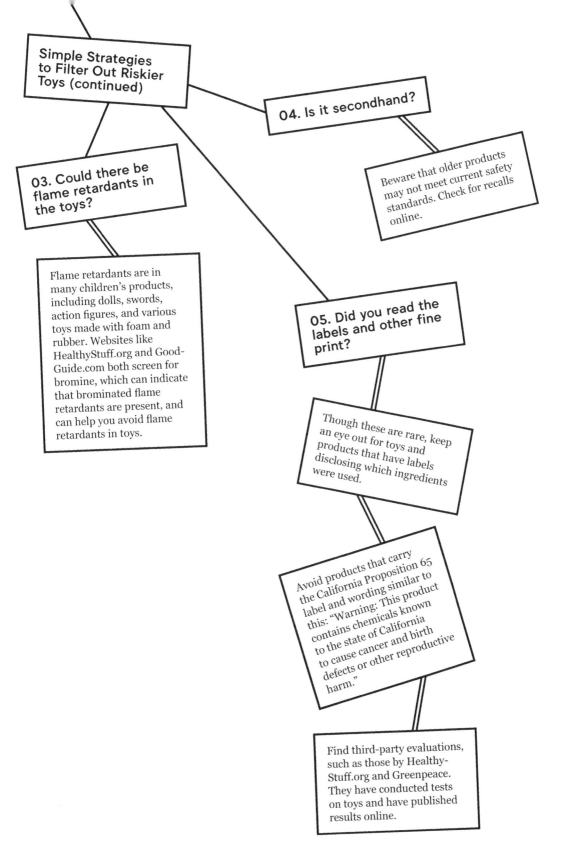

Simple Strategies to Filter Out Riskier Toys (continued)

04. Is it secondhand?

Beware that older products may not meet current safety standards. Check for recalls online.

03. Could there be flame retardants in the toys?

Flame retardants are in many children's products, including dolls, swords, action figures, and various toys made with foam and rubber. Websites like HealthyStuff.org and Good-Guide.com both screen for bromine, which can indicate that brominated flame retardants are present, and can help you avoid flame retardants in toys.

05. Did you read the labels and other fine print?

Though these are rare, keep an eye out for toys and products that have labels disclosing which ingredients were used.

Avoid products that carry the California Proposition 65 label and wording similar to this: "Warning: This product contains chemicals known to the state of California to cause cancer and birth defects or other reproductive harm."

Find third-party evaluations, such as those by Healthy-Stuff.org and Greenpeace. They have conducted tests on toys and have published results online.

Simple Strategies to Reduce Your Children's Exposures

01. Wash kids' hands often!
Try to wash your children's hands before they eat; after they've touched dusty surfaces; after they've played with soft plastic materials, electronics, or arts and crafts supplies; and after they've been outside.

02. Notice what they frequently put in their mouths
Make sure items that kids put in their moths often (such as teethers and toys) are made of safer materials (such as unpainted wood or stainless steel).
Be mindful that some children chew window sills, crib railings, and other painted surfaces.

03. Examine their diet
Refer to the Simple Strategies in chapter III.2. Children's diets tend to include more plastic-wrapped cheeses, juice boxes, and other packaged foods.

04. What is their sleep environment like?
Refer to Simple Strategies in chapter III.3 and relevant tips in this chapter to create the healthiest bedroom environment that you can. Also refer to part IV for great tips on improving indoor air quality.

05. What is slathered on their skin?
Products that are pure enough to eat are the safest, such as organic coconut oil and olive oil. Refer to the Simple Strategies for Children's Personal Care Products.

06. Toys
Refer to the Simple Strategies of five key questions to pursue.

07. Minimize popular Materials of Concern (Chapter II.3) in children's products.

Plastics

Avoid vinyl and brightly colored plastics that young children might put in their mouths. Avoid plastic that is visibly deteriorating.

Polyurethane foam

Avoid when possible (in upholstered furniture, toys, etc.), especially if exposed and crumbling.

Paints

Consider what toxicants may be in them, especially because children chew or mouth toys and crib railings.

Wood

Products made of solid wood—not pressed wood or plywood—are ideal. Be sure they are treated with nontoxic finishes. Finishes of natural oils or beeswax are the safest. If you're unsure whether a product contains pressed or solid wood, look at the edges. If you see layers of wood, it's most likely pressed wood and may have been made with formaldehyde-releasing glues.

Textiles

When buying toys, apparel, or gear that are made with textiles or leather, be aware of toxic dyes. Some, such as azo dyes, which are common in the textile and leather industries, may form carcinogenic compounds after inhalation, or through absorption by the skin or gastrointestinal tract. Choose toys made of wood and other natural materials, or products that carry eco-labels, in order to avoid these harmful dyes. Products with healthier textiles, such as dolls or stuffed animals, may have a European eco-label like Oeko-Tex. Synthetic leather and other rubbery, flexible items often contain vinyl: They may be found in kids' baseball gloves, balls, bracelets, and other items with rubbery and flexible textures.

Chapter III.6
Miscellaneous

OVERVIEW

Household Repeat Offenders and repeat issues continue to affect us through additional products both inside and outside the home, such as cars, pets, and more. This chapter spotlights miscellaneous stuff that I wish I knew sooner in caring for my family.

IN THIS CHAPTER:
— Cars
— Electromagnetic fields
— Exercise stuff
— Holidays and parties
— Home office and children's "work" areas
— Outdoor considerations
— Packaging
— Pets

Cars

OVERVIEW

Chemicals used in car interiors can release toxicants into air and dust, contaminating surface areas such as steering wheels, dashboards, and seats.

Most exposure to toxic compounds in our cars are through inhalation of dust and vapors. There are several studies that have addressed the concentration of VOCs, brominated flame retardants, and hydrocarbons in car interiors. A good number of these compounds, including benzene, toluene, and xylene, were detected at levels that exceeded quality standards for indoor and outdoor air. At times, in-vehicle VOC concentrations were 2 to 3 times higher than levels found in other means of transportation, and they were also higher than what is found in residential settings. In a study conducted by Scientific Instrument Services, more than 50 VOCs were identified in an air sample from a new car. Exposure can be significant since people spend approximately 5.5 percent of their time in their automobiles (Ecology Center 2012b).

The WHO recognizes interior air pollution of vehicles as a significant threat to human health (Ecology Center 2012b). Furthermore, the electrical nature of modern cars and their metal bodies may concentrate EMFs in the car's interior. Some people are sensitive to this, and may experience adverse reactions.

HOUSEHOLD REPEAT OFFENDERS

Toxicants
— Chlorine
— Lead
— Phthalates

Ingredients
— Chemical flame retardants, such as PBDEs and other brominated flame retardants (BFRs). For some BFRs, car exposures add almost 30 percent to total daily exposure (Ecology Center 2012b).
— Solvents
— Synthetic colors

Materials
— Conventional textiles
— Polyurethane foam
— Plastics, including vinyl

ADDITIONAL OFFENDERS
— EMFs
— Hydrocarbons
— Other heavy metals: Antimony, chromium, cobalt, copper, nickel, mercury, and tin
— Particulate matter
— VOCs, such as benzene, toluene, and styrene

REPEAT ISSUES
— Trails of Contamination throughout our Homes

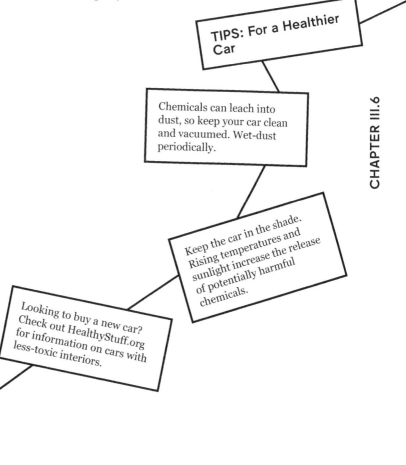

TIPS: For a Healthier Car

Chemicals can leach into dust, so keep your car clean and vacuumed. Wet-dust periodically.

Keep the car in the shade. Rising temperatures and sunlight increase the release of potentially harmful chemicals.

Looking to buy a new car? Check out HealthyStuff.org for information on cars with less-toxic interiors.

Ask passengers to switch mobile devices to airplane mode. Even better: Turn them off! The metal body of a car may trap EMFs, concentrating passengers' exposures.

Electromagnetic Fields (EMFs)

OVERVIEW

Electromagnetic fields (EMFs) or electromagnetic radiation (EMR) broadly describes electric and magnetic forces that are created both naturally and artificially by wired and wireless technologies, as chapter I.14 explained. Electric fields are produced by electric charges, and magnetic fields are produced by and surround any electrical device that is plugged in and turned on. Each of our homes has its own unique electromagnetic fields.

Since the human body has its own internal electrical systems (for example, our hearts and brains are regulated by bioelectrical signals), there is debate about whether artificial EMFs can disrupt these biological processes. Some experts believe that exposure to artificial EMFs can sometimes cause discomfort and disease. A study published in 1975 found that exposure to very weak microwave radiation breaches a critical protector of the brain: the regulatory interface known as the blood–brain barrier (Frey 2012).

Never before have we been surrounded by as much EMFs as we are today. It begins at a young age, and it's chronic. Further, it is intensifying as more public and private spaces set up wireless services, and we work more than ever in front of computers or with laptops on our bodies for hours. Cancer and other illnesses can develop over decades. The wireless industry has not existed long enough for us to have sufficient data to know whether these chronic exposures are safe.

In the US, there are no federal standards limiting occupational or residential exposure to power line EMFs. Some states set standards for the width of right-of-ways under high-voltage transmission lines because of the potential for electric shock.

Governments and schools have taken, or are recommending, precautionary measures. Examples include Australia, Austria, Germany, the UK, Canada, Ireland, India, France, Israel, Sweden, and several US states including California, Colorado, Hawaii, New York, Ohio, Texas, and Wisconsin.

HOUSEHOLD REPEAT OFFENDERS

Toxicants
— Electromagnetic fields: They are classified as possible carcinogens (IARC 2011)

REPEAT ISSUES
— Current exposures are unprecedented.
— Disclosure is lacking on the degree of EMF exposure caused by various devices and what the potential health risks are.
— Exposures at typical levels are linked to adverse health effects, including DNA damage, reproductive harm, neurotoxicity, Alzheimer's disease, and autism (Sage 2014).
— Safe levels of exposure and unique vulnerabilities are not fully understood.
— The examples of others indicate growing concern, as governments around the world are taking precautionary measures.
— Unintentional Potential Effects: EMFs may weaken the blood–brain barrier, rendering the brain more vulnerable to other toxicants.

POSSIBLE HEALTH EFFECTS
The IARC and the World Health Organization (WHO) have classified radiofrequency energy as "possibly carcinogenic to humans" (IARC 2011). This is the same classification given to lead, engine exhaust, DDT, and jet fuel. Chapter I.14 discusses potential health threats.

POSSIBLE SOURCES OF EXPOSURE
Electrical and electronic appliances and power lines: Cabled alarm clocks, televisions, cabled computers and computer monitors, appliances, hair dryers, power lines, electrical wiring, other electronics, and other cabled appliances. Wireless devices: Cell phones, cordless phones, Wi-Fi routers, wireless laptops, handheld devices, baby monitors, surveillance systems, wireless utility meters (smart meters), cellular antennas and towers, and broadcast transmission towers.

Turn off your wireless devices at night. If you can't, then put them into airplane mode, which turns off the device's ability to search for and receive signals. This stops the device from emitting radio-frequency radiation.

Turn wireless devices to airplane mode whenever you don't need the connectivity and whenever children are handling them.

Reduce your use of cell phones, cordless phones, and wireless products. Limit your children's use as well.

TIPS: Use Airplane Mode Often

KEY TIP: Reduce Your Use

TIPS: Protect Your Restorative Sleep

TIPS: Consult the Experts

Sleep time should be radiation-free. Turn Wi-Fi routers and cell phones off at night so your body can rest and rejuvenate. Even if your phone is not in use, it will emit radiation if it is turned on. If you must have your phone near you at night, then turn it to airplane mode.

The EWG ranks phones by radiation levels and has links for consumers who want to get involved by telling the FCC and FDA to update their cell phone radiation standards. Go to ewg.org/cellphone-radiation.

Minimize technology (Wi-Fi or cable-connected) in your bedroom, especially connected to things near your head or headboard. Things to reconsider include your clock radio, electric blanket, heated waterbed, bedside lamp, television, remote control, electrical wiring, cordless telephone, or computer.

For wired or wireless electronics that must stay in your bedroom, like an electric clock, place them at least a few feet away from the bed.

Avoid baby monitors. There are currently no radiation-free baby monitors sold in the US. Try to avoid a DECT monitor, which operates at more or less the same frequency as a cell phone. If you must have a monitor, be sure to position the transmitter as far from the baby as possible.

Check out the website from Environmental Health Trust, which was founded by epidemiologist and phone radiation expert Devra Davis PhD MPH. It has great information on EMFs.

Some believe that if your mattress contains innersprings, then your bed could expose you to more EMFs. So, in addition to minimizing technology in your bedroom, you could consider a mattress that's free of metal.

Wear bras that have no metal underwire.

TIPS: Healthier Uses

TIPS: Create Space

Reduce your family's chronic exposure to your wireless router by keeping it as far away from people as possible (for instance, in an unoccupied room). Radiation dissipates the farther you get from the source, so create distance between you and your other electronics too.

Use cables rather than wireless connections wherever possible. Ideally, wire your home computers, and avoid cordless phones and wireless baby monitors, among other electronics.

Cell phone manufacturers must provide instructions regarding the safest ways to use and carry their products, which depends on how much EMFs the devices emit. These guidelines aren't always easy to find, so read manufacturers' instructions carefully.

Keep cell calls short; duration of the exposure matters.

Use a headset to keep the cell phone far from your head and your body. This can lower exposure to the brain by 90 percent, but it can also expose other areas of the body.

If headphones aren't available, then use your phone's speaker function. Keep the phone a hand's distance away from your head (Davis 2010).

Sending texts generates less radiation (Davis 2010). Just don't text while driving.

Choose to carry your phone in a handbag or a hip holster, and consider purchasing a radiation-blocking pouch for your devices. Choices can be found at LessEMF.com and PongResearch.com.

Use speakerphone/headset. A Blue Tube headset is radiation-free and can be found on Amazon. Bluetooth is not recommended, as it can also be a source of significant EMF exposure.

Minimize the time you place a wireless laptop on your lap.

Avoid cordless phones at home. Cordless phones transmit full-power microwave radiation 24/7, whether the phone is being used or not. This is usually the biggest source of microwave radiation within the home. If you must have one in the home, do not speak on it for long periods. Let your children use a corded phone instead. Don't keep a cordless phone in the bedroom, where sleep should be restorative.

Avoid placing the laptop on your body, especially if you're pregnant. One study of EMFs' influence on the body, including on that of the fetus, recommended that "laptop" be renamed "to not induce customers towards an improper use" (Bellieni et al 2012). Some companies sell products, like pads and fabrics, that claim to reduce your exposure to EMFs from laptops, when used properly.

Have children avoid putting cell phones to their heads. According to experts, "When used by children, the average RF energy deposition is two times higher in the brain and up to ten times higher in the bone marrow of the skull, compared with mobile phone use by adults" (Landrigan and Etzel 2014).

TIPS: Reduce Radiation Exposure from Medical Imaging

Ask questions. Is a medical imaging test the best option? Can radiation be limited without compromising diagnostic quality? In what ways will the exam improve your (or your child's) health care? Are there other options for effective testing methods that do not use ionizing radiation? What measures have been taken to minimize the risks? What additional steps are needed to complete the imaging study (like the use of a contrast agent, sedation, or advance preparation; FDA 2014c)?

If imaging is required for your child, ask your physician to recommend an imaging center that uses appropriate pediatric techniques.

Check credentials. The FDA (2014d) recommends that you inquire if the facility has American College of Radiology accreditation, if the technologists have the proper credentials, and if the results will be interpreted by a board-certified radiologist or pediatric radiologist.

Try not to use your cell phone in an elevator, plane, or bus, where the signal will bounce off the metal interior and expose others to your phone's EMFs.

Avoid using cell phones in areas with weak signals or when in a vehicle moving at high speed. In such circumstances the phone will continually attempt to connect to a new tower/antenna, and this means it is emitting more radiation (Gupta 2012).

TIPS: Avoid Wireless Use In Certain Circumstances

Switch sides of your head regularly while using a cell phone, to spread out your exposure.

If you notice adverse changes in your health, then experiment with reducing your exposure to EMFs or, even better, take a vacation from technology and see if you feel better.

TIPS: Take Breaks

Electromagnetic Fields (EMFs): Electronics

REPEAT OFFENDERS

Toxicants
— Lead
— Mercury
— PCBs
— PBDEs
— Phthalates
— Tris flame retardants

Ingredients
— Chemical flame retardants

Materials
— Plastics, including vinyl

REPEAT ISSUES
— Electromagnetic fields
— Toxicants that leach into air and dust
— Trails of Contamination throughout our Homes

TIPS: Electronics

Buy conservatively. The more electronics we buy, the more we contaminate our Homes with persistent toxicants. When tossed in a landfill, the toxic components of electronics leach into the groundwater; when incinerated, they pollute the air and can harm workers. Then they travel the world and make their way into our food web.

Discontinue your support of manufacturers that are not committed to the phase out of PVC and other toxic ingredients in their production. Turn to Greenpeace's Greener Electronics Guide for guidance on these manufacturers.

Copy machines and certain printers can generate air-polluting ozone, so ask questions before you buy.

Rather than send unwanted electronics to landfills, consider places that would be happy to accept them as donations, like schools. If disposing, then drop off at a place that will recycle them.

Buy electronic gear from companies that have pledged to responsibly recycle it at the end of its useful life.

Prevent young children from playing with or mouthing electronics.

Flame retardants are added to electronics because electronics generate heat that can lead to fire when housed in flammable plastic. These chemicals may release particulates that settle in keyboard dust, mazes of electrical wires, and thick carpeting.

One type of flame retardant, known as Deca PBDE, is banned in some states but is commonly used in many electronics, including cell phones, computers, fax machines, remote controls, video equipment, printers, photocopiers, toner cartridges, scanners, and electronic components (EWG 2008d).

Many companies have committed to avoiding PBDEs. Ask for PBDE-free products when considering your purchases.

A—Z

Electromagnetic Fields (EMFs): Medical Imaging

OVERVIEW

While the development of medical imaging has provided invaluable benefits, there is increasing concern that its prevalence poses risk. Once relatively rare, medical imaging tests are now routine. According to the National Council on Radiational Protection and Measurements, our exposure to medical radiation increased more than sixfold between the 1980s and 2006 (Redberg and Smith-Bindman 2014). And "Americans now are estimated to receive nearly half of their total radiation exposure from medical imaging and other medical sources, compared with only 15 percent in the early 1980s," according to the PCP (Reuben 2010).

Medical imaging has been tied to various concerns, including a slightly greater risk of cancer later in life (just one CT scan can result in cancer-causing radiation exposure; Redberg and Smith-Bindman 2014). According to the FDA (2014c), "Radiation-induced cancer risks depend on the radiation dose, the patient's age at exposure, the sex of the patient (women are more radiosensitive than men), and the organ irradiated."

Children have a unique vulnerability to the effects of medical imaging. Their smaller bodies absorb more radiation, and they have a longer remaining life span over which to develop cancer than do adults. A 2009 study estimated that, compared with a 40-year-old patient, the risk of cancer from an imaging test doubles for patients under 20 years old (Smith-Bindman et al. 2009). To a developing fetus, the potential effects of radiation from medical imaging include childhood cancer, prenatal death, intrauterine growth restriction, small head size, mental retardation, and organ malformation (McCollough et al. 2007).

REPEAT ISSUES

— Radiation
— Safety standards are not yet fully understood.
— Unintentional Potential Effects
— Unique vulnerabilities

SPECIAL CONCERNS

— Exposure is unprecedented

Exercise Stuff

REPEAT OFFENDERS

Toxicants
— Phthalates
— PFCs
— Triclosan

Materials
— Conventional textiles
— Plastics, including vinyl

REPEAT ISSUES
— Carcinogens
— Endocrine disruptors
— Neurotoxins
— Trails of Contamination

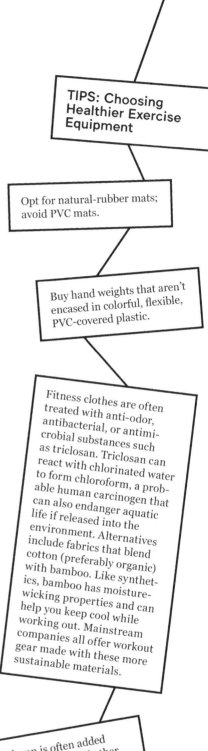

TIPS: Choosing Healthier Exercise Equipment

Opt for natural-rubber mats; avoid PVC mats.

Buy hand weights that aren't encased in colorful, flexible, PVC-covered plastic.

Fitness clothes are often treated with anti-odor, antibacterial, or antimicrobial substances such as triclosan. Triclosan can react with chlorinated water to form chloroform, a probable human carcinogen that can also endanger aquatic life if released into the environment. Alternatives include fabrics that blend cotton (preferably organic) with bamboo. Like synthetics, bamboo has moisture-wicking properties and can help you keep cool while working out. Mainstream companies all offer workout gear made with these more sustainable materials.

Triclosan is often added to towels, socks, and other fabric items. So read labels critically. Clues include items that have antimicrobial properties.

Holidays and Parties

HOUSEHOLD REPEAT OFFENDERS

Toxicants
— Heavy metals, including lead
— Phthalates

Ingredients
— Chemical flame retardants, like polybrominated diphenyl ethers (PBDEs) and other brominated flame retardants (BFRs) in costumes and accessories
— Preservatives
— Solvents
— Synthetic colors
— Synthetic fragrance

Materials
— Plastics, including vinyl

Additional Offenders
— Artificial sugars
— Chromium
— Cobalt
— Nickel
— Toluene

PRODUCTS OF CONCERN
— Candy and other treats
— Christmas trees
— Costumes
— Face paints
— Hair spray
— Holidays string lights
— Lipstick and other costume makeup
— Nail polish
— Temporary tattoos

Face paints
— Seek costumes that do not require face paint. Toxic chemicals in face paints may include lead, nickel, cobalt, and chromium, which are capable of causing skin sensitization and contact dermatitis.
— If your child insists, then consider homemade face paint. Effective recipes can be found online.
— Also avoid lipstick, which can contain lead.
— Nail polish can contain toxic solvents including dibutyl phthalate and toluene, which are linked to hormone disruption and cancer.
— Avoid products with fragrance, which may contain allergens and hormone-disrupting chemicals.

Face masks
— Masks and fake teeth may seem fun, but they may contain toxic chemicals; e.g., endocrine-disrupting phthalates if vinyl is a component.
— If masks are essential, then consider creating your own from simple materials. I have seen many children wearing masks made from cardboard, and they look great!
— Visit CosmeticsDatabase.com to research safer products.

Hair spray
Avoid colored hair spray; kids may inhale the toxic chemicals that these sprays commonly contain. Alternatives include a hat, wig, or some other creative solution that avoids paints and glues.

Christmas lights
— Lead may be in the vinyl that insulates the electrical wires of many Christmas lights.
— Healthier alternatives may be lights that comply with the Restriction of Hazardous Substances (ROHS) standard, which limits lead levels to no more than 1,000 parts per million.
— Other toxicants used in Christmas lights are most likely not listed on the label. So wear gloves when handling lights, especially old ones.

Toxic trees
Artificial Christmas trees are commonly made with PVC. Choose a freshly cut or live tree instead. Buy a Christmas tree that has been grown without pesticides, if possible.

Candy
— Healthier candy options are organic and do not contain GMOs or artificial dyes, sugars and preservatives.
— Instead of candy, give out nonfood items like stickers, school supplies (pencils, erasers, rulers), or even toothbrushes that you can decorate.

Home Office and Children's "Work" Areas

OVERVIEW

Conditions and sources that pollute indoor air quality—lack of ventilation, use of conventional cleaning products, construction materials, electronics, and off-gassing of carpets—apply to the home office and children's arts and crafts area as well. In fact, offices may have exacerbated factors. For example, they tend to have more electronics that can leach toxicants into air and dust and may create EMFs. And creative spaces tend to have more products, like paints, that emit toxicants.

HOUSEHOLD REPEAT OFFENDERS

Toxicants
— Formaldehyde
— PFCs

Ingredients
— Adhesives
— Artificial colors
— Heavy metals
— Solvents

Materials
— Paints
— Plastics, including vinyl
— Synthetic textiles
— Woods

REPEAT ISSUES
— Carcinogens, hormone disruptors, and neurotoxins
— Indoor air quality, including dust
— EMFs

PRODUCTS OF CONCERN
— Common sources of toxicants in a home office are cleaning products, interior furnishings, electronics, and office supplies.

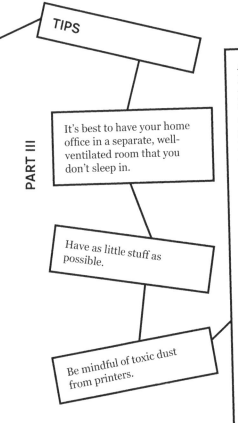

TIPS

It's best to have your home office in a separate, well-ventilated room that you don't sleep in.

Have as little stuff as possible.

Be mindful of toxic dust from printers.

Add plants to your space! Plants are natural air purifiers. They can absorb formaldehyde, benzene, and other chemicals. They won't filter everything, but every little bit helps. To be most effective, use a lot. A NASA study recommends 15 to 18 good-size houseplants in six- to eight-inch-diameter containers to improve air quality in an average 1,800-square-foot house. A few to consider that are easy to find and keep alive are: Boston fern (filters the most unwanted chemicals); Peace lily (alcohols, acetone, formaldehyde, benzene, trichloroethylene); Aloe vera (formaldehyde); Ficus (formaldehyde); Spider plant (carbon monoxide); Bamboo palm (formaldehyde, benzene, and trichloroethylene); and rubber plant (formaldehyde). For more, check out *How to Grow Fresh Air: 50 Houseplants That Purify Your Home or Office*, by B. C. Wolverton.

Refer to Tips Reports 1 and 2 for other tips to improve indoor air and fight dust.

Refer to key products of concern in part III (see above).

Home Office and Children's "Work" Areas: Office, School, and Art Supplies

OVERVIEW
What's the concern?
Office, school, and art supplies are chemical-filled and largely unregulated. Studies are finding hazardous materials in them, such as lead, phthalates, BPA, and cadmium. A study published in August 2012 found toxic phthalates in 75 percent of children's back-to-school supplies, including popular-brand vinyl lunch boxes, backpacks, three-ring binders, raincoats, and rain boots (Schade 2012). The levels detected would be illegal if found in toys.

HOUSEHOLD REPEAT OFFENDERS

Toxicants
— BPA
— Heavy metals, like lead and cadmium
— Phthalates

Ingredients
— Adhesives
— Chemical flame retardants in electronics. Read about the effects of PCBs, PBDEs, and Tris flame retardants in chapter II.1. Also see chapter I.13, Track Record of Substitutes.
— Fragrance
— Solvents
— Synthetic colors

Materials
— Paints
— Plastics, including vinyl

REPEAT ISSUES
— Carcinogens
— Contamination of indoor air and dust
— Hormone disruptors
— Neurotoxins

PRODUCTS OF CONCERN
— Correction fluids
— Paints
— Pens, permanent markers, and crayons
— Toner and ink cartridges

TIPS: Office Supplies

Office supplies—toner and ink cartridges, correction fluids, permanent markers, etc.—contain solvents and other ingredients that may pollute your indoor air and dust. To be safe, avoid those with strong vapors.

Crayons are usually made of petroleum-based ingredients, such as parafin wax and color pigments. It's hard to know what other toxicants may be in crayons, but tests have occasionally identified threatening ones:
— Asbestos has been detected in crayons, even as recently as in 2015 (Saltzman and Hatlelid 2000; Worland 2015).
— In the 1990s, the CPSC recalled crayons after finding lead in some that were imported from China.
   I reiterate to my toddler that she shouldn't eat the crayons and to all my children that they should wash their hands after playing with crayons.

Don't let your kids write on their skin with pens, since the ink may contain a harmful dye or solvent.

Look for water-based permanent markers and correction fluid to reduce VOCs. Find water-based, solvent-free adhesive tapes. And opt for traditional white glues and glue sticks, which tend to be safer than other versions.

The dust from toners for laser printers is quite toxic; when inhaled it can lead to respiratory issues. Most new printers and copiers use the comparatively safer ink jet technology. If you have an old printer, be careful when changing the toner or removing excess toner. You may want to wear a mask. Wipe up dust with a damp cloth, and wash your hands afterward. Always return your empties, and buy refilled ink cartridges rather than new ones. Some companies now offer soy ink as an alternative to petroleum-based versions.

TIPS: Crayons

TIPS: General Guidelines

Get to know the ingredients of art supplies because claims on labels can be misleading. "Nontoxic" doesn't necessarily mean what it says. Ingredients in art supplies that pose a concern include solvents in paints and markers, heavy metals in pigments, and VOCs in paints and glues.

Look for supplies made with natural pigments and materials (for instance, opt for beeswax and soy wax rather than petroleum-derived paraffin wax).

Avoid fragranced products.

If something smells strong and emits fumes—like permanent ink, rubber cement, and many paints—don't let your children use it.

Stick to watercolor paints, less likely than oil-based paints to contain VOCs.

Carefully watch young children who might be tempted to put things like markers in their mouths.

Simpler is better: Think crayons and pencils rather than markers. Encourage your children to make cards and collages using construction and scrap paper and to create papier-mâché sculptures using cornstarch or wheat flour paste.

Always wash hands after making an art project, especially if paint or ink has gotten on the skin.

Bottom line: If it's edible, it's probably safe.

Minimize unnecessary exposure to vinyl. This section contains tips on key categories. The CHEJ's website has many great reports on how to find safer, PVC-free supplies.

TIPS: Modeling Clays

Find clays made without PVC and phthalates.

Minimize unnecessary exposure to polymer clays. Some are made with PVC and can have high levels of phthalates. Even after washing, phthalate residues were found on the hands of children and adults who had worked with polymer clay. This sort of clay requires oven baking to harden, and when the clay was baked, phthalates migrated into the air, raising the possibility of exposure by inhalation.

Make your own play dough out of flour, water, oil, salt, and cream of tartar. Recipes abound online. For color, use the water you boiled beets in or blueberry juice instead of synthetic dye. There are USDA-certified organic natural food-grade dyes, which are also easy to find online.

TIPS: School Supplies

Cut down on plastic to avoid PVCs in notebooks, binders, packaging materials, paper clips, and backpacks. Instead, select products (and, ideally, their packaging) that are made from recycled materials like paper with high post-consumer recycled content, paperboard, and glass.

Avoid single-use disposable packaging.

Avoid products that bear the number "3" or the letters "PVC" within a triangular recycling symbol. That symbol indicates that the product is made with polyvinyl chloride. If neither symbol is on the product, speak with the manufacturer and inquire what it's made of.

Choose plain-looking notebook dividers that are made from only paper or manila. Avoid dividers with plastic (including on the tabs).

Forgo notebooks with metal spirals that are encased in colored plastic. Better choices include notebooks with uncovered metal spirals. Similarly, stick to plain metal paper clips.

Choose organizers and address books that are made with sustainably harvested wood, metal, or paper covers.

Avoid backpacks that have shiny plastic designs. While they may be fun, they typically contain PVC, and may even contain lead.

Use cardboard, fabric-covered, or polypropylene binders.

TIPS: Consider the Unique Circumstances of Your Occupation

Certain workers, including artists, have higher incidences of some diseases than other people in the population due to exposure to hazardous chemicals or materials. So take precautions.

If you're working with toxic materials at home, set up your home office in a space that doesn't share air with the rest of the home. An outbuilding is best.

Educate yourself on the safety of the materials you're working with. Be mindful of solvents. If you're unsure of what a material contains and if it doesn't have ingredients listed on the label, look up its material safety data sheet (MSDS) online.

If harmful substances contaminate your clothes or shoes, then remove them before entering your home, especially if you have young children. You don't want to hug your kids with contaminated clothing.

Outdoor Considerations

HOUSEHOLD REPEAT OFFENDERS

Toxicants
— Heavy metals, like arsenic, lead
— Pesticides
— PFCs
— Phthalates

Ingredients
— Preservatives used in wood
— Synthetic colors

Materials
— Conventional textiles
— Paints
— Plastics, including vinyl
— Woods

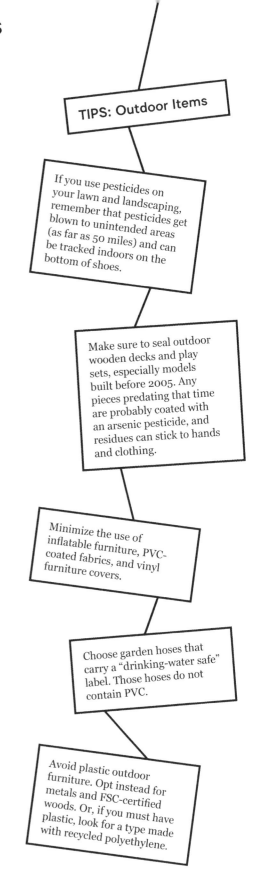

TIPS: Outdoor Items

If you use pesticides on your lawn and landscaping, remember that pesticides get blown to unintended areas (as far as 50 miles) and can be tracked indoors on the bottom of shoes.

Make sure to seal outdoor wooden decks and play sets, especially models built before 2005. Any pieces predating that time are probably coated with an arsenic pesticide, and residues can stick to hands and clothing.

Minimize the use of inflatable furniture, PVC-coated fabrics, and vinyl furniture covers.

Choose garden hoses that carry a "drinking-water safe" label. Those hoses do not contain PVC.

Avoid plastic outdoor furniture. Opt instead for metals and FSC-certified woods. Or, if you must have plastic, look for a type made with recycled polyethylene.

Packaging Materials

HOUSEHOLD REPEAT OFFENDERS
— Phthalates
— Toxicants

Materials
— Plastics, including vinyl

REPEAT ISSUES
— Carcinogens
— Hormone disruptors
— Neurotoxins
— Trails of Contamination

TIPS: For Less Toxic Trails of Contamination

Avoid products that bear the number "3" or the letters "PVC" within a triangular recycling symbol. That symbol indicates that the product is made with polyvinyl chloride. If neither symbol is on the product, speak with the manufacturer and inquire what the product is made of.

Try to avoid products that are packaged in unlabeled plastics (like clamshells and blister packs), which are often PVC.

Products that are packaged with easily recycled materials, such as paper with high postconsumer recycled content, glass, and metal, are good choices.

Minimize single-use disposable packaging whenever possible. Bring your own reusable bag to avoid the use of unnecessary packaging materials.

Pets

HOUSEHOLD REPEAT OFFENDERS

Toxicants
— Pesticides
— Phthalates

Ingredients
— Synthetic fragrance

Materials
— Plastics, including vinyl

REPEAT ISSUES
— Carcinogens
— Contamination of indoor air and household dust
— Hormone disruption
— Neurotoxins

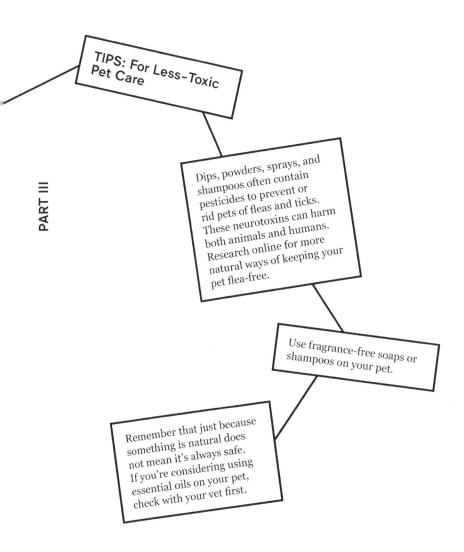

TIPS: For Less-Toxic Pet Care

Dips, powders, sprays, and shampoos often contain pesticides to prevent or rid pets of fleas and ticks. These neurotoxins can harm both animals and humans. Research online for more natural ways of keeping your pet flea-free.

Use fragrance-free soaps or shampoos on your pet.

Remember that just because something is natural does not mean it's always safe. If you're considering using essential oils on your pet, check with your vet first.

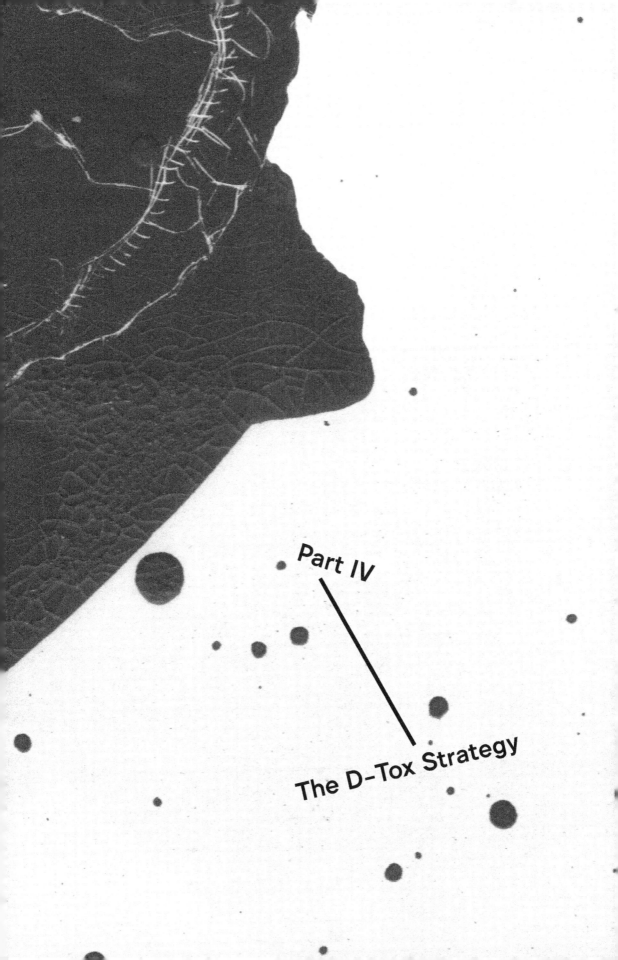

Part IV

The D-Tox Strategy

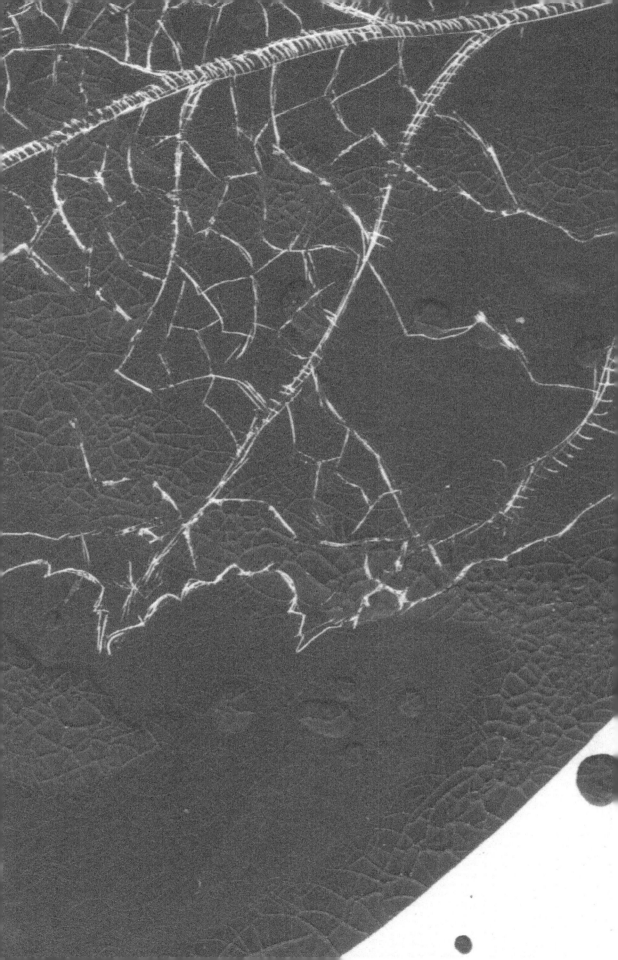

Introduction

The term "D-Tox" is meant to break away from the preconceived notions that "detox" carries. Some associate detox with dieting and juicing. Others think of breaking drug addiction. In this book, "D-Tox" means to "edit" your life with the intention of reducing your Trails of Contamination throughout our Homes, while "detox" means to purify.

"Edit" means to streamline all aspects of your life. This should be done at a pace that is comfortable for you so that you continue to feel successful in making changes.

This chapter considers and prioritizes the information given throughout parts I, II, and III, and discusses the top 10 most effective tips, or goals.

While the content in parts II and III will be invaluable in helping you redecorate a room for a new nursery, make healthier purchases, and select which healthy changes to incorporate next, the 10 tips in this chapter are the key ones that you can focus on daily. Most cost little or nothing.

D-Tox, baby! Our Homes depend on it.

IN THIS CHAPTER:
10 Tips to Focus Your D-Tox Strategy
While these tips are classic ideas, they deserve more popularity. The Tip Reports share science that underscores their impact.

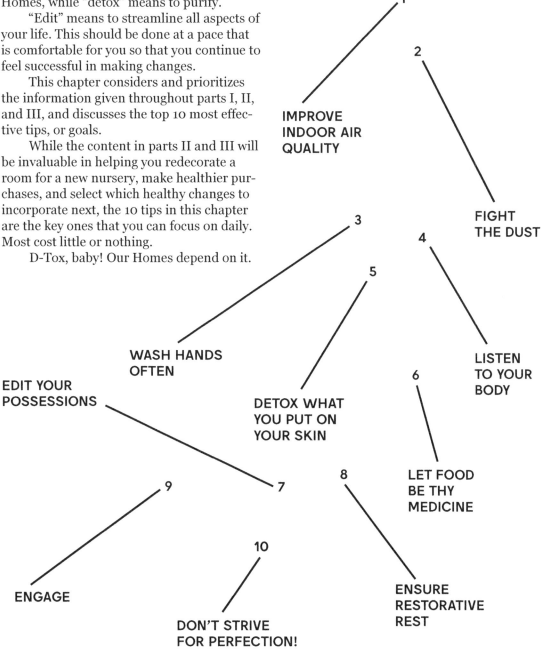

1 — IMPROVE INDOOR AIR QUALITY

2 — FIGHT THE DUST

3 — WASH HANDS OFTEN

4 — LISTEN TO YOUR BODY

5 — DETOX WHAT YOU PUT ON YOUR SKIN

6 — LET FOOD BE THY MEDICINE

7 — EDIT YOUR POSSESSIONS

8 — ENSURE RESTORATIVE REST

9 — ENGAGE

10 — DON'T STRIVE FOR PERFECTION!

Tip Report #1

Improve

Indoor Air Quality

Overview

I thought that outdoor air would be more polluted than indoor air. After all, outdoor air is contaminated frequently by vehicle and industry emissions. Whereas indoor air is protected by walls, roofs, and ventilation systems and has few sources of toxic emissions. As it turns out, I was wrong.

> Indoor levels of pollutants may be two to five times higher, and occasionally more than 100 times higher, than outdoor levels. (EPA 2009)

Levels of certain indoor pollutants like formaldehyde, chloroform, and styrene can range from two to 50 times higher than outdoor levels (Sutton 2011).

Why is indoor air so polluted?

Indoor air can be contaminated by natural sources, such as radon and mold, but it can also be polluted from unnatural sources that are emitted from various household items, like cleaning products, furniture, mattresses, carpets, and paints. Many household products are made of petroleum-based, synthetic materials that release gases, a process known as off-gassing.

Further, buildings are constructed to seal in air more tightly than ever, which helps control temperature and humidity. While this is more planet-friendly because it's more energy efficient, it's not as healthy for indoor residents. It reduces the amount of fresh air in the home, and it forces toxic emissions from household products to accumulate.

POSSIBLE HEALTH EFFECTS

The CPSC warns that some health effects stemming from poor indoor air quality may manifest immediately, while others may manifest either years after exposure or after long or repeated periods of exposure. Effects can include respiratory disease, heart disease, and cancer. They can be severely debilitating or fatal. The CPSC urges us to improve the indoor air quality in our homes even if symptoms are not noticeable (CPSC 2015c).

TERMS TO KNOW

Building-related illness

This term describes symptoms that are proven to be caused by specific indoor environmental agents, or from specific sources within a building (Seltzer 1994).

Sick building syndrome (SBS)

This encompasses symptoms that cannot be linked to specific pollutants or sources within a building. They include headache, irritation of the eye, nose, and throat, dry cough, dry or itchy skin, dizziness and nausea, difficulty in concentrating, fatigue, and sensitivity to odors. Symptoms typically occur inside the building but cease or diminish outside (Asthma and Allergy Foundation of America 2015).

POSSIBLE SOURCES OF EXPOSURE

01. Combustion

Sources include cooking (using gas and wood stoves, burning foods, grilling), fireplaces, tobacco smoke, unvented kerosene and gas space heaters, automobile exhaust, and candles.

— Cooking: Cooking with gas can be one of the most significant sources of indoor air pollution (Magaziner, Bonvie, and Zolezzi 2003).

— Cigarette smoke: Cigarette smoke contains more than 7,000 chemical compounds; according to the CDC, hundreds are toxic and about 70 can cause cancer. Some of these chemicals include formaldehyde, benzene, arsenic, lead, and carbon monoxide (CDC 2011).

— Fireplaces: Fireplaces can release toxic fumes. Burning wood can release formaldehyde, carbon monoxide, sulfur dioxide, polycyclic aromatic hydrocarbons, and sometimes dioxins. Burning wood is known to increase the risk of lung infections and to harm developing children (Hollender and Zissu 2010). Learn more at epa.gov/burnwise.

02. Interior furnishings

Along with building materials, these can contribute to indoor air pollution. Common culprits include paints, wallpaper, furniture, carpets, mattresses, and vinyl shower curtains. For example, formaldehyde is often released from building materials and wood products. Indoor formaldehyde levels depend on the source, the temperature, the humidity, and the amount of ventilation in a room (CPSC 2013).

03. Cleaning products

These can be a major source of indoor air pollution.

04. Natural sources

These can emit gases, like radon, that enter via the basement and rise to higher levels in the home.

05. Pollutants from outdoors

Toxic fumes and dust can enter the home through windows, doors, plumbing vents, building exhausts, electrical outlets, and other openings. We also bring toxicants home in other inadvertent ways, even on our newly cleaned clothes!

06. Dry cleaning

Dry-cleaned items can release highly toxic chemicals into the air, such as trichloroethylene or perchloroethylene ("perc"), the primary cleaning solvent for approximately 95 percent of dry cleaning facilities in the US (Bader 2009). If they are in an enclosed environment such as a car or closet, then levels of these toxic fumes will be more concentrated.

07. Personal care products

Various grooming products (such as hair spray, perfume, cologne, and nail polish) can pollute indoor air with the chemicals they emit.

08. Unintentional toxic fumes

Unintentional Toxicants can be created when fumes from various products combine.

HOUSEHOLD REPEAT OFFENDERS
These contaminate air

This section lists some common toxicants that pollute indoor air, as well as the ingredients, materials, and products that emit them. By focusing on improving your indoor air quality, you'll reduce your exposures to these toxicants as well as others.

Toxicants
— Benzene
— Chlorine
— Formaldehyde
— Methylene chloride
— Polycyclic aromatic hydrocarbons (PAHs)

Ingredients
— Fragrance: A common ingredient in personal care products, it can contain hundreds of chemicals that emit VOCs. One study detected 133 VOCs from 25 products, averaging 17 per product. Approximately 18 percent of those 133 VOCs are recognized as toxic or hazardous under US law, and every product emitted at least one of these compounds (Steineman et al. 2010). Emissions from "organic," "green," or "natural" products were not less harmful (Potera 2011).
— Petroleum-based ingredients

Materials
— Synthetic textiles, especially vinyl
— Polyurethane foam

PRODUCTS OF CONCERN
— Air fresheners: Can emit toxic phthalates and VOCs.
— Art and office supplies: Some, such as paint and glue, contain solvents; others, like binder covers, are made of harmful plastics and are common sources of contaminants.
— Candles: These can release formaldehyde, soot, and PAHs into air. High levels of PAHs have been found in churches after candles or incense were burned (*National Geographic* 2008).
— Carpets: Can emit VOCs. When mice were exposed to 300 carpet samples in a toxicology lab in 1992, the mice had neurotoxic reactions, some severe, and 25 percent died. Some carpet samples were new and some were up to 12 years old (Bader 2009; Gram 1993).
— Cleaning products: May contain solvents and fragrances that are common sources of contaminants.
— Interior wall paints: May off-gas for up to 3.5 years (Chang 2001). Paints used to color products are also a concern.
— Mattresses: Have been found to emit anywhere from 39 to 61 VOCs. While most emissions generally occur in the first 60 days, the off-gassing never completely stops (Bader 2009).
— Personal care products: These contain solvents and fragrances that are common sources of air contaminants.
— Upholstered furniture: Cushioning materials, fabrics, fabric treatments, and wood adhesives are common sources of air contaminants.

ADDITIONAL OFFENDERS

— Carbon monoxide: A deadly gas (CPSC 2015a)

— Chloroform: A VOC and probable human carcinogen that poses other adverse health risks (ATSDR 1997)

— Nitrogen dioxide: A highly reactive gas that poses various adverse health risks (EPA 2014e)

— Perc: A likely human carcinogen that also poses non-cancer risks from chronic exposure, including damage to the nervous, immune, and reproductive systems, specific organs, and overall development (EPA 2015c). Exposure from inhalation occurs in the home from dry-cleaned products.

— Radon: An odorless gas and the second-leading cause of lung cancer; exposure at home is a worldwide health risk (EPA 2015d).

— Styrene: A VOC and anticipated human carcinogen (ATSDR 2012)

SPECIAL CONCERNS

— Toxicants outside the home: May influence the air quality inside the home. Examples of this include car exhaust from a nearby garage, or fumes from stored products with off-gassing solvents, like paints and automobile fluids.

— Unknown Potential Effects: Chronic inhalation and low doses make it difficult to know exactly how dangerous specific chemicals are.

— Unintentional Toxicants: These can be created unknowingly, such as secondary air pollutants.

— Unique vulnerabilities: Vary by age, sex, and individuals.

Tips—Improve Indoor Air Quality

01. Reduce sources of combustion

Ban smoking at home.

Reduce fireplace use.

Never burn printed paper or particleboard.

Install a carbon monoxide detector near the fireplace.

Remember that toxicants from combustion can enter a building from a nearby garage, and make adjustments accordingly. For example, refrain from leaving a car running in a garage.

Open windows when cleaning (but not on days when smog and ozone levels are high, as ozone can aggravate asthma symptoms).

Open windows in bathrooms when heat and humidity increase from a shower or bath, or when personal care products or cleaners have the greatest opportunity to off-gas fumes. If no windows are available, think of creative ways to ventilate.

02. Edit your possessions
Dispose of what's unnecessary. Be selective in what you bring home. Refer to Tip Report 7 for more tips.

03. Ventilate often and during key times
Facilitate fresh air exchange often, even in the winter!

Consider that gases will disperse throughout an interior and that certain areas may be more polluted than others. Concentrations of fumes will generally be higher in a small room than in a large one.

Remember that air pressure in a home can influence chemical dispersion. A vented attic, for example, may attract warm air from the lower floors. This may draw toxic gases like radon and carbon monoxide up from the basement.

Open windows to ventilate when there is combustion, such as when cooking, using a fireplace, or smoking (if smoking must occur at home).

Ventilate during home improvement projects or installation of new interior furnishings. Proper ventilation is especially important if you have recently painted, installed new carpeting, or renovated. After certain activities, like paint stripping, indoor pollution levels have been found to be 1,000 times higher than outside levels (EPA 1988). Products that contain VOCs affect indoor air quality the most during installation and immediately after.

04. Add indoor houseplants

Houseplants have been shown to detoxify indoor air. In the 1970s, in researching indoor air for a possible moon base, NASA scientists—led by B. C. Wolverton PhD, an environmental scientist working with the US military—detected more than 300 volatile organic chemicals (VOCs) inside a spacecraft they tested. The off-gassing of spacecraft materials was the suspected source. Eventually, Wolverton discovered that houseplants help filter common pollutants such as ammonia, formaldehyde, and benzene (Wolverton 1997). If you have pets, however, be aware that some houseplants are poisonous to pets.

Peace lilies and snake plants are easy to find, harder to kill, low-maintenance, and they detox air from indoor pollutants. (Snake plants are poisonous to cats.)

05. Consider air purifiers

Some people with allergies and chemical sensitivities find that air purifiers may reduce indoor levels of animal dander, dust, pollen, and certain toxic fumes like cigarette smoke and VOCs.

Confirm that the machine you buy is adequate for your space and will tackle your specific concerns. For example, a machine that is very effective in addressing cigarette smoke may not be the best one to address VOCs.

Choose HEPA (high-efficiency particulate air) filters, which are more effective in trapping the tiny particles that other purifiers may redistribute into the air.

Change the filters according to manufacturer instructions.

Avoid ozone filters. Ozone is a lung irritant that can cause adverse health effects even at low levels (EPA 2014d). Additionally, ozone filters do not remove dust, pollen, or most other allergens from the home.

07. Regulate humidity and temperature

Temperature, humidity, and light can affect the chemical nature of some substances, making them more harmful. Formaldehyde, for example, can be released more readily from products as temperature and humidity rise. The EPA (2012d), CPSC (2015c), and Mayo Clinic (2013) all recommend maintaining humidity between 30 and 50 percent for better indoor air quality. Those levels will discourage off-gassing as well as the growth of bacteria, mildew, dust mites, and mold.

06. Be mindful of off-the-shelf sprays and powders

Toxicants can easily be inhaled from sprays and powders, more so than from liquids and solids. Common products to be mindful of include air fresheners, talc and other powders, spray-on sunscreens, powders with nanoparticles, perfume/cologne, hair spray, and cleaning products.

08. Reevaluate the use of dry cleaning

Reduce buying clothes that require dry cleaning; wash by hand instead.

If you do have your clothes dry-cleaned, remove the plastic covers as soon as possible (discard them outside your home), and hang the clothes outside for an hour or two. This will reduce fumes from dry cleaning chemicals from accumulating in your home.

Consider less toxic methods, including "wet cleaning" or liquid CO_2 technology.

09. Be particularly careful during renovation projects
Home improvement and renovation projects can create indoor air pollution from paint fumes, wallpaper adhesives, carpets, sofas, mattresses, and so on.

Be aware of the toxicants you may be "awakening" in your home. Common concerns include lead in painted surfaces (especially in homes built before 1978) and asbestos behind walls or under the roof.

Plan to have polluting projects conducted when you and your family can stay elsewhere. The longer you're away, the more time VOCs have to off-gas and disperse.

If pregnant, delegate home improvement projects to others, and avoid being home while work is being done! Try to complete renovations before you conceive.

10. Remember the maintenance details

Clean air conditioner filters regularly, and replace per manufacturer's advice.

Wash window screens every spring.

Periodically test your home for radon.

Follow manufacturers' instructions for their products. For example, if instructed to let a product air out for two hours, do so!

Consider outdoor humidity levels. Humidity can encourage off-gassing, so on especially muggy days, it may be best to keep windows closed.

Cigarette Smoke

According to the American Lung Association (2015), "every year tobacco kills more Americans than did World War II—more than AIDS, cocaine, heroin, alcohol, vehicular accidents, homicide, and suicide combined."

Premature Deaths		
From cigarette smoke	From smoking or exposure to second hand smoke	480,000+ per year
	Additional people who live with a serious illness caused by smoking	8,600,000
From World War II	Soldiers, sailors, airmen, and marines who were killed in battle	292,000
	Members of US forces that died of other causes during WWII	114,000
From other causes	Alcohol	24,518
	AIDS	17,774
	Car accidents	34,485
	Drug use, both legal and illegal	39,147
	Murder	16,799
	Suicide	36,909

Cigarette fumes can be absorbed by clothes, furniture, cars, and other materials. Later, they can be released under various conditions. This is considered third-hand smoke.

Did You Know?

Tip Report #2

Fight

the Dust

Overview

House dust is known for triggering asthma and allergy attacks in some people. However, it is less known for exposing us to toxicants. In fact, dozens of toxicants have been identified in household dust, including arsenic, lead, phthalates, chemical flame retardants, and a number of pesticides (Roberts et al. 2009; Stapleton et al. 2009).

Once these toxicants are indoors, they do not degrade as easily as they would outdoors. Without sun, wind, water, and bacteria to break them down, they persist for longer periods of time in your carpets and other indoor areas (Roberts et al. 2009). Dust is then inhaled, absorbed, and ingested.

Children, who play on the floor and put things in their mouths, generally have much higher levels of these chemicals in their bodies than do their parents (Callahan and Roe 2012).

In fact, infants are estimated to ingest twice as much dust and are up to ten times more vulnerable than adults are to dust exposure (Roberts et al. 2009).

Major sources of pollutants include the bottoms of shoes and consumer products—interior furnishings, electronics, plastics, and more. Frequent exposure to the biological and chemical contaminants found in dust can have both short-term and long-term health effects. In addition to triggering asthma and allergies in some, dust may also contribute to endocrine disruption, reproductive impairment, and certain cancers and may cause lasting damage to the nervous and respiratory systems.

Dr. Dust
John W. Roberts, who passed away in 2008, contributed a great deal to research on dust. While he was an expert on air pollution, he was so distinguished in his contributions to understanding and fighting house dust that he was sometimes referred to as "Dr. Dust." In addition to publishing many enlightening articles, Roberts was instrumental in developing the HVS3 vacuum cleaner, which is used as a standard method for collecting dust for the analysis of pollutants (*Seattle Times* 2008). He was also one of the founders of the Master Home Environmentalist program, which sends trained volunteers to residents' homes to improve indoor air quality at no cost to residents. In 2005 the program earned the EPA's Children's Environmental Health Excellence Award.

In "Monitoring and Reducing Exposure of Infants to Pollutants in House Dust," Roberts et al. (2009) noted that "over 100 potentially toxic metals, pesticides, other carcinogens, other neurotoxins, allergens, and EDCs have been identified in house dust."

HOUSEHOLD REPEAT OFFENDERS
These contaminate dust
This section briefly summarizes the toxicants you can reduce in your home by fighting the dust; and the key ingredients, materials, and products that emit toxicants into dust.

Toxicants
— Coal tar: A carcinogen that contains an estimated 10,000 compounds (EWG 2015d; Franck 1963). It is a by-product of coal and is used in a variety of commercial and consumer products.

— Firemaster® 550: Found in dust and poses various health risks (Hawthorne 2012). It was introduced into commerce to replace PBDEs as a flame retardant, even though its impact on human and environmental health was not understood.

— Heavy metals, like arsenic, cadmium, and lead: May concentrate in house dust at levels 2 to 32 times higher than concentrations in outside garden soil (Roberts et al. 2009; Rasmussen, Subramanian, and Jessiman 2001). For children, household dust is a common source of lead exposure (Roberts et al. 2009; Davies et al. 1990; Lanphear et al. 1996; EPA 1997).

— Other metals, including aluminum, chromium, cobalt, copper, iron, and manganese, have been detected in common house dust.

— PAHs and PCBs: Commonly detected in household dust. One study found that PCB concentrations in dust can increase the risk of non-Hodgkins lymphoma (Roberts et al. 2009; Colt et al. 2005). Other studies found that babies' exposure to BaP, a type of PAH which is found in house dust, may contribute to asthma and impair mental development (Roberts et al. 2009; Miller et al. 2004; Perera et al. 2006).

— PBDEs: House dust may account for up to 82 percent of our PBDE exposure (Roberts et al. 2009; Lorber 2008). Although phased out in the mid-2000s, PBDEs are thought to enter American homes through foreign-made products, such as sofas manufactured in China (Betts 2008).

— Pesticides: Have been detected in dust samples from hundreds of homes in the US (Roberts et al. 2009; Colt et al. 2004). Some, like DDT, have been banned for decades.

— PFCs: Linked with lower birth weight and smaller size in infants, elevated cholesterol, abnormal thyroid hormone levels, liver inflammation, and a weakened immune system (EWG 2015g). The indoor environment can account for up to 50 percent of total ingestion (Haug et al. 2011).

— Phthalates: Known endocrine disruptors, and some are also probable carcinogens (EPA 2007b). One study of dust from 70 homes nationwide found that phthalates made up 89 percent of the total concentration of the 44 toxins identified (McDonald 2007; Costner, Thorpe, and McPherson 2005). "Typically, pesticide concentrations in vacuumable house dust are 10 to 100 times higher than those found in outdoor surface soil" (Roberts et al. 2009).

— Tris flame retardants: Have been detected in the household dust of 96 percent of homes in a Boston-area study (Stapleton et al. 2009). They became a popular replacement for PBDEs, when the latter were phased out of production in the US.

Ingredients

— Chemical flame retardants: Found in various products, chemical flame retardants are a family of many different types, such as PBDEs and tris flame retardants. Researchers at the Silent Spring Institute tested household dust for 49 chemical flame retardants and detected 44 (Dodson et al. 2012).

— Endocrine disrupting chemicals (EDCs): Found in various household and food materials have been detected house hold dust. One study conducted by researchers at the Silent Spring Institute found that of the 89 organic compounds identified as EDCs, 66 were detected in the dust of 120 homes (Roberts et al. 2009; Rudel et al. 2003).

Materials

— Plastics: May contain chemical flame retardants that can escape their products and enter people's bodies via household dust (Schreder 2012).

— Polyurethane foam: Contains chemical flame retardants that can escape their products, accumulating in household dust and entering people's bodies (Schreder 2012).

— Synthetic textiles: May contain chemicals, including flame retardants and stain and water guards, that can escape their products, and accumulate in house dust and people's bodies (Schreder 2012).

— Vinyl: Found in the home as PVC flooring and wall material, vinyl was associated with higher concentrations of phthalates (BBzP and DEHP) in house dust, according to one Swedish study (Bornehag et al. 2005).

ADDITIONAL OFFENDERS

— Allergens, like those originating from dust mites and rodents, have been detected in dust.

— Auto exhaust particles, like lead, can contaminate nearby soil and dust.

— Bacteria and viruses: Found in dust, attributed to traces of saliva and tracked-in bird, rodent, cat, and dog feces (Roberts et al. 2009; Benenson 1985; McCaustland et al. 1982). Bacteria can create endotoxins, which are linked to asthma (Roberts et al. 2009; Thorne et al. 2005).

— Mold: Can collect in house dust. Along with dampness, mold can have an effect similar to that of secondary tobacco smoke, contributing to child asthma, allergies, bronchitis, and other health problems (Roberts et al. 2009; Brunekreef et al. 1989; Institute of Medicine 2000). Children are more vulnerable to the effects of mold exposure than are adults (Roberts et al. 2009; Selgrade et al. 2006).

— Workplace contaminants: Can inadvertently be brought home, where it settles in the dust. In a study of 28 countries and 36 states, the National Institute for Occupational Safety and Health identified a variety of workplace contaminants that posed risks to workers' families, including asbestos, lead, mercury, arsenic, cadmium, estrogenic substances, asthmagens and allergens, infectious agents, and pesticides (CDC 2014b).

PRODUCTS OF CONCERN

— Carpets: Accumulate dust that contains pesticide residues, which are guarded by the carpet from sunlight, rain, temperature extremes, and some microbial action and therefore may persist for years (Roberts et al. 2009).

— Children's sleepwear: May contain chemical flame retardants that can be released into air and dust. Snug-fitting, organic cotton pajamas that are labeled as non-flame-retardant are the best alternative to combat harmful exposures.

— Electronics: Can leach chemicals such as flame retardants that settle in dust.

— Upholstered furniture: Can contain flame retardants that settle in dust. Furniture is even more of a concern if the fabric covering is ripped.

SPECIAL CONCERNS

— Banned chemicals are still found in dust, even those that were regulated decades ago.

— It doesn't matter if you don't use pesticides yourself: They are still likely to be present in your household dust because they can be tracked into the home on shoes.

Tips—Fight the Dust

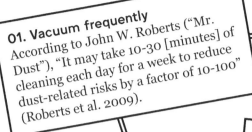

01. Vacuum frequently
According to John W. Roberts ("Mr. Dust"), "It may take 10-30 [minutes] of cleaning each day for a week to reduce dust-related risks by a factor of 10-100" (Roberts et al. 2009).

Consider a vacuum cleaner that detects dirt on your floors and carpets.

Remember that for crawling babies, high-traffic common areas like hallways and kitchens may be particularly polluted. Focus on these areas when you clean.

Choose a model that uses a HEPA filter.

02. Wet-dust after vacuuming
Use a wet microfiber cloth to dust hard surfaces after vacuuming, as vacuuming can stir up dust. A microfiber cloth captures more dust, and wetting it reduces the amount of particles that can recirculate into the air. Change or clean your microfiber cloth every 10 minutes to maintain efficiency, "Dr. Dust" recommends (Roberts et al. 2009).

03. Think twice about buying carpets for the home
Carpets are reservoirs for dust, as substances are sometimes hard to eliminate through normal vacuuming. Contaminants in carpets may include lead, mercury, pesticides, pollen, and more (Roberts et al. 2009).

04. Implement a "no shoes" policy at home

Studies indicate that leaving shoes at the door may keep out toxicants including PAHs from yard soil or residues from garage floors (Schantz et al. 2007), coal tar from driveways and parking lots (Mahler et al. 2010), and pesticides from lawn care (Nishioka et al. 1996). These can enter homes on the bottom of shoes. Research has found that wiping shoes on a mat and leaving them at the door can reduce lead dust and other toxicants by 60 percent (Turner, Gibson, and Reed 2010).

If "no shoes" is impossible, use a large, commercial-grade doormat, and wipe your feet twice before entering the home. A pesticide-tracking study showed that doormats could reduce pesticide residues on carpets by 25 percent and total carpet dust by 33 percent. According to dust researcher John Roberts, effective cleaning and use of doormats may reduce an infant's dust exposure by 90 to 98 percent (Washington Toxics Coalition 2000).

Consider your pets' feet as well. They can contbute to household dust, so rinse them off whenever possible!

05. Isolate certain dirty laundry

If you work or spend time in areas with toxicants, then consider leaving shoes and contaminated clothes outside the home. For example, if you work in landscaping, then your shoes and clothes can collect and bring home pesticides.

06. Ventilate

VOCs and SVOCs (volatile and semi-volatile organic compounds) can migrate from household products and into the air and will settle on surfaces and dust particles. Combat this process by ventilating your home, especially when off-gassing products are first brought into the house.

07. Streamline your possessions

Many products, including electronics and items that contain polyurethane foam (e.g., upholstered furniture, mattresses, and toys), generate dust that contains harmful toxicants. Declutter your space to limit household exposure!

08. Keep in mind that infants and toddlers get the highest dose of dust

According to experts, babies' vulnerability to house dust is 10 times greater than that of adults. Dust is the main source of infant exposure to allergens, lead, and PBDEs and a major source of exposure to pesticides, PAHs, bacteria, arsenic, cadmium, chromium, phthalates, phenols, other EDCs, mutagens, and carcinogens. For the very young, contact with these pollutants is linked with higher rates of asthma, loss of intelligence, ADHD, and cancer (Roberts et al. 2009).

09. Think critically about your environment

Old buildings, homes, schools, or hotels may contain higher levels of lead, PCBs, PBDEs, and other banned pollutants.

Think critically about the best times to open windows for fresh air since unique exposures occur in areas with high vehicle traffic, farming activity, or proximity to a Superfund site.

10. Pregnant? Be extra mindful

Detected in dust, chemical flame retardants can cross the placenta and enter breast milk (Mazdai et al. 2003). Prenatal exposure to one type, PBDE, is linked with adverse birth outcomes such as decreased birth weight, length, and chest circumference (Rao et al. 2007) and cryptorchidism, or undescended testicles (Main et al. 2007). It may impair a child's neurodevelopment as well (Eskenazi et al. 2013).

Tip Report #3

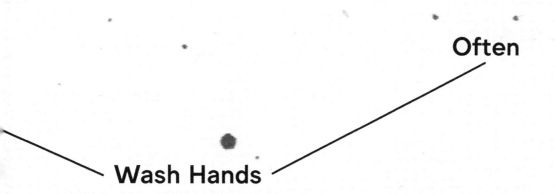

Overview

The hygiene hypothesis proposes that exposures to bacteria and germs in childhood may strengthen the immune system. While experts continue to study this theory, those familiar with the toxicants in dust advocate frequent hand washing. For example, Heather Stapleton PhD, one of the nation's leading authorities on chemical flame retardants found in households, has recommended it as an important step in reducing one's exposure to those chemicals (Hawthorne 2012).

Toxicants found in dust, as well as chemicals (like phthalates and lead) in toys and other items, can end up on your fingers. For years doctors have widely recommended frequent hand washing to battle the microbes that cause infectious diseases like the flu. Toxicants are just another reason to wash your hands often, especially before eating.

Dust has more than just allergens
Studies have detected dozens of toxicants—pesticides, carcinogens, neurotoxins, endocrine disruptors, and more—in dust (Roberts et al. 2009; Butte and Heinzow 2002; Rudel et al. 2003).

HOUSEHOLD REPEAT OFFENDERS
These contaminate hands
Below are some common toxicants that may be reduced by washing hands more frequently. Descriptions of these toxicants can be found in Tip Report 2: Fight the Dust. Special concerns that may motivate your family to wash hands more often are noted below.

Toxicants from Dust
— Banned chemicals, like PCBs
— Chemical flame retardants, including PBDEs, Tris flame retardants, and Firemaster® 550 chemicals
— Coal tar
— Endocrine disrupting chemicals, such as phthalates
— Heavy metals, like lead, arsenic, and cadmium
— PAHs
— Pesticides
— Unintentional Toxicants

Additional Toxicants
— Allergens
— Auto exhaust particles
— Bacteria
— Mold
— Other metals, including aluminum, chromium, cobalt, copper, iron, and manganese
— Phenols
— Workplace contaminants

Special Concerns
— Semi-volatile organic compounds (SVOCs): These stick to surfaces or dust particles, which can then be transferred to hands. They include several types of phthalates and flame retardants.
— Toxic residues: Formed from various sources, such as cleaning products and pesticides, they settle on surface areas and in dust, which can be picked up on hands.
— Unique vulnerabilities

Tips—Wash Hands Often

01. Wash with organic soap and water
Avoid antibacterial products. Read more about antibacterials in chapter III.1 and about triclosan in chapter II.2.

02. Be especially diligent with children
Experts suggest that children are ten times more vulnerable to the hazards in house dust than are adults (Roberts et al. 2009). Wash children's hands after they have crawled, played outside, and used toys, electronics, and art supplies. Do the same before they eat and sleep, too!

03. Use edible moisturizers
Given how often I wash my hands and prepare snacks and meals for the kids, I moisturize with organic coconut oil or olive oil. Both are safe enough to eat so safe enough to rub off on their meals and snacks!

Tip Report #4

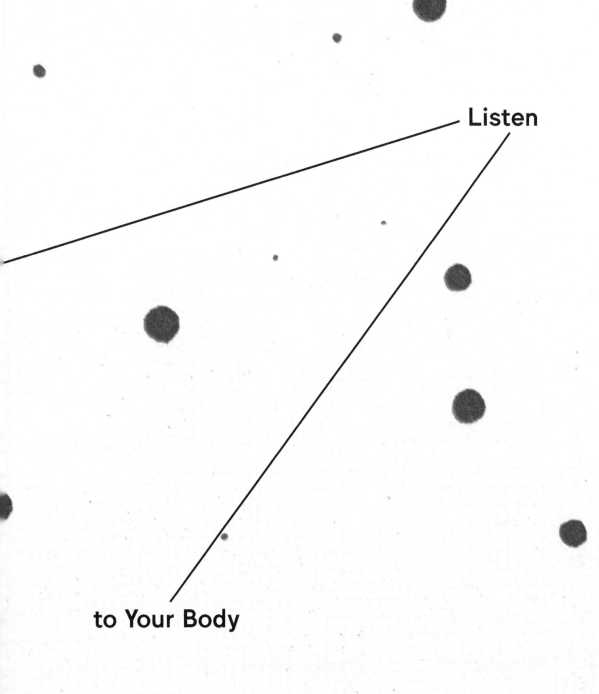

Listen

to Your Body

Overview

After years of adopting simple changes, my body has a new radar for toxic fumes. I recognize the "clean" smell of a new car or new carpet as potentially unhealthy. When my children open new toys, certain odors will lead me to add that product to my mental list of things that I will discreetly move out of our home.

I also listen to changes in my body, such as an escalating heart rate, rapid breathing, and nausea. Those sensations inspire me to get up and start sniffing around our apartment.

For months I avoided entering my children's bedroom after bedtime for fear of waking them. However, after becoming aware of subtle changes in my body, I felt moved to go to their room in the middle of the night. There I discovered fumes from a neighbor's smoking.

In another example, changes in my heart rate and sensations in my body led me to discover that a door to the attic of our home had been left open. Our builder later explained that my body was probably reacting to fumes from exposed insulation materials in the attic. After closing the attic door, I stopped experiencing the symptoms.

Needless to say, these experiences led me to place new reliance on my senses and to always investigate unusual sensations.

Over time, as you D-Tox and sharpen your senses, your journey on a cleaner path will become more organic too. You'll start noticing that you do not feel well around unhealthy environmental factors and when you eat less-healthy foods. So, in reducing the body burdens of your family, every change—no matter how seemingly small—is advancing you and your family toward greater health.

HOUSEHOLD REPEAT OFFENDERS
These may cause the body to react

The ingredients, materials, and products below may cause reactions in our bodies that signal toxic exposures. These offenders are capable of triggering acute health effects, like nausea, dizziness, and headache. They are explained in parts II and III.

Ingredients
— Adhesives
— Fragrances
— Solvents

Materials
— Conventional textiles
— Plastics
— Polyurethane foam
— Wood products

PRODUCTS OF CONCERN
— Air fresheners
— Building materials
— Candles
— Cleaning products
— Conventional carpets
— Conventional mattresses

SPECIAL CONCERNS
— Children may be more vulnerable to the health effects of chemical exposures, and they may have trouble communicating their symptoms, which makes it hard to pinpoint an environmental source for their ailments.

Tips—Listen to Your Body

01. Learn your scents and use your nose
Notice the common scents of chemicals, including those in nail polish (and polish remover), paints, adhesives, glues, new carpets, and some conventional cleaning products. Remembering and looking out for these chemical smells, and your body's reaction to them, can alert you to fumes that may be potentially harmful.

02. Don't ignore your symptoms
It can be easy to think of headaches, nausea, dizziness, and other symptoms as things that just happen sometimes. However, they may indicate that an environmental toxicant (or a cocktail of them) is having an impact on your health. Don't ignore your body's signals!

03. Think critically
When you're feeling unusual symptoms, consider whether toxic exposures may play a role. For example, when you experience sneezing or stuffiness, then explore whether dust could be the cause.

Tip Report #5

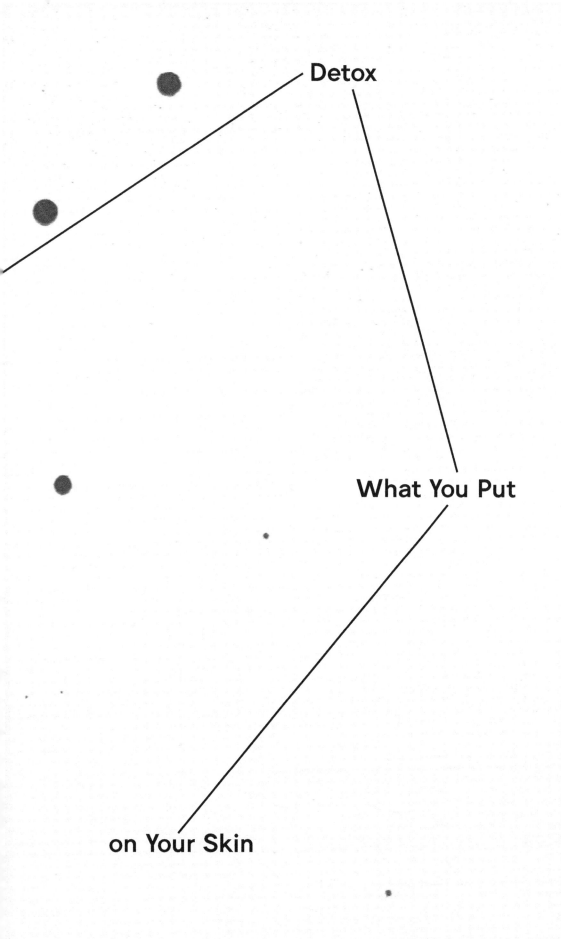

Detox

What You Put

on Your Skin

Overview

In 2009 I met a 35-year-old woman who told me about her successful battle with breast cancer. She met with the best breast cancer physician in Manhattan, who gave her a list of consumer products, including personal care products, to avoid since a number of ingredients from these products had been found in women with breast cancer. This was when I first realized that our consumer products could be absorbed into our blood, tissues, and organs. It was an important turning point in my perspective on health, forever changing the way I thought about the products that would sit on my skin.

As a result, I avoid the use of unnecessary products, and have significantly reduced my use of toxic products (using some, like nail polish and perfume, for special occasions). There are an estimated 10,500 ingredients in personal care products (EPA 2012b; EWG 2015v). So this is a high impact area of your life to detox.

HOUSEHOLD REPEAT OFFENDERS
These may penetrate skin

Below are some of the common toxicants and ingredients (as well as products that contain them) that make personal care products troublesome.

Toxicants
— Formaldehyde
— Heavy metals like lead
— Parabens
— Phthalates

Ingredients
— Fragrance
— Preservatives, like parabens, formaldehyde, and sodium benzoate
— Solvents and VOCs
— Synthetic colors including coal tar
— Unintentional by-products, like 1,4 dioxane and dioxins

PRODUCTS OF CONCERN
— Cosmetics
— Deodorants
— Insect repellents
— Perfumes and colognes
— Moisturizers
— Sunscreens

REPEAT ISSUES
— Lack of disclosure of product ingredients
— Many ingredients are petroleum based
— No required unbiased safety testing
— What little is known causes concern, such as the presence of carcinogens, EDCs, and developmental toxins.

Tips—Detox What You Put on Your Skin

01. Read ingredient labels
Before you buy a new product, examine the label, picking one ingredient of concern (like "fragrance" or "parabens") to use as a filter.

02. Consider the Simple Strategies in chapter III.4
These strategies are the "cleanest" ones that worked for me when pregnant and nursing. I didn't follow them all the time but whenever I reasonably could. After pregnancy and nursing, when my children's exposures weren't so dependent on mine, I started using more conventional products to make my hair look better. You can cherry pick for your preferences. Small changes are helpful!

03. Invest in your diet and sleep
Exercise and drink lots of water. They may improve your complexion enough that your desire for skin products decreases.

04. Minimize unnecessary sun exposure
Reducing your sun exposure will reduce your need for sun protection lotions and cosmetics, as well as protect your skin which will reduce your desire for additional beauty products that will fight or camouflage the sun's damaging effects.

Tip Report #6

Let the Food

be Thy Medicine

Overview

Hippocrates coined the saying "Let food be thy medicine." Several millennia later, science continues to prove him wise! A commonly overlooked consideration with diet, however, is the presence of toxicants in our food. Depending on what it is and how it's made, food can be contaminated during preparation, cooking, or storage. Or, if the food item is an animal, then it may have created its own toxic body burden from the organisms it ate during its lifetime as well as its own environment.

HOUSEHOLD REPEAT OFFENDERS:
These contaminate food

Food is a major source of exposure to some toxicants. Below are some of the common toxicants you can reduce your exposure to by avoiding the listed ingredients, materials, and products.

Toxicants
— BPA and phthalates: Leach from food containers
— Pesticides, including DDT: Farming practices and bioaccumulation from our polluted environment result in pesticides being in our food.
— Heavy metals: Are detected in our food supply. Contamination can occur unintentionally from our polluted environment and through the process of bioconcentration.
— PFCs: Leach into food from nonstick surfaces like pots and pans as well as from delivery and takeout containers.
— Unintentional Toxicants, such as dioxins

Ingredients
— Artificial additives, including artificial sugars, colors, and preservatives

Materials
— Plastics: Can leach toxicants such as BPA, phthalates, and styrene.
— Nonstick surfaces: Can leach highly persistent and toxic chemicals.

PRODUCTS OF CONCERN
— Animal proteins, such as dairy, eggs, meat, poultry, and seafood
— Cooking tools and storage containers
— Processed or packaged foods, including baby food

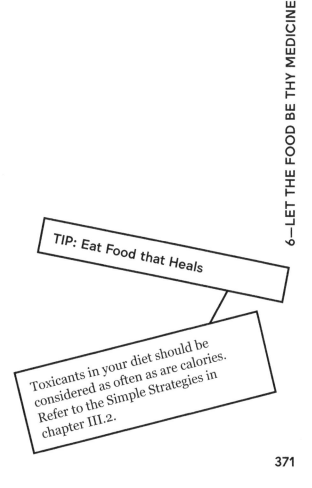

TIP: Eat Food that Heals

Toxicants in your diet should be considered as often as are calories. Refer to the Simple Strategies in chapter III.2.

Tip Report #7

Edit

Your Possessions

Overview

Most products in your home contribute toxicants to indoor air and house dust, and provide surface areas where contaminated air can be absorbed or dust can reside. So less stuff is physically healthier!

By "edit your possessions," I mean review, streamline (declutter), and prioritize what should be replaced. Most important, buy less and buy mindfully. Consider what you're contributing to landfills and garbage patches in the oceans. Also, less stuff is just better for your wallet, sense of order, and mental, emotional, and spiritual clarity. It's a win-win tip!

Most household products contaminate indoor air and dust, as Tip Reports 1 and 2 explain. In fact, this is worth repeating:

"The concentration of pollutants in house dust may be 2 to 32 times higher than that found in the soil near a house. Reducing infant exposures... may reduce lifetime health costs, improve early learning, and increase adult productivity." (Roberts et al. 2009)

SIX REASONS TO STREAMLINE YOUR POSSESSIONS

01. Less stuff means fewer sources of pollutants in your home
Many things off-gas VOCs, SVOCs, and hazardous air pollutants or contribute toxicants to dust. Having fewer things in the home means there is less opportunity for off-gassing.

02. More stuff makes it harder to fight dust
When there is more to vacuum under and around, dust is harder to control.

03. Most products contain petroleum-based ingredients
These burden our planet. If we decrease demand for unnecessary products, manufacturers will produce less of those things, eventually reducing the contamination throughout our homes and bodies.

04. Organization encourages serenity
Decluttering one's home is mentally and emotionally cleansing.

05. Buying less makes money available for healthier purchases
Buying less frees up funds to invest in a healthier diet. It also reduces garbage that goes into our landfills and oceans.

06. Product ingredients may have unforeseen interactions
Below are examples of how reactions among common products can create toxic fumes. These Unintentional Toxicants and Unintentional Potential Effects are another reason to have less at home.

— Bleach should not be mixed with any acid, as the mixture can create toxic fumes such as chloroform, which the EPA has classified as a probable human carcinogen (EPA 2000a). Acid can be found in tile and toilet bowl cleaners. Vinegar is also an acid.

— Dishwasher detergent can react with food residues to create chloroform.

— Air fresheners and personal care products can release compounds that combine with other substances to create Unintentional Potential Effects. For example, *National Geographic*'s (2008) *Green Guide* mentions terpenes, ingredients found in pine-scented cleaners, lemon-scented air fresheners, and personal care products such as men's aftershave and women's foundation makeup. When terpenes react with ozone, generated by air purifiers or supplied by outdoor smog, this can create harmful VOCs and ultrafine particles that can trigger allergies, asthma, and other respiratory illnesses.

Tips—Edit Your Possessions

01. Minimize your demand for plastics

Whenever possible, choose products that don't use plastics or support plastics that can be recycled. Recycle. And reduce your demand of new shopping bags by bringing your own reuseable bags.

02. Minimize polyurethane foam

Made mostly of petroleum-based ingredients, polyurethane foam is so flammable that chemical flame retardants must be added to products that contain it. In recent years, researchers have proved that these chemical flame retardants pose serious health risks, leach from their products, reside in dust, and enter our bodies (Lunder 2012). Polyurethane foam is present in many popular household products, including toys, upholstered furniture, mattresses, carpets, and nursing pillows.

03. Minimize electronics

Since electronics can heat up to high temperatures and are made of flammable materials, chemical flame retardants are added. Dust from TVs, computers, and other electronics can easily redistribute these chemicals throughout our Homes.

04. Avoid buying pesticides

Pest-control chemicals can become a component of dust. And children are prone to accidental poisoning. It is estimated that for most people, 80 percent of exposure to pesticides happens indoors (EPA 2012c).
— Pesticides can be brought indoors on our clothes or tracked in on the bottoms of our shoes.
— Pesticides can enter our homes through wind and collect on surface areas, to be released or taken up by hands.
— Pesticide residues can easily make their way into bedding, clothing, and food.
— Pesticides persist longer indoors than outdoors, where they are removed from the effects of sunlight, flowing water, wind, and microbes.

05. Consider having fewer carpets

Carpets are reservoirs of dust. A home with bare floors and a few area rugs can have one-tenth of the dust found in a home with wall-to-wall carpet, according to Dr. Dust (*BBC* 2001). Area rugs that you can wash and lay out to dry in the sun are good choices.

Tips—Edit Your Possessions

06. Beware of products with potentially toxic VOC emissions

Common culprits are paints and interior furnishings.

— Limit your exposure to products that contain solvents. Avoid petroleum-based solvents, which should be labeled "DANGER: Harmful or fatal if swallowed." Seek water-based or other natural-based solvents instead. Buy just what you need to avoid waste and storage.

— Choose zero-VOC products, which are usually labeled as such. But even zero-VOC items can emit small amounts levels of toxic compounds.

— Carefully evaluate "fast drying" and "streak free" labels, often used on products containing solvents.

07. Buy limited quantities

Purchase only as much as you intend to use right away, especially high-VOC products that you use only occasionally, like paints, paint strippers, and kerosene or gasoline for lawn mowers.

08. Seek third-party certifications

For indoor air quality, certification programs mainly assess formaldehyde and other VOC emissions. The GREEN-GUARD® Environmental Institute (GEI), an industry-independent nonprofit organization that certifies products for low emissions, offers a comprehensive evaluation that tests for more than 10,000 VOCs. Note that few certification programs test for other chemicals of potential concern, such as semi-volatile organic compounds (like perfluorinated chemicals), hazardous air pollutants, chemical flame retardants, or endocrine disruptors (like phthalates).

09. Beware of "nontoxic" claims

Be skeptical when you see this claim because nothing is truly nontoxic.

10. Consider whether claims of safety are based on proof of safety, or on lack of proof of harm

In many instances, no one has investigated for harm or there is insufficient information to draw a conclusion. That's why it's important that consumers become more informed and think critically.

11. Find helpful resources
Use online databases and smartphone apps to make informed choices.
— Cleaning products: ewg.org/guides/cleaners
— Personal care products: ewg.org/skindeep/
— Other consumer products, including toys, cars, children's products, pets, apparel, accessories, and home improvement: HealthyStuff.org/

12. Visit my website: NontoxicLiving.tips
Each year, products improve and research uncovers more relevant information. My website, NontoxicLiving.tips, is the most current pathway to stay updated on products I prefer.

14. Re-prioritize your budget
Information in parts II and III will help you decide what you'll spend less on, such as electronics, furniture, or toys. The opportunities are endless.
— To simplify my shopping list, I use the timeless strategy of cleaning with a short list of trusted ingredients: vinegar, baking soda, castile soap, and hydrogen peroxide. In addition to saving money, this reduces the potential sources of harmful off-gassing, Unintentional Toxicants, and Unintentional Potential Effects.
— Invest in the quality of your diet. If you eat more plant-based and nutrient-dense foods, your skin, energy, and sleep could improve so much that you won't desire as many personal care products. Experiment with a diet that has fewer chemicals in it.
— The potential payoff from investing in a healthier diet is immeasurable. It can decrease your risk of disease, disorders, and discomfort, increase your energy, improve your skin and sleep, and liberate you to enjoy life more.

13. Follow the Simple Strategies in part III
Each of the chapters in part III offers tips on common household products of concern. While there are tips on how to buy healthier "off-the-shelf" products, there are also "Simple Strategies," basic plans that we can focus on when we get overwhelmed by so much information and so many options. I followed these Simple Strategies when I was pregnant, nursing, and when my children were most vulnerable because I was comfortable with their track record of safety.

15. Jog, don't sprint
The tips in this chapter are a great way to start editing your possessions, but remember to pace yourself. Small changes can have big impacts, and overwhelming yourself may lead to frustration and, worse, quitting.

Tips—Properly Care for Your Things

01. Follow directions
Read and follow label instructions. Potentially hazardous products typically have warnings that can help reduce the user's exposure. For instance, if a product label instructs you to use an item in a well-ventilated area, do so outside or in a room with an exhaust fan. At the very least, open windows to maximum fresh air exchange.

02. Mix mindfully
Be cautious when combining household products. Again, read labels carefully! Mixing products can create toxic by-products, as when certain cleaning products are used together. The attached boxes provide two examples.

01. Ammonia and chlorine, found in various cleaning products, can create a deadly gas (*National Geographic* 2008).

02. The popular trio of diethanolamine (DEA), triethanolamine (TEA), and monoethanolamine (MEA), used in liquid soaps, body washes, and shampoos, can react with other ingredients called nitrites (used as preservatives) to create nitrosamines. These compounds, which have caused cancer in laboratory animals, can be absorbed through the skin (*National Geographic* 2008).

03. Store properly
Don't store high-VOC products that you don't need. When you must store them (like paints, kerosene, etc), then choose a well-ventilated area that is also safely out of children's reach.

04. Dispose mindfully!
Safely discard partially used containers of old or unneeded chemicals. Find out if your local government or an organization in your community offers responsible collection of toxic household wastes.

Tips—To Reduce Demand for Pesticides

01. Detox your diet
Prioritize your budget for organic foods, especially those that are higher on the food chain (meat, dairy, etc.). Use the EWG's lists of the "Clean Fifteen" and the "Dirty Dozen," which rank produce items by their level of pesticide contamination. Download a free smartphone app, or view the lists online at ewg.org/foodnews/.

02. Manage pests naturally
Household pests can be addressed through a variety of ways that don't require pesticides. Prevention is key. Clean your home often, especially the kitchen! If pests become an issue, search online for nontoxic solutions. Outdoors, explore the feasibility of organic lawn care.

For example, plagued by fruit flies during some seasons, I use a mixture of wine and rotting fruit in a container beneath a funnel. They can't escape!

03. Consider the impact of your purchases
There's more than one way to reduce demand for pesticides. For example, in addition to the tips above, when you buy products that use cotton, choosing products that use organic (rather than conventional) cotton would support agricultural practices that avoid pesticides. The Simple Strategies in part III provide other options to reduce our Trails of Contamination.

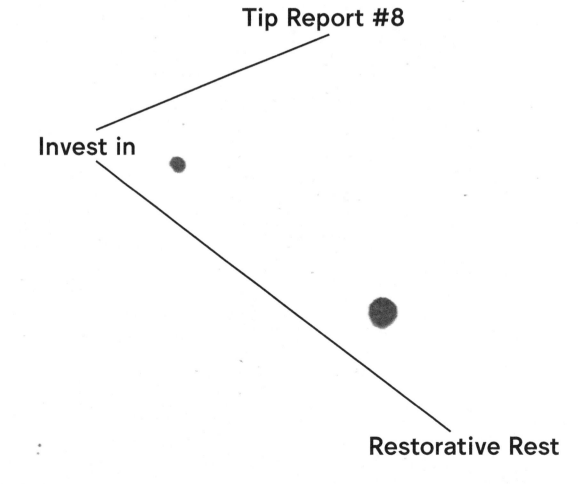

Tip Report #8

Invest in

Restorative Rest

Overview

A growing body of science attests to the powers of sleep. It is no longer viewed as a luxury but as essential to health as exercise and a nourishing diet.

Emerging data suggest that insufficient sleep can have a significant impact on chronic disease risk, health problems, perception, judgment, learning, and memory (Division of Sleep Medicine at Harvard Medical School 2007a; 2007b). In October 2013, a study funded by the National Institute of Neurological Disorders and Stroke found that the brain may rid itself of toxic molecules during sleep (Xie et al. 2013).

You may already have an effective sleep routine, but protecting yourself from toxicants while you sleep will help your nights be even more restorative. Detoxing your sleep environment and minimizing electromagnetic fields will free up your body's resources to repair and reboot.

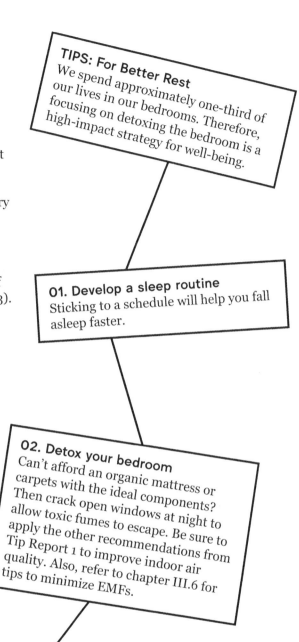

TIPS: For Better Rest
We spend approximately one-third of our lives in our bedrooms. Therefore, focusing on detoxing the bedroom is a high-impact strategy for well-being.

01. Develop a sleep routine
Sticking to a schedule will help you fall asleep faster.

02. Detox your bedroom
Can't afford an organic mattress or carpets with the ideal components? Then crack open windows at night to allow toxic fumes to escape. Be sure to apply the other recommendations from Tip Report 1 to improve indoor air quality. Also, refer to chapter III.6 for tips to minimize EMFs.

03. Avoid technology before bedtime
It's best to turn off the TV or computer a few hours before sleeping. The blue light that is emitted from video displays can confuse your circadian rhythms and keep you awake.

Tip Report #9

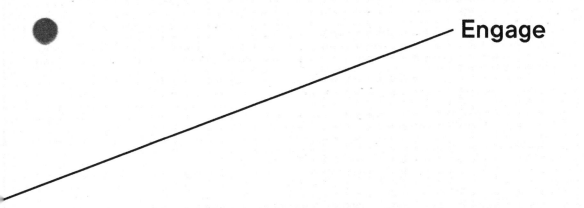

Engage

Overview

This book is full of alarming facts and each of us will be changed by different ones. For me, the one that motivated me most to create this book during an intensely busy time in my life is the chemical contamination of cord blood and breast milk.

I was upset to learn that breast milk can have among the highest concentrations of certain toxicants. For example, concentrations of organochlorine pollutants in breast milk was typically 10 to 20 times higher than those in cow's milk (Steingraber 2001). As a result, a nursing infant, who is at the peak of our food chain (WHO 2008), can be exposed to a substantial portion of its total lifetime exposure to certain chemicals during the first few months of life (Schettler et al. 2000). In many cases, breastfeeding exposes infants to levels of POPs that exceed the tolerable daily intake defined for lifelong exposure (Polder, Gabrielsen, et al. 2008; Polder, Thomsen, et al. 2008).

Regardless, breastfeeding is still the ultimate nourishment for children. Infant formula is contaminated as well and it does not offer the innate benefits that breastfeeding offers (Schettler et al. 2000).

This unfortunate truth is what motivates me to engage in possible solutions. Parents should have the option to nourish their newborns with uncontaminated milk. However, change can only occur if more people are aware and engaged.

CONTAMINANTS FOUND IN BREASTMILK FROM AROUND THE WORLD

Made from a mother's fat storage, breast milk shares a mother's lifelong accumulation of toxicants with her nursing baby (EWG 2003).
— Cable-insulating ingredients
— Dry cleaning fluids
— Flame retardants: PCBs and PBDEs
— Gasoline vapors
— Pesticides: DDT, dieldrin, heptachlor, and fungicides
— Wood preservatives: Termite poisons, moth-proofing agents, and toilet deodorizers
— Unintentional by-products: Dioxins from manufacturing and garbage incineration

(Steingraber 2001; NRDC 2005; and Williams 2005)

FORMULA IS CONTAMINATED TOO

One FDA assessment estimated that formula-fed infants had 12.5 times more BPA exposure than adults per pound of body weight; the likely explanation is the presence of BPA in some infant formula (banned in 2013) and baby bottles. The EWG estimated infant exposure may have been up to twice the FDA's estimate (EWG 2008b).

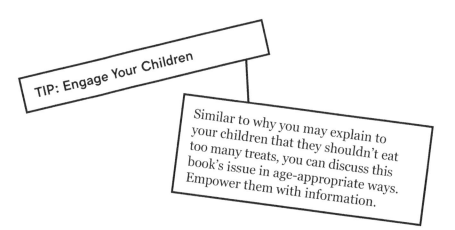

TIP: Engage Your Children

Similar to why you may explain to your children that they shouldn't eat too many treats, you can discuss this book's issue in age-appropriate ways. Empower them with information.

Tips—To Help the Cause

01. Spread the word
The more collective awareness we can achieve, the more likely we can create healthy change.

02. Support meaningful petitions
Sign and start petitions to let businesses and elected officials know that you want laws that are more protective of public health. For help in starting a petition, visit Change.org.

03. Exercise your political power
From the past, we have seen that regulation of toxic chemicals can be effective in reducing human exposure. One of the best examples of legislation "gone right" pertains to lead, a notorious neurotoxin. Between 1976 and 1995, the period during which lead was phased out of gasoline, blood level concentrations decreased more than 90 percent (WHO 2010; CDC 1997; Jones et al. 2009). As citizens we can advocate for better laws. Visit Safer Chemicals.org to learn what you can do.

— Contamination from PCBs and POPs has decreased in both humans and wildlife since bans and restrictions were placed on these chemicals. Some scientists believe this has helped decrease the "frequency of disorders in humans and wildlife" (WHO and UNEP 2013).

— Blood levels of PFOS and PFOA have significantly fallen, by approximately 32 percent and 25 percent, respectively, in test samples collected in 2003 and 2004. The CDC concluded that the decrease was likely the result of a phaseout of these chemicals by manufacturers (Calafat et al. 2007).

— Prevalence of PBDEs in blood began to dwindle in the early 2000s, following the phaseout of PBDEs (WHO and UNEP 2013).

04. Take control of your own health
Experts are focused on their area of specialty, which doesn't always fit your needs. *You* can become the leader of your own health. Start by becoming more curious and informed. Leave your convictions open to evolution as credible new research emerges.

05. Be selective in the experts you trust
If you persist in your research, you can find physicians whose perspective resonates with yours. Know what you do not know, and consider what the experts still do not know. Give weight to what your informed instincts say, and use this insight to ask probing questions to find the experts who are best suited to your unique situation.

06. Use your purchasing power to help create positive change
Buy consciously. By doing so, we're telling businesses and government that we care enough about our health and planet to pay the premium. As the eco-friendly market grows, more businesses will want to compete, which will lower the prices for these types of products. Manufacturers responded to parents' concerns over BPA and phased it out *before* the FDA banned it from baby bottles!

07. Support worthwhile efforts
Give your support to organizations that are fighting for this cause. Visit NontoxicLiving.tips to see a list of my favorites.

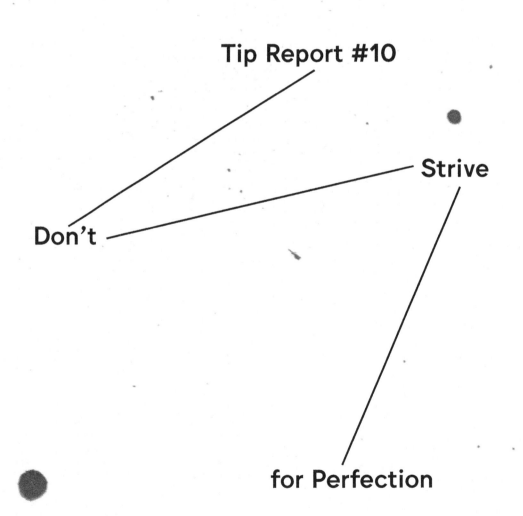

Tip Report #10

Don't Strive for Perfection

Overview

As you Edit your life, set achievable goals and create an overall positive trend at your own pace, no matter how small the change or how slowly you progress. Drastic changes will burn you out and lead you to feel failure, and then you'll give up. That's not productive! Focus on positive trends.

Reward yourself for your baby steps, and don't criticize your daily performance. Gaining awareness is already a challenge. As the EPA urges on its website on climate change: "Small steps add up, if we all do our part" (EPA 2014f).

While our understanding of environmental harms will improve, the most practical and effective solutions are timeless. Our collective body of science continues to prove the wisdom of how people of my grandparents' generation lived. *It's back to basics, baby!*

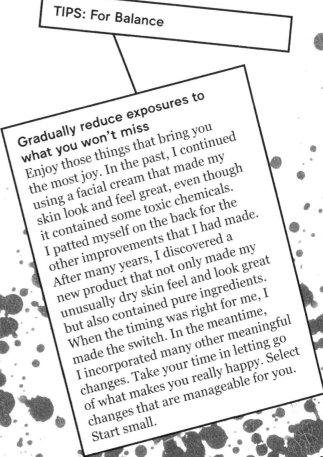

TIPS: For Balance

Gradually reduce exposures to what you won't miss

Enjoy those things that bring you the most joy. In the past, I continued using a facial cream that made my skin look and feel great, even though it contained some toxic chemicals. I patted myself on the back for the other improvements that I had made. After many years, I discovered a new product that not only made my unusually dry skin feel and look great but also contained pure ingredients. When the timing was right for me, I made the switch. In the meantime, I incorporated many other meaningful changes. Take your time in letting go of what makes you really happy. Select changes that are manageable for you. Start small.

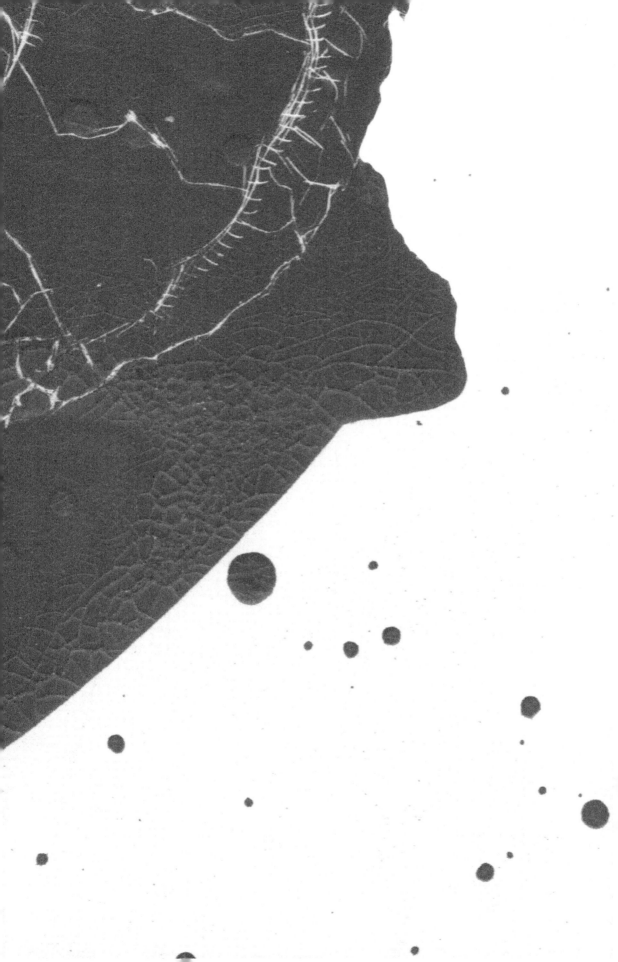

Appendix

How to Use This Book

A to Z of D-Toxing: The Ultimate Guide to Reducing Our Toxic Exposures is a reference book that is meant to nurture curiosity with each reading session, intriguing you to revisit the book when you feel ready to learn more. For me, it took repeated exposures to the messages in this book before I could be receptive to them. Therefore, I appreciate that we each have our own timetable for being ready to "hear" this information.

The book contains four main parts. For ease of reference, chapter numbers begin with a roman numeral to indicate in which part—such as I, II, or III—it is located. The chapter numbers reset in each part; for example, the first chapter in part II is identified as chapter II.1. Part IV is its own chapter.

If you're the type of person who likes details, then parts II and III will be of interest to you. If you prefer less information and just want high impact strategies, then refer to part IV. Part IV contains ten simple ideas that I focus on, even while knowing all the particulars.

PART I: WHY YOU SHOULD REDUCE YOUR TOXIC EXPOSURES

Part I is an overview of how our deteriorating environment affects our Homes: our built environments, our bodies, and our planet. It contains 15 chapters.

Chapters I.1 through I.9 provide a science-based overview of the prevalence of, and threats from, toxicants in our Homes. Chapters I.10 through I.14 spotlight relevant track records of governments and other authoritative organizations in dealing with these toxicants; the complexities of proving harm and our responses to such proof; the safety of substitute chemicals; and the risks of choosing a reactive rather than precautionary approach.

Part I ends with chapter I.15, which underscores the power of now. We're learning that it's never too late to improve our wellness. The emerging field of epigenetics is proving how diet and other *choices* affect our gene expression. And pregnant women have a unique opportunity to position their children's health for better outcomes.

PART II: HOUSEHOLD REPEAT OFFENDERS

Part II introduces Household Repeat Offenders, the common denominators that occur among a wide range of household products. In the same way that various foods share common ingredients (like wheat and sugar), various household products share common toxicants, ingredients, and materials. Part II profiles those that I encountered most often and that are of concern.

Recognizing these offenders helped me drown out greenwashing noise so I could home in on potential sources of toxicants. For example, solvents contain a variety of toxicants. They are found in many products, such as cleaners, fragrances, paints, markers, air fresheners, nail polish, adhesives, and wood items. Becoming familiar with the detailed tips provided throughout part III furthered my understanding of where these Household Repeat Offenders might reside, and reviewing them continues to further sharpen my critical thinking.

PART III: TIPS FOR PRODUCTS OF CONCERN

Part III contains all the tips that I gathered during my research. They are organized into six chapters: Cleaning Products, In the Kitchen, Interior Furnishings, Personal Care Products, Children's Stuff, and Miscellaneous.

Within these categories I profile key products that pose concern, as well as the Household Repeat Offenders from part II and other "offenders" that may be in them. Formaldehyde and vinyl, for example, are profiled in the part II. In part III, you'll see them listed as Household Repeat Offenders in the profiled products that may contain them, such as mattresses and furniture.

Incorporating these tips will help you to reduce your unnecessary exposures to unhealthy chemicals in the air you breathe, the food you eat, and the materials you come in contact with every day. Start with the easiest steps, then revisit the book when you're ready for more change. For my favorite products and latest tips, visit my website, NontoxicLiving.tips, which I will update as time fosters better information and better products.

PART IV: THE D-TOX STRATEGY
Given all that I've learned about toxicants in my life, my D-Tox strategy is simple. Part IV shares the top 10 goals that I strive to achieve every day. Most of them cost little or nothing, and they are the most impactful ideas to focus on.

I began my research with the goal of reducing to zero my family's exposure to toxicants. As I learned more, I realized this was unrealistic because our environment is so polluted. More realistic, yet still meaningful, is the goal of *minimizing* the body burdens of my loved ones and myself.

Today I manage this by focusing on positive progress over a long period of time, rather than aiming for perfection at every moment. I minimize chemical exposure in high-impact areas that I can control, such as in the home. I relax at low-impact times, or when it's impractical to control things (like at birthday parties). Or when I'm just too tired! The goal should be to create a positive trend at your own pace.

OTHER NOTES
Defined terms
Inspired by the way defined terms are used in legal documents (strange as that seems), whenever I capitalize a term, like Homes, that's a signal that I have given the term a specific meaning that is explained in the chapter that introduces it. While this makes some sections harder to read, this approach allows me to communicate more precisely and concisely about this highly complex subject.

The defined terms are included in the Terms to Know and Index sections, located on the next few pages.

In-text citations
This book uses in-text (author and date) citations; in other words, it notes the author of the source from which the information was taken, along with the date of publication so you can quickly see how current the information is. I chose this format because I found myself wishing for this type of disclosure of sources when I started reading about toxicants in our Homes. There were inconsistent "facts" and a lot of information that I had never heard before, so I was skeptical of the health warnings that I encountered. As I sought the best available material, in-text citations from credible sources would have saved me a lot of time. Moreover, if you're able to access more holistic and progressive health care providers, then this book's transparency of sources should help your communication with them.

While names of authors will not be meaningful to most readers and the average reader will not be able to make sense of the opinion of author/scientist A versus the opposing opinion of author/scientist B, upon review of the Works Cited sections, you'll notice that many authors were published in peer-reviewed medical journals, government reports and websites, leading advocacy groups, and respected popular publications like the *New York Times*. It may be helpful to know that tremendous effort was invested in obtaining unbiased, credible sources whenever possible. When not possible, I relied on the next best available option.

Studies will continually emerge to update the data and refine our understanding. However, the key message, which won't become outdated, is that environmental factors play a bigger role in our health than has historically been appreciated. In addition, the D-Tox Strategy and Simple Strategies should endure as helpful guidance even amid new information.

Acronyms

Acronyms for key organizations that are used throughout the book are below.

CDC
US Centers for Disease Control and Prevention

CEHC
Children's Environmental Health Center at Mount Sinai Hospital, NYC

CHEJ
Center for Health, Environment & Justice

CPSC
Consumer Product Safety Commission

EEA
European Environmental Agency

EPA
US Environmental Protection Agency

EWG
Environmental Working Group

FSC
Forest Stewardship Council

FDA
US Food and Drug Administration

IARC
International Agency for Research on Cancer

IPCC
Intergovernmental Panel on Climate Change

MAB
CNA Corporation's Military Advisory Board

NASA
National Aeronautics and Space Administration

NRDC
Natural Resources Defense Council

PCP
President's Cancer Panel

POPs
United Nations Stockholm Convention on Persistent Organic Pollutants

TEDX
The Endocrine Disruption Exchange

WHO
World Health Organization

UNEP
United Nations Environment Programme

Terms to Know

This list is a combination of a glossary, list of abbreviations, and the author's Defined Terms. Acronyms for organizations can be found in the Appendix.

1,1,1-trichloroethane
A chlorinated solvent that was banned in 1996 after scientists learned that it was harming the ozone layer.

ADHD
See *Attention-deficit hyperactivity disorder*.

Allergen
A substance that induces an adverse immune response.

Allergy
A hypersensitive response by the body's immune system to an allergen that is consumed, inhaled, or touched. There are many different types of allergies, ranging from mild to severe.

Arsenic
An element that occurs in two forms, organic and inorganic. The inorganic form causes cancer.

Arthritis
A disorder of the musculoskeletal system that causes inflammation. There are over 100 types of arthritis.

Asbestos
A heat-resistant mineral fiber, found in soil and rocks, that is used in insulation and as a fire retardant.

Asbestosis
A lung disease, caused by inhaling asbestos fibers, that leads to lung tissue scarring.

Asthma
A lung disease that causes the airways to narrow and become inflamed. It can be inherited or acquired.

Attention-deficit hyperactivity disorder (ADHD)
A neurodevelopmental disorder that affects both children and adults.

Autoimmune disease
A condition in which the body's immune system fights healthy cells. There are more than 80 types of autoimmune disease.

BBB
See *Blood-brain barrier*.

Benzene
A chemical found in coal, oil, cigarette smoke, gasoline, and some adhesives. It is a carcinogen.

Bioaccumulation
A state in which a substance is ingested or absorbed at a greater rate than it is eliminated.

Bioconcentration
The accumulation of a chemical in the body to levels that are greater than that found in the surrounding environment.

Biomagnification
The increasing concentration of a substance as it ascends the food chain.

Biomonitoring
The measurement of exposure to certain toxic substances in the environment, usually through the analysis of blood and urine.

Birth defect
An abnormal physical or biochemical change to the fetus that can be inherited or caused by the environment.

Bisphenol-A (BPA)
A chemical commonly found in plastics, canned goods, and some types of paper (such as cash register receipts). It is an endocrine disruptor.

Bisphenol-S (BPS)
A chemical often used in place of BPA. It has been found to disrupt estrogen.

Blood-brain barrier (BBB)
A semipermeable membrane that protects the brain. It is more developed in adults than in infants.

Body burden
The total amount of a chemical that has accumulated in the body.

BPA
See *Bisphenol–A*.

BPS
See *Bisphenol-S*.

Brain cancer
Cancer that affects the brain's ability to function. It can either originate in the brain or develop in another part of the body and migrate (metastasize) to the brain.

Building-related illness
A disorder caused by being in a building with sealed windows and internal air circulation, such as an office or home. Legionnaires' disease and occupational asthma are some examples of this disorder.

By-product
A product created during the production or breakdown of another substance.

C8
See *Perfluorooctanoic acid*.

Cadmium
A metal found in zinc. It is used in pigment, batteries, and nuclear reactors, and is a known carcinogen.

Carcinogen
A substance that causes cancer.

CFC
See *Chlorofluorocarbons*.

Chlorofluorocarbons (CFC)
A group of chemicals that contain chlorine, fluorine, and carbon. The US and other countries banned their use because they deplete the ozone layer.

Chronic illness
A disease or disorder that develops over a period of time and is rarely cured completely. Examples include respiratory diseases, diabetes, and arthritis.

Colitis
Inflammation of the colon that triggers diarrhea and abdominal pain. Examples include ulcerative colitis and microscopic colitis.

Computed tomography (CT)
A noninvasive medical imaging test that uses computer processed X-rays to obtain cross-sectional images of the body. It is sometimes called computerized tomography or computed axial tomography (CAT).

Corporate Interests
The business goal of protecting revenues in the face of emerging evidence of harm.

Crohn's disease
A condition in which the gastrointestinal tract suffers from chronic inflammation.

Cryptorchidism
A condition in which one or both testicles has not descended by the time of birth.

CT
See *Computed tomography*.

DDT
A pesticide, banned by the US in 1972, that is still found in the environment. Some countries continue to use it to combat malaria-carrying mosquitoes.

Developmental disability
A chronic disability that originates before the age of 22 and can affect learning, behavior, or the body. Examples include hearing loss, learning disability, or blindness.

Developmental neurotoxicant
A toxicant that damages the developing brain and nervous system, either before or after birth. See *Toxicant*.

Developmental toxicant
A toxicant that interferes with physical and mental development prenatally and in early childhood. See *Toxicant*.

Diabetes
A disease that causes the body to either not produce insulin, or to use it improperly, resulting in above normal blood glucose levels.

Diacetyl
A chemical, which has a buttery taste, that has been used as an artificial flavoring. Inhalation of diacetyl can damage the respiratory system.

Dioxins
Chemical compounds that are considered to be Persistent Organic Pollutants (POPs). They are potent at minuscule levels.

D-Tox
The process of reducing your Trails of Contamination throughout your Homes (whereas "detox" means to purify).

D-Tox Strategy
The 10 goals to focus on, each of which has its own Tip Report in part IV.

EDC
See *Endocrine disrupting chemical*.

Edit
The act of constantly streamlining and revising your life to D-Tox.

EHS
See *Electromagnetic hypersensitivity*.

Electromagnetic field (EMF)
The field of energy that encircles an electrically charged device. Examples include computers, radio towers, and power lines.

Electromagnetic hypersensitivity (EHS)
An illness caused by exposure to electromagnetic fields. It is also called electromagnetic sensitivity (EMS).

Electromagnetic radiation
A type of energy that includes ultraviolet light, radio waves, X-rays, microwaves, and gamma rays.

EMF
See *Electromagnetic field*.

Endocrine disrupting chemical (EDC)
A chemical that interferes with natural hormone activity and undermines normal cell metabolism, reproduction, development, and behavior.

Endocrine system
The system of glands that create and release hormones, which the body uses to regulate growth, metabolism, sexual development, and sexual function. The endocrine system includes the adrenals, hypothalamus, ovaries, parathyroids, pineal body, pituitary, testes, and thyroid.

Endocrine toxicant
A toxicant that affects the endocrine system. Cadmium is an example of an endocrine toxicant. See *Toxicant*.

Endometriosis
A disorder in which the endometrial tissue that lines the uterus grows outside it.

Epigenetics
The study of changes to a gene that affects its function, but not its structure.

Estrogenic
Having the characteristics of estrogen.

Exposure
Contact with a substance.

Fetal origins
The study of the relationship of adult-onset diseases or disorders to the prenatal period.

Fetotoxicity
Toxic effects on the fetus.

Flame retardants
Chemicals that inhibit or delay the spread of fire.

Formaldehyde
A chemical used in building materials and household products. It is a carcinogen that is also naturally occurring.

Genetically modified organism (GMO)

An organism whose genetic material has been purposefully modified to obtain a specific trait or product.

Genotoxic

A toxicant that damages genetic material. See *Toxicant*.

Glycol ethers

Chemicals used as solvents or as an ingredient in cleaners, paints, or cosmetics. Some glycol ethers are reproductive toxins and neurotoxins.

GMO

See *Genetically modified organism*.

HAPs

See *Hazardous air pollutants*.

Hay fever

An upper respiratory response to allergens, such as pollen, dust mites, or animal dander. It is another name for allergic rhinitis.

Hazardous air pollutants (HAPs)

Airborne pollutants thought to cause cancer or other health issues. They are also called toxic air pollutants or air toxins. Examples include benzene, dioxin, and methylene chloride.

HEPA filter

See *High efficiency particulate air filter*.

High efficiency particulate air (HEPA) filter

A type of filter, usually made of submicron glass fibers, that removes fine particles from the air.

Homes

Our built environments, our bodies, and our planet.

Hormone

A chemical substance that controls the activity of specific cells or organs. Hormones are both naturally and synthetically produced.

Household Repeat Offenders

Common toxicants, ingredients, and materials of concern that are commonly found in various household products. They are profiled in part 2.

HVAC

Heating, ventilation, and air-conditioning system.

Hypertension

A condition in which the pressure of the blood in the blood vessels is high enough to cause health problems, including stroke and heart disease. It is also called high blood pressure.

Hypospadias

An abnormality in which the urethra opens on the underside of the penis rather than at the tip.

IAQ

See *Indoor air quality*.

Immunotoxicant

A toxicant that affects the immune system. See *Toxicant*.

In utero

In the uterus.

Indoor air pollutant

A biological or chemical toxin or toxicant found indoors. Examples include animal dander, pollen, carbon monoxide, and tobacco smoke.

Indoor air quality

The quality of the air inside a building as defined by the level of indoor air pollutants and ventilation.

Ingredients of Concern

Ingredients that are profiled in chapter II.2. They are Household Repeat Offenders.

Lead

A naturally occurring element found deep within the earth. Lead has been used for centuries in materials such as paints, cosmetics, and bullets. A neurotoxin, it has been banned from some consumer products, such as paint, but it is still in a number of others.

Lead poisoning

Poisoning caused by the accumulation of lead in the body, often over a period of months or years.

Leukemia

Cancer that causes the body to make a high number of abnormal white blood cells. These cells are unable to ward off infection, and they hinder the bone marrow's ability to create red blood cells and platelets.

Life Cycle

The trajectory of a substance's existence, from its design, creation, and use to its disposal and breakdown or persistence.

Lymphoma

Cancer of the lymphatic system that begins in the cells of the immune system.

Magnetic resonance imaging (MRI)

An imaging procedure that uses powerful magnetic fields, as well as radio waves, to create images of the body's organs and internal structures.

Manipulative Business Strategies

Six business strategies that have manipulated consumer demand and delayed regulation while evidence of harm emerges. These tactics were pioneered by the tobacco companies and adopted by others. Profiled in chapter 1.12.

Material Safety Data Sheet (MSDS)

Safety and health information about certain products or chemicals that workers may handle on the job. It is also called a Safety Data Sheet (SDS).

Materials of Concern

Materials that are profiled in chapter II.3. They are Household Repeat Offenders.

Melanoma

Cancer that originates in the cells that create melanin, the pigment that colors eyes, hair, and skin. Melanoma can occur in the eyes, skin, and mucous membranes. Most cases are caused by ultraviolet ray exposure, whether from the sun or from a manufactured source, such as a tanning bed.

Mercury

A naturally occurring element found in air, water, soil, and rocks. It is a central nervous system toxin.

Mesothelioma
Cancer of the mesothelium, which is the cellular layer lining the internal organs and body walls. It can develop in workers who have had prolonged exposure to asbestos.

Metabolize
To break down, use, and excrete substances brought into the body.

Methylene chloride (METH)
A chemical that is often used as a solvent. It is a carcinogen.

Methylmercury
A type of mercury. It has been used to treat seed grain, but it can also develop in water and accumulate in the bodies of predator fish, such as tuna. It is a neurotoxin.

Microbiome
The community of microorganisms that inhabit the body.

Mold
A type of fungus that grows in warm, moist conditions both indoors and outdoors. There are thousands of mold species.

MRI
See *Magnetic resonance imaging*.

MSDS
See Material Safety Data Sheet.

Mutagen
A substance that causes changes in the genetic structure.

Neurobehavioral disorders
Disorders that involve transient or permanent damage to the brain. Examples include stroke, dementia, and multiple sclerosis.

Neurodevelopmental disorders
Disorders that affect the function of the neurological system and brain. Examples include autism, cerebral palsy, and learning disabilities.

Neurotoxicant
A toxicant that affects the central and peripheral nervous system. See *Toxicant*.

Obesity
A condition in which there is an excess of body fat.

Off-gassing
The release of gasses into the atmosphere from materials or products.

Organic compounds
Chemical compounds that contain carbon.

Organochlorine pesticides
A class of pesticides, many of which are no longer in use. DDT is an example of an organochlorine pesticide.

PAHs
See *Polycyclic aromatic hydrocarbons*.

Parabens
Preservatives added to cosmetics, personal care products, and pharmaceuticals to prevent the growth of microorganisms. Parabens mimic estrogen and have the potential to act as endocrine disruptors. Examples include methylparaben, propylparaben, and butylparaben.

PBB
See *Polybrominated biphenyl*.

PBDE
See *Polybrominated diphenyl ether*.

PBT
See *Persistent, bioaccumulative, and toxic*.

PCB
See *Polychlorinated biphenyl*.

Perc
See *Perchloroethylene*.

Perchloroethylene
A chemical commonly used in dry cleaning processes, it is also in matches, fireworks, and rocket fuel. It now pervades our environment and has been found to be a contaminant in drinking water. It is an endocrine disruptor.

Perfluorocarbons (PFCs)
Synthetic chemicals used in stain treatments and as refrigerants. Examples include perfluorooctane sulfonate (PFOS) and perfluorooctanoic acid (PFOA). Also called perfluorinated chemicals, perfluorochemicals, fluorocarbons, perfluorinated compounds, they are likely carcinogens.

Perfluorooctane sulfonate (PFOS)
Fluorinated, organic compound previously used in industrial and commercial products but no longer manufactured in the US. They persist in the environment and may be an endocrine disruptor.

Perfluorooctanoic acid (PFOA)
A synthetic chemical often used in water- and stain-repellent treatments. Also called C8, there is a "probable link" between C8 and a variety of adverse health effects, such as kidney cancer, testicular cancer, high cholesterol, ulcerative colitis, and thyroid disease.

Persistent, bioaccumulative, and toxic (PBT)
Toxic pollutants that persist in the environment and have the capability to bioaccumulate in the food chain.

Persistent organic pollutants (POPs)
Toxic, carbon-based chemicals that remain in the environment for a long time and travel long distances. They can accumulate and pass through different species by way of the food chain.

Pesticide
A chemical designed to kill insects, animals, microorganisms, plants, or fungi. There are many different types of pesticides so their health effects vary by the type. Possible adverse health effects include neurotoxicity, cancer, and endocrine disruption.

Petroleum distillate
A synthetic chemical extracted from oil.

PFCs
See *Perfluorocarbons*.

PFOA
See *Perfluorooctanoic acid*.

Phthalates
A family of chemicals used in plastics, personal care products, building materials, medical equipment and products, and cleaning products. They are considered to be endocrine disruptors.

Polybrominated biphenyl (PBB)
Flame retardants discontinued in 1976 but still found in the environment. The health effects on humans are not known but they are suspected carcinogens and endocrine disruptors.

Polybrominated diphenyl ethers (PBDE)
Flame retardants, some uses of which were phased out in the mid-2000s in the US. They are still found in households and continue to be detected in global biomonitoring studies. Studies on humans are limited, but emerging. In animal studies, PBDEs have been found to adversely affect various processes, including those of the thyroid gland, liver, nervous system, and the immune system.

Polychlorinated biphenyl (PCB)
Flame retardants, banned by the US in 1979, that do not break down easily and can persist for a long time in the environment. They may cause various adverse effects, including those on the immune, nervous, reproductive, and endocrine systems.

Polycyclic aromatic hydrocarbons (PAHs)
Chemical compounds that both exist naturally in the environment and are also manufactured unintentionally. They can occur when coal, garbage, gas, or oil are incompletely burned. They persist in the environment and are reasonably anticipated to be carcinogenic.

Polyvinyl chloride (PVC)
A plastic that often contains phthalate. It has many uses, including pipes, children's toys, and shower curtains.

POP
See *Persistent organic pollutants.*

PPB
Parts per billion.

PPM
Parts per million.

PPT
Parts per trillion.

Precocious puberty
Puberty that starts before the age of 8 in girls and 9 in boys.

Premature birth
Birth that occurs at least three weeks before the due date.

Primary air pollutant
A pollutant that is released directly into the air from a particular source.

Pro-industry Research
Scientific research that was directly or indirectly conducted or influenced by a sponsoring industry to yield results that support Corporate Interests.

Proposition 65
A California law that requires the State to publish a list of chemicals known to cause cancer, birth defects, or other reproductive harm. Since it was first published in 1987, approximately 800 chemicals have been identified. Businesses are required to warn Californians if products contain significant amounts of these listed chemicals. This list must be updated annually.

PVC
See *Polyvinyl chloride.*

Reproductive toxicant
A toxicant that threatens the development and function of reproductive organs. See *Toxicant.*

SBS
See *Sick building syndrome.*

Secondary air pollutant
An air pollutant emitted when other pollutants react in the atmosphere.

Semivolatile organic compound (sVOC)
An organic compound that can convert to gas or vapor in environments above room temperature. Examples include phenols and polycyclic aromatic hydrocarbons (PAHs).

Sick building syndrome (SBS)
Symptoms that occupants experience while in a specific building that diminish or disappear when they leave.

SIDS
See *Sudden infant death syndrome.*

Simple Strategies
Five strategic plans to detox cleaning products, interior furnishings, kitchen items, personal care products, and children's products. They are found in part III.

Sources
Refers to the literary, scientific, and legal sources listed in chapter 1.12 that detail the use of Manipulative Business Strategies.

Styrene
A chemical used in the manufacture of rubber, some types of plastics, and resins. It can cause central nervous system issues, such as headaches, dizziness, or confusion.

Sudden Infant Death Syndrome (SIDS)
The sudden, unexpected death of an apparently healthy infant during sleep. It is also called crib death.

sVOC
See *Semivolatile organic compound.*

Synthetic
A substance artificially created to imitate a natural product.

TBBPA
See *Tetrabromobisphenol A.*

TBT
See *Tributyltin.*

TCA
See *1,1,1-trichloroethane.*

Tetrabromobisphenol A (TBBPA)
A fire retardant used in consumer electronics and children's products. It is suspected to be an endocrine disruptor.

Tip Reports
The 10 key tips presented part IV. Each has its own report.

Toxicant
A poison that is introduced into the environment through human activities, such as through manufacturing or as an unintentional by-product. Pesticide is an example of a toxicant.

Toxicants of Concern
Toxicants that are profiled in chapter II.1. They are Household Repeat Offenders.

Toxicology
The branch of science that deals with poisons and their effects.

Toxin
A poison found naturally in the environment. It can be generated by animals, microorganisms, plants, or insects.

Trails of Contamination
The contamination of our planet, built environments, and bodies throughout the Life Cycle of a toxicant or material.

Triclosan
An agent used to kill bacteria. It is an ingredient in disinfectants, toothpastes, and other products. It can cause endocrine disruption, and it may make bacteria resistant to antibiotics.

Tris
A class of flame retardants. Phased out for use in children's sleepwear in the 1970s, it is still used in products, such as upholstered furniture or crib mattresses. It is thought to be a carcinogen and is suspected of contributing to other adverse health effects, including neurotoxicity and reproductive effects.

Type I diabetes: A type of diabetes that primarily affects children, adolescents, and young adults. Formerly called juvenile diabetes, it causes the body to not be able to produce insulin. See *Diabetes*.

Type II diabetes: A type of diabetes that often occurs later in life. Formerly called adult onset diabetes or noninsulin-dependent diabetes, it causes the body to either not produce enough insulin or not use it properly. See *Diabetes*.

Unintentional By-products
Compounds that are inadvertently created during manufacturing, combustion, and breakdown through metabolism or natural biodegradation. This is introduced in chapter I.4.

Unintentional Potential Effects
The possible biological and chemical effects of toxicants that are not fully understood. Effects vary by many factors, such as dosage, timing of exposure, and unique vulnerabilities. These are discussed in chapter I.8.

Unintentional Toxicants
Unintended toxic compounds that result from various combinations of other compounds—parent, by-products, or other types. This is introduced in chapter I.4.

VOC
See *Volatile organic compound*.

Volatile Organic Compound (VOC)
An organic compound that can convert easily to gas or vapors. Examples include formaldehyde, gasoline, or benzene. Health effects depend on various factors, such as length of exposure and exposure dosage. Examples of health effects include nausea, dizziness, cancer, organ (liver and kidney) damage, and damage to the central nervous system.

Web of Influence
One of the six Manipulative Business Strategies that are discussed in chapter I.12

All works cited, in addition to relevant website addresses, are available through NontoxicLiving.tips.

AARDA 2014. American Autoimmune Related Diseases Association. 2014. "In Focus: Vol 22, No 1., March 2014." Accessed August 30.

Adams, Kohlmeier, and Zeisel 2010. Adams, Kelly M., Martin Kohlmeier, and Steven H. Zeisel. 2010. "Nutrition Education in US Medical Schools: Latest Update of a National Survey." *Academic Medicine* 85(9): 1537-42.

Adler and Rehkopf 2008. Adler, Nancy E. and David H. Rehkopf. 2008. "US Disparities in Health: Descriptions, Causes and Mechanisms." *Annual Review of Public Health* 29: 235-52.

Affective and Clinical Neuroscience Laboratory 2014. Affective and Clinical Neuroscience Laboratory. 2014. "Northwestern Symposium on Mind and Society. Happiness as a Skill: The Brain's Ability to Change Itself through Mental Training." Last modified September 26.

American Cancer Society 2010. American Cancer Society. 2010. *Cancer Facts and Figures 2010.* Atlanta, GA: American Cancer Society.

American Cancer Society 2014. American Cancer Society. 2014. "Press Releases: Otis Brawley Responds to IARC Classification of Cell Phones as Possible Carcinogenic." Accessed October 29.

American Chemical Society 2004. American Chemical Society. 2004. "Flame Retardants Found on Supermarket Shelves." *ScienceDaily,* September 8.

American Chemical Society 2012. American Chemical Society. 2012. "Widespread Exposure to BPA Substitute is Occurring from Cash Register Receipts, Other Paper." *ScienceDaily,* July 11.

American Chemistry Council 2014. American Chemistry Council. 2014. "TSCA Modernization." Accessed October 15.

American College of OB/GYN 2013. The American College of Obstetricians and Gynecologists. 2013. "Exposure to Toxic Environmental Agents." *Fertility and Sterility* 100(4): 931-4.

Associated Press 2014. Associated Press. 2014. "Beijing Air Pollution at Dangerously High Levels." *New York Times,* January 15.

Association for Packaging and Processing Technologies 2013. Association for Packaging and Processing Technologies. 2013. *Executive Summary and Industry Perspective.* Reston, VA: The Association for Packaging and Processing Technologies.

ATSDR 2004. Agency for Toxic Substances and Disease Registry. 2004. "Toxic Substances Portal – Polybrominated Biphenyls (PBBs) and Polybrominated Diphenyl Ethers (PBDEs)." Last modified September.

ATSDR 2010. Agency for Toxic Substances and Disease Registry. 2010. *Toxicological Profile for Chlorine.* Atlanta, GA: US Department of Health and Human Services, Public Health Service.

ATSDR 2012. Agency for Toxic Substances and Disease Registry. 2012. *Toxicological Profile for Cadmium.* Atlanta, GA: US Department of Health and Human Services, Public Health Service.

Aubrey 2014. Aubrey, Allison. 2014. "Exercise and Protein May Help Good Gut Bacteria Get Their Groove On." *The Salt by NPR* (blog), June 13.

Axelrad et al. 2013. Axelrad, Daniel, Kristen Adams, Farah Chowdhury, Louis D'Amico, Erika Douglass, Gwendolyn Hudson, Erica Koustas, et al. 2013. *America's Children and the Environment, Third Edition.* Washington, DC: United States Environmental Protection Agency.

Baldwin 2012. Baldwin, Shawn. 2012. "LIBOR Liabilities: How Litigation Will Drive Down Banks Profitability for Years to Come..." *Forbes,* October 29.

Barker et al. 1989. Barker, D. J., C. Osmond, J. Golding, D. Kuh, and M. E. Wadsworth. 1989. "Growth In Utero, Blood Pressure in Childhood and Adult Life, and Mortality from Cardiovascular Disease." *British Medical Journal* 298(6673): 564-7.

Barrett 2006. Barrett, Julia R. 2006. "Endocrine Disruptors: Bisphenol A and the Brain." *Environmental Health Perspectives* 114(4): A217.

Barry 2009. Barry, Carolyn. 2009. "Plastic Breaks Down in Ocean, After All – and Fast." *National Geographic News,* August 20.

BBC 2014. BBC. 2014. "What Would Happen If Bees Went Extinct?" *BBC Future,* May 4.

Bein 2010. Bein, Barbara. 2010. "Nutrition Education in US 'Precarious,' Say Researchers." *American Academy of Family Physicians News,* October 20.

Bero 2005. Bero, Lisa A. 2005. "Tobacco Industry Manipulation of Research." *Public Health Reports* 120: 200-8.

Bero 2013. Bero, Lisa A. 2013. "Tobacco Industry Manipulation of Research." In *Late Lessons from Early Warnings: Science, Precaution, Innovation,* edited by David Gee, Philippe Grandjean, Steffen Foss Hansen, Sybille van den Hove, Malcolm MacGarvin, Jock Martin, Gitte Nielsen, David Quist, and David Stanners, 151-78. Copenhagen, Denmark: European Environment Agency.

Berry 2013. Berry, Ian. 2013. "Pesticides Make a Comeback. Many Corn Farmers Go Back to Using Chemicals as Mother Nature Outwits Genetically Modified Seeds." *Wall Street Journal,* May 21.

Bethell et al. 2011. Bethell, C. D., M. D. Kogan, B. B. Strickland, E. L. Schor, J. Robertson, and P. W. Newacheck. 2011. "A National and State Profile of Leading Health Problems and Health Care Quality for US Children: Key Insurance Disparities and across-State Variations." *Academy Pediatrics* 11(3 Suppl): S22-33.

Bhasin et al. 2013. Bhasin, Manoj K., Jeffery A. Dusek, Bei-Hung Chang, Marie G. Joseph, John W. Denniger, Gregory L. Fricchione, Herbert Benson, and Towia A. Libermann. 2013. "Relaxation Response Induces Temporal Transcriptome Changes in Energy Metabolism, Insulin Secretion and Inflammatory Pathways." *PLoS One* 8(5): e62817.

Bienkowski 2012. Bienkowski, Brian. 2012. "EPA Responds to Scientists' Concerns, Initiates New Effort for Low-Dose, Hormone-Like Chemicals." *Environmental Health News,* December 13.

Bienkowski 2013. Bienkowski, Brian. 2013. "BPA Replacement Alters Hormones at Low Doses, Study Finds." *Environmental Health News,* January 17.

Bienkowski and *Environmental Health News* **2013.** Bienkowski, Brian and Environmental Health News. 2013. "EPA Defends Chemical Testing of Low-Dose Hormone Effects." *Scientific American,* June 28.

Biggs et al. 2001. Biggs, Jennifer L., Raja R. Bhagavatula, Ralph S. Blanchard, Bryan C. Gillespie, Lee R. Steeneck, and Kimberley A. Ward. 2001. *Overview of Asbestos Issues and Trends.* Washington, DC: American Academy of Actuaries.

Bilbrey 2014. Bilbrey, Jenna. 2014. "BPA-Free Plastic Containers May Be Just as Hazardous." *Scientific American,* August 11.

BioInitiative Working Group 2014a. BioInitiative Working Group. 2014. "BioInitiative 2012: A Rational for Biologically-Based Exposure Standards for Low-Intensity Electromagnetic Radiation." Accessed October 29.

BioInitiative Working Group 2014b. BioInitiative Working Group. 2014. "New Studies Show Health Risks from Wireless Tech." Last modified April 11.

BIWG and NPPTAC 2005. Broader Issues Work Group (BIWG) and National Pollution Prevention and Toxics Advisory Committee (NPPTAC). 2005. *How Can EPA More Efficiently Identify Potential Risks and Facilitate Risk Reduction Decision for Non-HPV Existing Chemicals? Draft.* United States Environmental Protection Agency.

Blum 2014. Blum, Deborah. 2014. "A Rising Tide of Contaminants." *Well by the New York Times* (blog), September 25.

Bowers 2012. Bowers, Simon. 2012. "Global Profits for Tobacco Trade Total $35bn as Smoking Deaths Top 6 Million." *Guardian,* March 22.

Bowker 2003. Bowker, Michael. 2003. *Fatal Deception: The Terrifying True Story of How Asbestos Is Killing America.* New York: Touchstone.

Boyle et al. 2011. Boyle, Coleen A., Sheree Boulet, Laura A. Schieve, Robin A. Cohen, Stephen J. Blumberg, Marshalyn Yeargin-Allsopp, Susanna Visser, and Michael D. Kogan. 2011. "Trends in the Prevalence of Developmental Disabilities in US Children, 1997-2008." *Pediatrics* 127(6): 1034-42.

Braun et al. 2014. Braun, Joseph M., Amy E. Kalkbrenner, Allan C. Just, Kimberly Yolton, Antonia M. Calafat, Andreas Sjödin, Russ Hauser, Glenys M. Webster, Aimin Chen, and Bruce Lanphear. 2014. "Gestational Exposure to Endocrine-Disrupting Chemicals and Reciprocal Social, Repetitive, and Stereotypic Behaviors in 4- and 5-Year-Old Children: The HOME Study." *Environmental Health Perspectives* 122(5): 513–20.

Breslow 2014. Breslow, Jason M. 2014. "Labor Dept. Warns of 'Alarming' Rise in Cell Tower Deaths." *PBS Frontline,* February 13.

Brownell and Warner 2009. Brownell, Kelly D. and Kenneth E. Warner. 2009. "The Perils of Ignoring History: Big Tobacco Played Dirty and Millions Died. How Similar Is Big Food?" *Milbank Quarterly* 87(1): 259-94.

Bunge and Gasparro 2014. Bunge, Jacob and Annie Gasparro. 2014. "Food Industry Sues Vermont Over Label Law for Genetically Modified Products." *Wall Street Journal,* June 12.

Bunim 2012. Bunim, Juliana. 2012. "Blood-Brain Barrier Less Permeable in Newborns Than Adults after Acute Stroke." *University of California, San Francisco News,* July 10.

C8 Science Panel 2012. C8 Science Panel. 2012. "C8 Science Panel Final Quarterly Newsletter." Last modified November.

CA EPA 1999. California Environmental Protection Agency, Air Resources Board Research Division. 1999. *Common Indoor Sources of Volatile Organic Compounds: Emission Rates and Techniques for Reducing Consumer Exposures. Contract No. 95-302, Final Report.* Sacramento, CA: California Environmental Protection Agency, Air Resources Board.

Caione 2009. Caione, Paolo. 2009. "Prevalence of Hypospadias in European Countries: Is It Increasing?" *European Urology* 55(5): 1027-9.

Callahan and Hawthorne 2012. Callahan, Patricia and Michael Hawthorne. 2012. "New Calif. Standards Could Reduce Flame Retardants." *Chicago Tribune,* June 19.

Callahan and Roe 2012a. Callahan, Patricia and Sam Roe. 2012. "Big Tobacco Wins Fire Marshals as Allies in Flame Retardant Push." *Chicago Tribune,* May 8.

Callahan and Roe 2012b. Callahan, Patricia and Sam Roe. 2012. "Chemical Makers Fan the Flames of Fear." *Chicago Tribune,* May 12.

Callahan and Roe 2012c. Callahan, Patricia and Sam Roe. 2012. "Playing with Fire." *Chicago Tribune,* May 6.

Campaign for Safe Cosmetics 2014a. Campaign for Safe Cosmetics. 2014. "European Laws." Accessed September 19.

Campaign for Safe Cosmetics 2014b. Campaign for Safe Cosmetics. 2014. "Nonprofits: Endorse the Campaign." Accessed October 7.

Campbell and Campbell 2006. Campbell, T. Colin and Thomas M. Campbell II. 2006. *The China Study: The Most Comprehensive Study of Nutrition Ever Conducted. The Startling Implications for Diet, Weight Loss, and Long-Term Health.* Dallas, TX: BenBella.

Carroll et al. 2002. Carroll, Stephen J., Deborah Hensler, Allan Abrahamse, Jennifer Gross, Michelle White, Scott Ashwood, and Elizabeth Sloss. 2002. *Asbestos Litigation Costs and Compensation: An Interim Report.* Santa Monica, CA: RAND.

Carson [1962] 2002. Carson, Rachel. (1962) 2002. *Silent Spring.* New York: First Mariner Books.

CAS 2014. Chemical Abstracts Service, a Division of the American Chemical Society. 2014. "CAS REGISTRY and CAS Registry Number FAQs." Accessed October 21.

Cavagnaro 2007. Cavagnaro, Andrew T. 2007. *Autism Spectrum Disorders: Changes in the California Caseload an Update: June 1987 – June 2007.* Sacramento, CA: California Health and Human Services Agency.

CBS News Staff 2012. CBS News Staff. 2012. "FDA Bans BPA from Baby Bottles, Sippy Cups." *CBS News,* July 17.

CDC 2012a. Centers for Disease Control and Prevention. 2012. "Key Findings: Trends in the Prevalence of Developmental Disabilities in US Children, 1997 – 2008." Last modified August 14.

CDC 2012b. Centers for Disease Control and Prevention. 2012. "Meditation and Health." Last modified April 2.

CDC 2012c. Centers for Disease Control and Prevention. 2012. "National Biomonitoring Program: Environmental Chemicals." Last modified October 19.

CDC 2013a. Centers for Disease Control and Prevention. 2013. "Blood Lead Levels in Children Aged 1-5 Years – United States, 1999-2010." Last modified April 5.

CDC 2013b. Centers for Disease Control and Prevention. 2013. "NCHS Data Brief: Trends in Allergic Conditions among Children: United States, 1997-2011." Last modified May 2.

CDC 2013c. Centers for Disease Control and Prevention. 2013. "Toys." Last modified October 15.

CDC 2014a. Centers for Disease Control and Prevention. 2014. "An Alcohol-Free Pregnancy Is the Best Choice for Your Baby." Accessed November 13.

CDC 2014b. Centers for Disease Control and Prevention. 2014. "Childhood Obesity Facts." Last modified August 13.

CDC 2014c. Centers for Disease Control and Prevention. 2014. "Chronic Diseases and Health Promotion." Last modified May 9.

CDC 2014d. Centers for Disease Control and Prevention. 2014. "Frequently Asked Questions About Cell Phones and Your Health." Accessed October 29.

CDC 2014e. Centers for Disease Control and Prevention. 2014. "Smoking and Tobacco Use: Fast Facts." Last modified April 24.

CEHC 2014a. Mount Sinai Children's Environmental Health Center. 2014. "Children and Toxic Chemicals." Accessed September 18.

CEHC 2014b. Mount Sinai Children's Environmental Health Center. 2014. "Importance of Children's Environmental Health." Accessed October 22.

Center for Investigating Healthy Minds 2014. Center for Investigating Healthy Minds at the Waisman Center. 2014. "Center for Investigating Healthy Minds." Accessed December 5.

CHEJ 2014a. Center for Health, Environment and Justice. 2014. "Environmental Justice and the PVC Chemical Industry." Accessed September 22.

CHEJ 2014b. Center for Health, Environment and Justice. 2014. "Top Ten Reasons Your School Should Go PVC-Free." Accessed September 22.

Chemical Industry Archives 2009. Chemical Industry Archives: A Project of Environmental Working Group. 2009. "Fiction #1: 'You'd Have to Drink 500 Bathtubs to Get a Dose That Caused Any Harm in Animal Studies." Last modified March 27.

Chen 2010. Chen, Pauline W. 2010. "Teaching Doctors About Nutrition and Diet." *New York Times,* September 16.

Choi and Friso 2010. Choi, Sang-Woon and Simonetta Friso. 2010. "Epigenetics: A New Bridge between Nutrition and Health." *Advances in Nutrition* 1(1): 8-16.

Chudler 2014. Chudler, Eric H. 2014. "The Blood Brain Barrier ('Keep out')." *Neuroscience For Kids, on University of Washington Faculty Web Server* (blog), accessed September 2.

CIA 2013. Central Intelligence Agency. 2013. *The World Factbook 2013-2014.* Washington, DC: Central Intelligence Agency.

CIRS 2011. Chemical Inspection and Regulation Service. 2011. "Global Chemical Inventories 2011." Last modified November.

CIRS 2014a. Chemical Inspection and Regulation Service. 2014. "Australian Inventory of Chemical Substances (AICS)." Accessed November 24.

CIRS 2014b. Chemical Inspection and Regulation Service. 2014. "Canada DSL/NDSL." Accessed October 14.

CIRS 2014c. Chemical Inspection and Regulation Service. 2014. "China Existing Chemical Inventory – IECSC." Accessed October 14.

CIRS 2014d. Chemical Inspection and Regulation Service. 2014. "Japanese Existing and New Chemical Substances Inventory (ENCS.)" Accessed October 14.

CIRS 2014e. Chemical Inspection and Regulation Service. 2014. "Korea Existing Chemicals Inventory (KECI)." Accessed October 14.

CIRS 2014f. Chemical Inspection and Regulation Service. 2014. "National Existing Chemical Inventory in Taiwan." Accessed October 14.

CIRS 2014g. Chemical Inspection and Regulation Service. 2014. "Philippine PICCS." Accessed November 24.

CIRS 2014h. Chemical Inspection and Regulation Service. 2014. "US TSCA Inventory." Accessed October 14.

Cisco 2014. Cisco.com. 2014. "Cisco Visual Networking Index: Global Mobile Data Traffic Forecast Update, 2013 – 2018." Last modified February 5.

Clapp et al. 2014. Clapp, Richard, Polly Hoppin, Jyotsna Jagai, and Sara Donahue. 2014. "Perfluorooctanoic Acid." *Defending Science* (blog), accessed November 21.

Cohen 2001. Cohen, Sheldon. 2001. "Social Relationships and Health: Berkman and Syme (1979)." *Advances in Mind-Body Medicine* 17: 2-59.

Cohn et al. 2007. Cohn, Barbara A., Mary S. Wolff, Piera M. Cirillo, and Robert I. Sholtz. 2007. "DDT and Breast Cancer in Young Women: New Data on the Significance of Age at Exposure." *Environmental Health Perspectives* 115(10): 1406-14.

Colborn, Dumanoski, and Myers 1997. Colborn, Theo, Dianne Dumanoski, and John Peterson Myers. 1997. *Our Stolen Future: Are We Threatening Our Fertility, Intelligence, and Survival? – A Scientific Detective Story.* New York: Plume.

Collaborative on Health and the Environment – Washington 2014. The Collaborative on Health and the Environment – Washington. 2014. "Developmental and Neurobehavioral Disabilities." Accessed August 27.

Collegium Ramazzini 2010. Collegium Ramazzini. 2010. "Asbestos Is Still with Us: Repeat Call for a Universal Ban." *Archives of Environmental and Occupational Health* 65(3): 121-6.

Colon et al. 2000. Colon, Ivelisse, Doris Caro, Carlos J. Bourdony, and Osvaldo Rosario. 2000. "Identification of Phthalate Esters in the Serum of Young Puerto Rican Girls with Premature Breast Development." *Environmental Health Perspectives* 108(9): 895-900.

Committee on Nutrition in Medical Education 1985. Committee on Nutrition in Medical Education. 1985. *Nutrition Education in US Medical Schools.* Washington, DC: National Academy Press.

ComScore 2014. ComScore. 2014. "ComScore Reports December 2013 US Smartphone Subscriber Market Share." Last modified February 4.

Cone 2009a. Cone, Marla. 2009. "Autism Increase Not Caused Only by Shifts in Diagnoses; Environmental Factors Likely, New California Study Says." *Environmental Health News,* January 9.

Cone 2009b. Cone, Marla. 2009. "Scientists Find 'Baffling' Link Between Autism and Vinyl Flooring." *Environmental Health News,* March 31.

Cone 2012a. Cone, Marla. 2012. "Long-Awaited Dioxins Report Released; EPA Says Low Doses Risky But Most People Safe." *Environmental Health News,* February 17.

Cone 2012b. Cone, Marla. 2012. "Low Doses, Big Effects: Scientists Seek 'Fundamental Changes' in Testing, Regulation of Hormone-Like Chemicals." *Environmental Health Perspectives,* March 15.

Cone and *Environmental Health News* 2012. Cone, Marla and Environmental Health News. 2012. "Children May Be Exposed to Higher Chemical Concentrations Than Their Mothers." *Scientific American,* January 26.

Consumer Reports 2012. Consumer Reports. 2012. "Arsenic in Your Food. Our Findings Show a Real Need for Federal Standards for This Toxin." Last modified November.

Consumer Reports 2014a. Consumer Reports. 2014. "FDA Data Show Arsenic in Rice, Juice, and Beer. Here's an Overview of Some Significant Developments Regarding Arsenic in Food in the Last Year." Last modified February 6.

Consumer Reports 2014b. Consumer Reports. 2014. "The Risky Chemical Lurking in Your Wallet. New Research Finds That the BPA in Cash Register Receipts Can Be Absorbed through Skin." Last modified March 29.

Cook 2008. Cook, Ken. 2008. "10 Americans." Presentation given at Tides Momentum Conference, San Francisco, CA. Presentation given and filmed July 21. YouTube, 22:21. Posted May 2, 2011.

CPSC 2007. United States Consumer Product Safety Commission. 2007. "CPSC Delivers the ABC's of Toy Safety." Last modified November 20.

Crimmins, Preston, and Cohen 2011. Crimmins, Eileen M., Samuel H. Preston, and Barney Cohen, eds. 2011. *Explaining Divergent Levels of Longevity in High-Income Countries.* Washington, DC: National Academies Press.

Daneman et al. 2010. Daneman, Richard, Lu Zhou, Amanuel A. Kebede, and Ben A. Barres. 2010. "Pericytes Are Required for Blood-Brain Barrier Integrity during Embryogenesis." *Nature* 468(7323): 562-6.

Dashwood and Ho 2008. Dashwood, Roderick H. and Emily Ho. 2008. "Dietary Agents as Histone Deacetylase Inhibitors: Sulforaphane and Structurally Related Isothiocyanates." *Nutrition Reviews* 66(Suppl 1): S36–8.

Davidson and Asch 2011. Davidson, Peter and Rebecca G. Asch. 2011. "Plastic Ingestion by Mesopelagic Fishes in the North Pacific Subtropical Gyre." *Marine Ecology Progress Series* 432: 173-80.

Davis 2009. Davis, Donald R. 2009. "Declining Fruit and Vegetable Nutrient Composition: What Is the Evidence?" *HortScience* 44(1): 15-9.

Davis 2010. Davis, Devra. 2010. *Disconnect: The Truth About Cell Phone Radiation, What the Industry Has Done to Hide It, and How to Protect Your Family.* New York: Dutton.

Davis 2013. Davis, John. 2013. "Researchers Find Cancer Risks Double When Two Carcinogens Present at 'Safe' Levels." *Texas Tech Today by Texas Tech University*, June 28.

Davis, Epp, and Riordan 2004. Davis, Donald R., Melvin D. Epp, and Hugh D. Riordan. 2004. "Changes in USDA Food Composition Data for 43 Garden Crops, 1950 to 1999." *Journal of the American College of Nutrition* 23(6): 669-82.

Denison 2009. Denison, Richard. 2009. "EPA's New Chemicals Program: TSCA Dealt EPA a Very Poor Hand." *EDF Health by Environmental Defense Fund* (blog), April 16.

Department of Veteran Affairs 2013. United States Department of Veteran Affairs. 2013. "Birth Defects in Children of Vietnam and Korea Veterans." Last modified December 30.

Diamanti-Kandarakis et al. 2009. Diamanti-Kandarakis, Evanthia, Jean-Pierre Bourguignon, Linda C. Giudice, Russ Hauser, Gail S. Prins, Ana M. Soto, R. Thomas Zoeller, and Andrea C. Gore. 2009. "Endocrine-Disrupting Chemicals: An Endocrine Society Scientific Statement." *Endocrine Reviews* 30(4): 293–342.

Dingemans et al. 2008. Dingemans, M. M., A. de Groot, R. G. van Kleef, A. Bergman, M. van den Berg, H. P. Vijverberg, and R. H. Westerink. 2008. "Hydroxylation Increases the Neurotoxic Potential of BDE-47 to Affect Exocytosis and Calcium Homeostasis in PC12 Cells." *Environmental Health Perspectives* 116(5): 637-43.

Doe Run Company 2013. Doe Run Company. 2013. *Mining in the US.* St. Louis, MO: Doe Run.

Dolinoy, Huang, and Jirtle 2007. Dolinoy, Dana C., Dale Huang, and Randy L. Jirtle. 2007. "Maternal Nutrient Supplementation Counteracts Bisphenol A-Induced DNA Hypomethylation in Early Development." *Proceedings of the National Academy of Sciences of the United States of America* 104(32): 13056-61.

Drope and Chapman 2001. Drope, J. and S. Chapman. 2001. "Tobacco Industry Efforts at Discrediting Scientific Knowledge of Environmental Tobacco Smoke: A Review of Internal Industry Documents." *Journal of Epidemiology and Community Health* 55: 588-94.

Duke Medicine 2005. Duke Medicine News and Communications. 2005. "'Epigenetics' Means What We Eat, How We Live and Love, Alters How Our Genes Behave." Last modified October 26.

Duty et al. 2003. Duty, Susan M., Narendra P. Singh, Manori J. Silva, Dana B. Barr, John W. Brock, Louise Ryan, Robert F. Herrick, David C. Christiani, and Russ Hauser. 2003. "The Relationship between Environmental Exposures to Phthalates and DNA Damage in Human Sperm Using the Neutral Comet Assay." *Environmental Health Perspectives* 111(9): 1164-9.

***Economist* 2012.** Economist. 2012. "Focus: World GDP." *Economist,* October 9.

EEA 2001. European Environment Agency. 2001. *Late Lessons from Early Warnings: The Precautionary Principle 1986-2000. Report Number 22.* Copenhagen, Denmark: European Environment Agency.

EEA 2012. European Environment Agency. 2012. *The Impacts of Endocrine Disrupters on Wildlife, People and Their Environments—The Weybridge+15 (1996–2011) Report.* Copenhagen, Denmark: European Environment Agency.

EEA 2013. European Environment Agency. 2013. *Late Lessons from Early Warnings: Science, Precaution, Innovation. ISSN 1725–9177.* Copenhagen, Denmark: European Environment Agency.

Egner et al. 2014. Egner, Patricia A., Jian-Guo Chen, Adam T. Zarth, Derek K. Ng, Jin-Bing Wang, Kevin H. Kensler, Lisa P. Jacobson, et al. 2014. "Rapid and Sustainable Detoxification of Airborne Pollutants by Broccoli Sprout Beverage: Results of a Randomized Clinical Trial in China." *Cancer Prevention Research* 7(8): 813-23.

Endocrine Society 2014a. Endocrine Society. 2014. "AMA Adopts Endocrine Society Resolution Calling for New Policies to Decrease Public Exposure to Endocrine-Disrupting Chemicals." Accessed October 4.

Endocrine Society 2014b. Endocrine Society. 2014. "Common BPA Substitute, BPS Disrupts Heart Rhythms in Females." *ScienceDaily,* June 23.

Eng 2012. Eng, Monica. 2012. "Citizen Complaints Not Addressed by FDA. As It Stands, Ingredients in Microwave Popcorn Found to Pose Risk for Workers - But Consumer Issues Have Not Been Addressed." *Chicago Tribune,* August 25.

Environmental Health Association of Quebec 2014. Environmental Health Association of Quebec. 2014. "EMFS Recognition." Accessed October 29.

Environmental Health Trust 2014. Environmental Health Trust. 2014. "About Devra Lee Davis

PhD MPH: Founder and President of Environmental Health Trust." Accessed October 29.

EPA 1989. United States Environmental Protection Agency. 1989. "40 CFR Part 763. Asbestos: Manufacture, Importation, Processing, and Distribution in Commerce Prohibitions; Final Rule." *Federal Register* 54(132): 29460–513.

EPA 1994. United States Environmental Protection Agency. 1994. *Chemicals in the Environment: Chlorine (CAS No. 7782-50-5).* Washington, DC: United States Environmental Protection Agency.

EPA 1997. United States Environmental Protection Agency. 1997. "The Premanufacture Notification (PMN) Review Process." In *Chemistry Assistance Manual for Premanufacture Notification Submitters, EPA 744-R-97-003,* 5-43. Washington, DC: United States Environmental Protection Agency.

EPA 2005. United States Environmental Protection Agency. 2005. *Guidelines for Carcinogen Risk Assessment. EPA/630/P-03/001F.* Washington, DC: United States Environmental Protection Agency.

EPA 2006. United States Environmental Protection Agency. 2006. "5.0 Toxicology." Last modified May.

EPA 2009a. United States Environmental Protection Agency. 2009. "Buildings and Their Impact on the Environment: A Statistical Summary." Last modified April 22.

EPA 2009b. United States Environmental Protection Agency. 2009. "Speeches – By Date. Administrator Lisa P. Jackson, Remarks to the Commonwealth Club of San Francisco, As Prepared." Last modified September 29.

EPA 2010. United States Environmental Protection Agency. 2010. "HPV Chemical Hazard Data Availability Study." Last modified August 2.

EPA 2011a. United States Environmental Protection Agency. 2011. "DDT." Last modified April 18.

EPA 2011b. United States Environmental Protection Agency. 2011. "High Throughput Pre-Screening (HTPS) and Quantitative Structure Activity Relationships (QSAR)." Last modified August 11.

EPA 2012a. United States Environmental Protection Agency. 2012. "EPA Updates Science Assessment for Dioxins/Air Emissions of Dioxins Have Decreased by 90 Percent since the 1980s." Last modified February 17.

EPA 2012b. United States Environmental Protection Agency. 2012. "An Introduction to Indoor Air Quality (IAQ): Lead (Pb)." Last modified June 21.

EPA 2013a. United States Environmental Protection Agency. 2013. "Methylene Chloride (Dicholomethane)." Last modified October 18.

EPA 2013b. United States Environmental Protection Agency. 2013. "Testimony of James Jones Assistant Administrator Office of Chemical Safety and Pollution Prevention US Environmental Protection Agency before the Subcommittee on Environment and the Economy Committee on Energy and Commerce United States House of Representatives." Last modified November 13.

EPA 2014a. United States Environmental Protection Agency. 2014. *2012 Toxics Release Inventory, National Analysis Overview.* Washington, DC: United States Environmental Protection Agency.

EPA 2014b. United States Environmental Protection Agency. 2014. "Climate Change: Basic Information." Last modified March 18.

EPA 2014c. United States Environmental Protection Agency. 2014. "EPA Releases 2010 Toxics Release Inventory National Analysis." Last modified September 19.

EPA 2014d. United States Environmental Protection Agency. 2014. "Perfluorooctanoic Acid (PFOA) and Fluorinated Telomers." Last modified September 9.

EPA 2014e. United States Environmental Protection Agency. 2014. "Persistent Organic Pollutants: A Global Issue, a Global Response." Last modified June 12.

EPA 2014f. United States Environmental Protection Agency. 2014. "Summary of Key Points from *Climate Change Indicators in the United States, 2014.*" Last modified May.

EPA 2014g. United States Environmental Protection Agency. 2014. "Technical Factsheet on: ASBESTOS." Accessed October 16.

EPA 2014h. United States Environmental Protection Agency. 2014. "Technical Fact Sheet – Polybrominated Diphenyl Ethers (PBDEs) and Polybrominated Biphenyls (PBBs)." Last modified January.

EPA 2014i. United States Environmental Protection Agency. 2014. "TRI-Listed Chemicals." Last modified November 6.

EPA 2014j. United States Environmental Protection Agency. 2014. "Understanding PCB Risks." Last modified October 9.

Eriksen et al. 2014. Eriksen, Marcus, Laurent C. M. Lebreton, Henry S. Carson, Martin Thiel, Charles J. Moore, Jose C. Borerro, Francois Galgani, Peter G. Ryan, and Julia Reisser. 2014. "Plastic Pollution in the World's Oceans: More Than 5 Trillion Plastic Pieces Weighing over 250,000 Tons Afloat at Sea." *PLoS ONE* 9(12): e111913.

EU OSHA 2014. European Agency for Safety and Health at Work. 2014. "Regulation (EC) No 1907/2006-REACH." Accessed November 28.

European Commission 2014. European Commission. 2014. "List of Substances Prohibited in Cosmetic Products." Accessed September 19.

European Commission 2015. European Commission. 2015. "EU Calls on Industry to Register Chemicals in Preparation for New "REACH" Regulation on Chemicals and Their Safe Use." Last modified October 4.

EWG 1999. Environmental Working Group. 1999. "EPA Asbestos Materials Bans: Clarification." Last modified May 18.

EWG 2003a. Environmental Working Group. 2003. "Mother's Milk: Health Risks of PBDEs." Last modified September 23.

EWG 2003b. Environmental Working Group. 2003. "PFCs: Global Contaminants: PFCs Last Forever." Last modified April 3.

EWG 2004a. Environmental Working Group. 2004. "Asbestos: Think Again: Asbestos Is Still Not Banned." Last modified March 4.

EWG 2004b. Environmental Working Group. 2004. "Asbestos: Think Again: Industry Hid Dangers for Decades." Last modified March 4.

EWG 2005a. Environmental Working Group. 2005. "Body Burden: The Pollution in Newborns." Last modified July 14.

EWG 2005b. Environmental Working Group. 2005. "Body Burden: The Pollution in Newborns: Babies Are Vulnerable to Chemical Harm." Last modified July 14.

EWG 2008. Environmental Working Group. 2008. "EWG's Healthy Home Tips for Parents." Last modified October 11.

EWG 2010a. Environmental Working Group. 2010. "Off the Books: Industry's Secret Chemicals: Thousands of Chemical Names and Ingredients Kept Under Wraps at EPA." Last modified January 4.

EWG 2010b. Environmental Working Group. 2010. "Testimony of Kenneth A. Cook, President of the Environmental Working Group, before the Subcommittee on Commerce, Trade and Consumer Protection, US House of Representatives, Committee on Energy and Commerce." Last modified July 29.

EWG 2013a. Environmental Working Group. 2013. "EWG's Guide to Safer Cell Phone Use." Last modified August 27.

EWG 2013b. Environmental Working Group. 2013. "Oral Testimony of Heather White on the Regulation of New Chemicals, Protection of Confidential Business Information, and Innovation." Last modified July 11.

EWG 2013c. Environmental Working Group. 2013. "Real Chemical Reform Must Ban Asbestos." Last modified July 30.

EWG 2013d. Environmental Working Group. 2013. "Regulation of New Chemicals, Protection of Confidential Business Information, and Innovation." Last modified July 11.

EWG 2014a. Environmental Working Group. 2014. "The Asbestos Epidemic in America." Accessed November 28.

EWG 2014b. Environmental Working Group. 2014. "Cleaning Supplies: Secret Ingredients, Hidden Hazards." Accessed September 19.

EWG 2014c. Environmental Working Group. 2014. "Cleaning Supplies and Your Health." Accessed September 19.

EWG 2014d. Environmental Working Group. 2014. "Fact Sheets: Can Low Doses of Chemicals Hurt Me?" Accessed February 21.

EWG 2014e. Environmental Working Group. 2014. "Findings and Recommendations." Accessed November 26.

ExxonMobil 2014. ExxonMobil. 2014. *Summary Annual Report 2013.* Irving, TX: Exxon Mobil Corporation.

Falco 2012. Falco, Miriam. 2012. "CDC: US Kids with Autism Up 78 percent in Past Decade." *CNN,* March 29.

FCC 2012. Federal Communications Commission. 2012. "Radio Frequency Safety." Last modified June 25.

FDA 2013a. United States Food and Drug Administration. 2013. "FDA Continues to Study BPA." Last modified August 23.

FDA 2013b. United States Food and Drug Administration. 2013. "Select Committee on GRAS Substances (SCOGS) Opinion: Diacetyl." Last modified April 18.

FDA 2014. United States Food and Drug Administration. 2014. "Questions and Answers: Apple Juice and Arsenic." Last modified June 4.

Feinstein 2011. Feinstein, Dianne. 2011. "Ban Unsafe Chemical from Baby Bottles and Cups." *CNN,* July 14.

Foley 2015. Foley, Libby. 2015. "Chemical Industry Spending Surges to Support Sham Reform." *Enviroblog by Environmental Working Group,* March 6.

Fortune 2012. Fortune. 2012. "Fortune 500 2012: 1: Exxon Mobil Corporation." Accessed December 2.

Freuman 2012. Freuman, Tamara Duker. 2012. "Tending Your Inner Ecosystem. How to Boost the Friendly Bacterial in Your Gut." *US News,* September 5.

Fuchs 2014. Fuchs, Victor R. 2014. "Why Do Other Rich Nations Spend So Much Less on Healthcare?" *Atlantic,* July 23.

Galvez 2011. Galvez, Maida P. 2011. "EDs, Early Puberty, and Breast Cancer." Presentation given at Mount Sinai Children's Environmental Health Center's event titled *Birth Defects, Learning Disabilities, Obesity, and Breast Cancer: How Can We Avoid the Effects of Toxic Chemicals?*, New York Academy of Medicine, New York. Presentation given and filmed December 5. Vimeo, 9:56. Posted December 14, 2011.

GAO 2005. United States Government Accountability Office. 2005. *Chemical Regulation: Options Exist to Improve EPA's Ability to Assess Health Risks and Manage Its Chemicals Review Program. GAO 05-458.* Washington, DC: United States Government Accountability Office.

GAO 2009a. United States Government Accountability Office. 2009. "Observations on Improving the Toxic Substances Control Act." Last modified December 2.

GAO 2009b. United States Government Accountability Office. 2009. *Testimony before the Committee on Environment and Public Works, US Senate. Chemical Regulation: Observations on Improving the Toxic Substances Control Act. GAO-10-292T.* Washington, DC: United States Government Accountability Office.

Gersowitz, Libo, and Korek, PC 2014. Gersowitz, Libo, and Korek, P. C. 2014. "C8 Personal Injury Lawsuits for Toxic Chemical Exposure." Accessed September 29.

Gever 2010. Gever, John. 2010. "Weight Loss May Release Stored Toxins." *Medpage Today,* September 9.

Gilgoff 2010. Gilgoff, Dan. 2010. "Can Meditation Change Your Brain? Contemplative Neuroscientists Believe That It Can." *Belief Blog by CNN,* October 26.

Gillis 2014. Gillis, Justin. 2014. "Panel's Warning on Climate Risk: Worst Is Yet to Come." *New York Times,* March 31.

Glass 1975. Glass, W.I. 1975. "Dieldrin Poisoning: Case Report." *New Zealand Medical Journal* 81(534): 202-3.

Global Climate Change 2015. NASA: Global Climate Change: Vital Signs of the Planet. 2015. "Consensus: 97 percent of Climate Scientists Agree." Accessed June 24.

Grandjean and Landrigan 2014. Grandjean, Philippe and Philip J. Landrigan. 2014. "Neurobehavioural Effects of Developmental Toxicity." *The Lancet Neurology* 13(3): 330-8.

Gross 2013. Gross, Liza. 2013. "Flame Retardants in Consumer Products Are Linked to Health and Cognitive Problems." *Washington Post,* April 15.

Grube et al. 2011. Grube, Arthur, David Donaldson, Timothy Kiely, and La Wu. 2011. *Pesticides Industry Sales and Usage 2006 and 2007 Market Estimates.* Washington, DC: Biological and Economic Analysis Division, Office of Pesticide Programs, Office of Chemical Safety and Pollution Prevention, United States Environmental Protection Agency.

Haberman 2014. Haberman, Clyde. 2014. "The Head-Scratching Case of the Vanishing Bees." *New York Times,* September 28.

Halladay 2014. Halladay, Alycia. 2014. "What Do Scientists Mean When They Talk About 'Environmental Factors' That Cause Autism." *Autism Speaks* (blog), accessed November 13.

Hamers et al 2008. Hamers, Timo, Jorke H. Kamstra, Edwin Sonneveld, Albertinka J. Murk, Theo J. Visser, Martin J. Van Velzen, Abraham Brouwer, and Ake Bergman. 2008. "Biotransformation of Brominated Flame Retardants into Potentially Endocrine-Disrupting Metabolites, with Special Attention to 2,2',4,4'-Tetrabromodiphenyl Ether (BDE-47)." *Molecular Nutrition and Food Research* 52(2): 284-98.

Hamilton 2012. Hamilton, Jon. 2012. "Legal Battle Erupts Over Whose Plastic Consumers Should Trust." *Shots by NPR* (blog), July 30.

Harley et al. 2010. Harley, Kim G., Amy R. Marks, Jonathan Chevrier, Asa Bradman, Andreas Sjödin, and Brenda Eskenazi. 2010. "PBDE Concentrations in Women's Serum and Fecundability." *Environmental Health Perspectives* 118: 669-704.

Harvard Health Publications 2014. Harvard Health Publications. 2014. "How to Boost Your Immune System." Accessed November 6.

Harvard Medical School Family Health Guide 2004. Harvard Medical School Family Health Guide. 2004. "Benefits of Moderate Sun Exposure." Last modified June.

Harvard Women's Health Watch 2010. Harvard Women's Health Watch. 2010. "The Health Benefit of Strong Relationships." *Harvard Health Publications by Harvard Medical School,* December.

Hattis et al. 2001. Hattis, D., A. Russ, R. Goble, P. Banati, and M. Chu. 2001. "Human Interindividual Variability in Susceptibility to Airborne Particles." *Risk Analysis* 21(4): 585-99.

Hawthorne 2005. Hawthorne, Michael. 2005. "EPA Charges DuPont Hid Teflon's Risks." *Chicago Tribune,* January 18.

Hawthorne 2012. Hawthorne, Michael. 2012. "Danger for Kids' Pajamas, Safe for Sofas? Flame Retardant Removed from Sleepwear amid Health Concerns Is Increasingly Used in Furniture." *Chicago Tribune,* November 27.

Hawthorne 2014. Hawthorne, Michael. 2014. "Chemical Industry Fights for Flame Retardants." *Chicago Tribune,* August 29.

Hertz-Picciotto and Delwiche 2009. Hertz-Picciotto, Irva and Lora Delwiche. 2009. "The Rise in Autism and the Role of Age at Diagnosis." *Epidemiology* 20(1): 84-90.

HESIS and LOHP 2008. Hazard Evaluation System and Information Service (HESIS) and the Labor Occupational Health Program (LOHP). 2008. *Understanding Toxic Substances: An Introduction to Chemical Hazards in the Workplace.* Richmond, CA: Hazard Evaluation System and Information Service (HESIS) and the Labor Occupational Health Program (LOHP).

Hibbard 2012. Hibbard, Matthew. 2012. "Doe Run CEO Bruce Neil to Retire." *St. Louis Business Journal,* June 15.

Hong and Bero 2002. Hong, Mi-Kyung and Lisa A. Bero. 2002. "How the Tobacco Industry Responded to an Influential Study of the Health Effects of Secondhand Smoke." *BMJ* 325: 1413.

Hoshaw 2009. Hoshaw, Lindsey. 2009. "Afloat in the Ocean, Expanding Islands of Trash." *New York Times*, November 9.

Houlihan, Lunder, and Jacob 2008. Houlihan, Jane, Sonya Lunder, and Anila Jacob. 2008. "Timeline: BPA from Invention to Phase-Out." *Research by Environmental Working Group*, April 22.

HSPH 2014. Harvard School of Public Health. 2014. "Laura Kubzansky." Accessed November 5.

Hu 2001. Hu, Angang. 2001. "The Chinese Economy in Prospect." In *China, the United States, and the Global Economy*, edited by Shuxun Chen and Charles Wolf, Jr., 99-146. Santa Monica, CA: RAND.

Hume and Christensen 2014. Hume, Tim and Jen Christensen. 2014. "WHO: Imminent Global Cancer 'Disaster' Reflects Aging, Lifestyle Factors." *CNN,* February 4.

Hurt and Robertson 1998. Hurt, R. D. and C. R. Robertson. 1998. "Prying Open the Door to the Tobacco Industry's Secrets About Nicotine: The Minnesota Tobacco Trial." *The Journal of the American Medical Association* 280(13): 1173-81.

Huyghe, Matsuda, and Thonneau 2003. Huyghe, E., T. Matsuda, and P. Thonneau. 2003. "Increasing Incidence of Testicular Cancer Worldwide: A Review." *The Journal of Urology* 170(1): 5-11.

IARC 2011. International Agency for Research on Cancer. 2011. "Press Release: IARC Classifies Radiofrequency Electromagnetic Fields as Possibly Carcinogenic to Humans." Last modified May 31.

IARC 2014. International Agency for Research on Cancer. 2014. "Agents Classified by the *IARC Monographs,* Volumes 1-111." Last modified October 30.

ICOH 2014. The International Commission on Occupational Health. 2014. "ICOH Statement: Global Asbestos Ban and the Elimination of Asbestos-Related Diseases." Accessed October 16.

International Ban Asbestos Secretariat 2014. International Ban Asbestos Secretariat. 2014. "Current Asbestos Bans and Restrictions." Last modified January 27.

IPCC 2014. Intergovernmental Panel on Climate Change. Christopher B. Field, Vicente R. Barros, Michael D. Mastrandrea, Katharine J. Mach, Mohamed A. K. Abdrabo, W. Neil Adger, Yury A. Anokhin, et al. 2014. *Climate Change 2014: Impacts, Adaptation, and Vulnerability. Summary for Policymakers. Working Group II Contribution to the Fifth Assessment Report of the Intergovernmental Panel on Climate Change.* Geneva, Switzerland: Intergovernmental Panel on Climate Change.

IRC 2014. Insight Research Corporation. 2014. *The 2014 Telecommunications Industry Review: An Anthology of Market Facts and Forecasts 2013-2018.* Mountain Lakes, NJ: The Insight Research Corporation.

IRTA 2000. Institute for Research and Technical Assistance. 2000. *Cleaner Technologies Substitutes Assessment Case Studies: Mattress Manufacturing.* Santa Monica, CA: Institute for Research and Technical Assistance.

Jacobs and Johnson 2014. Jacobs, Andrew and Ian Johnson. 2014. "Pollution Killed 7 Million People Worldwide in 2012, Report Finds." *New York Times,* March 25.

Jirtle 2012. Jirtle, Randy. 2012. "Epigenetics. How Genes and Environment Interact." Presentation given at the NIH Director's Wednesday Afternoon Lecture Series, Bethesda, MD. Presentation given and filmed April 18. NIH VideoCasting, 58:00. Posted July 31, 2012.

Johnston 2012. Johnston, Ian. 2012. "Study: Plastic in 'Great Pacific Garbage Patch' Increases 100-Fold." *NBC News,* May 9.

Jones, Wills, and Kang 2010. Jones, Robert, Brandon Wills, and Christopher Kang. 2010. "Chlorine Gas: An Evolving Hazardous Material Threat and Unconventional Weapon." *Western Journal of Emergency Medicine* 11(2): 151-6.

JustLabelIt.Org 2014. JustLabelIt. Org. 2014. "GMO Labeling Isn't Dead: See Which States Are Leading the Fight." Accessed October 27.

Kaldveer 2014. Kaldveer, Zack. 2014. "Five Ways the FDA Has Failed Consumers on Genetically Engineered Foods." *Organic Consumers Association* (blog), accessed October 28.

Kerry 2014. Kerry, John. 2014. "John Kerry: Our Historic Agreement with China on Climate Change." *New York Times,* November 11.

Kim 2011. Kim, Andy. 2011. "Health and Human Services. Time to Ban BPA?" *Governing the States and Localities,* March.

Kluger 2010. Kluger, Jeffrey. 2010. "Flushed Away." *Time,* April 1.

Koike and Cardoso 2014. Koike, Marcia Kiyomi and Robert Cardoso. 2014. "Meditation Can Produce Beneficial Effects to Prevent Cardiovascular Disease." *Hormone Molecular Biology and Clinical Investigation* 18(3): 137-43.

Kortenkamp et al. 2011. Kortenkamp Andreas, Olwenn Martin, Michael Faust, Richard Evans, Rebecca McKinlay, Frances Orton, and Erika Rosivatz. 2011. *State of the Art Assessment of Endocrine Disrupters. Final Report. Project Contract No. 070307/2009/550687/SER/D3.* Brussels, Belgium: European Commission, Directorate-General for the Environment.

Landrigan 2010. Landrigan, Philip J. 2010. "What Causes Autism? Exploring the Environmental Contribution." *Current Opinion in Pediatrics* 22(2): 219-25.

Landrigran and Etzel 2014. Landrigan, Philip J. and Ruth A. Etzel, eds. 2014. *Textbook of Children's Environmental Health.* New York: Oxford University Press.

Lang 2006. Lang, Susan S. 2006. "'Slow, Insidious' Soil Erosion Threatens Human Health and Welfare as Well as the Environment, Cornell Study Asserts." *Cornell Chronicle by Cornell University,* March 20.

Latini et al. 2003. Latini, Giuseppe, Claudio De Felice, Giuseppe Presta, Antonio Del Vecchio, Irma Paris, Fabrizio Ruggieri, and Pietro Mazzeo. 2003. "In Utero Exposure to Di-(2-ethylhexyl) Phthalate and Duration of Human Pregnancy." *Environmental Health Perspectives* 111(14): 1783–5.

Layton 2008. Layton, Lyndsey. 2008. "Lawmakers Agree to Ban Toxins in Children's Items." *Washington Post,* July 29.

Lee 2011. Lee, Jaeah. 2011. "BPA Makes Little Girls Anxious and Depressed." *Mother Jones,* October 25.

Lee 2014. Lee, Stephanie M. 2014. "Flame-Retardant Maker Sues Over New Calif. Law." *SFGate,* January 17.

Leffall 2008. Leffall, LaSalle D., ed. 2008. *Meeting Summary. President's Cancer Panel. Environmental Factors in Cancer.* East Brunswick, NJ: National Cancer Institute.

Lent 2007. Lent, Tom. 2007. "USGBC: PVC Is Not a Healthy Building Material." *Healthy Building News by Healthy Building Network* (blog), March 9.

Letcher, Klasson-Wehler, and Bergman 2000. Letcher, Robert J., Eva Klasson-Wehler, and Ake Bergman. 2000. "Methyl Sulfone and Hydroxylated Metabolites of Polychlorinated Biphenyls." In *The Handbook of Environmental Chemistry: Volume 3 Anthropogenic Compounds Part K,* edited by Otto Hutzinger and Jaakko Paasivirta, 315-59. Berlin, Germany: Springer.

Liao, Liu, and Kannan 2012. Liao, Chunyang, Fang Liu, and Kurunthachalam Kannan. 2012. "Bisphenol S, a New Bisphenol Analogue, in Paper Products and Currency Bills and Its Association with Bisphenol A Residues." *Environmental Science and Technology* 46(12): 6515-22.

Lin 2010. Lin, Eugene C. 2010. "Radiation Risk from Medical Imaging." *Mayo Clinic Proceedings* 85(12): 1142-6.

Lioy 2006. Lioy, Paul J. 2006. "Employing Dynamical and Chemical Processes for Contaminant Mixtures Outdoors to the Indoor Environment: The Implications for Total Human Exposure Analysis and Prevention." *Journal of Exposure Science and Environmental Epidemiology* 16(3): 207-24.

Liu, Schade, and Simpson 2008. Liu, Jeannie, Michael Schade, and Heather Simpson. 2008. *Pass Up the Poison Plastic: The PVC – Free Guide for Your Family and Home.* Falls Church, VA: The Center for Health, Environment and Justice.

London et al. 2000. London, S. J., J. M. Yuan, F. L. Chung, Y. T. Gao, G. A. Coetzee, R. K. Ross, and M. C. Yu. 2000. "Isothiocyanates, Glutathione S-transferase M1 and T1 Polymorphisms, and Lung-Cancer Risk: A Prospective Study of Men in Shanghai, China." *Lancet* 356(9231): 724-9.

Lorber 2008. Lorber, Matthew. 2008. "Exposure of Americans to Polybrominated Diphenyl Ethers." *Journal of Exposure Science and Environmental Epidemiology* 18: 2-19.

Louis et al. 2013. Louis, Germaine M. Buck, Rajeshwari Sundaram, Enrique F. Schisterman, Anne M. Sweeney, Courtney D. Lynch, Robert E. Gore-Langton, Jose Maisog, Sungduk Kim, Zhen Chen, and Dana B. Barr. 2013. "Persistent Environmental Pollutants and Couple Fecundity: The LIFE Study." *Environmental Health Perspectives* 121(2): 231-6.

Lunder et al. 2010. Lunder, Sonya, Lotta Hovander, Ioannis Athanassiadis, and Ake Bergman. 2010. "Significantly Higher Polybrominated Diphenyl Ether Levels in Young US Children than in Their Mothers." *Environmental Science and Technology* 44(13): 5256-62.

Luntz Memorandum to Bush White House 2002. Frank Luntz Memorandum to Bush White House. 2002. "The Environment: A Cleaner Safer, Healthier America." Boston College.

Ma et al. 2002. Ma, Xiaomei, Patricia A. Buffler, Robert B. Gunier, Gary Dahl, Martyn T. Smith, Kyndaron Reinier, and Peggy Reynolds. 2002. "Critical Windows of Exposure to Household Pesticides and Risk of Childhood Leukemia." *Environmental Health Perspectives* 110(9): 955-60.

MAB 2014. CNA Military Advisory Board. 2014. *National Security and the Accelerating Risks of Climate Change.* Alexandria, VA: CNA Corporation.

Malaspina et al. 2008. Malaspina, D., C. Corcoran, K. R. Kleinhaus, M. C. Perrin, S. Fennig, D. Nahon, Y. Friedlander, and S. Harlap. 2008. "Acute Maternal Stress in Pregnancy and Schizophrenia in Offspring: A Cohort Prospective Study." *BMC Psychiatry* 8: 71.

Manikkam et al. 2012. Manikkam, Mohan, Rebecca Tracey, Carlos Guerrero-Bosagna, and Michael K. Skinner. 2012. "Dioxin (TCDD) Induces Epigenetic Transgenerational Inheritance of Adult Onset Disease and Sperm Epimutations." *PLoS ONE* 7(9): e46249.

Markets and Markets 2014. Markets and Markets. 2014. "Flame Retardant Market by Type (Aluminum Trihydrate, Antimony Oxide, Brominated, Chlorinated, Organphosphorous) and End-User Industry (Building and Construction, Electronics, Wire and Cables, Automotive) - Global Trends and Forecast to 2019." Last modified August.

Markowitz and Rosner 2002. Markowitz, Gerald and David Rosner. 2002. *Deceit and Denial: The Deadly Politics of Industrial Pollution (California/Milbank Books on Health and the Public).* Berkeley, CA: University of California Press.

Markowitz and Rosner 2013. Markowitz, Gerald and David Rosner. 2013. *Lead Wars: The Politics of Science and the Fate of America's Children.* Berkeley, CA: University of California Press.

Mascarelli 2010. Mascarelli, Amanda Leigh. 2010. "Before You Buy That Train Set, Do Your Homework." *Los Angeles Times,* November 22.

McCarthy 2015. McCarthy, Niall. 2015. "Air Pollution: Chinese and American Cities in Comparison." *Forbes,* January 23.

McGinn 2000. McGinn, Anne Platt. 2000. *POPs Culture.* Washington, DC: Worldwatch Institute.

McInergy to FCC and FDA 2013. Thomas K. McInergy, President of the American Academy of Pediatrics, to the Honorable Mignon L. Clyburn, Acting Commissioner of the Federal Communications Commission, and the Honorable Dr. Margaret A. Hamburg, Commissioner of the US Food and Drug Administration. 2013, August 29. FCC.gov.

Mead 2010. Mead, M. Nathaniel. 2010. "Cadmium Confusion: Do Consumers Need Protection?" *Environmental Health Perspectives* 118(2): A528-34.

Meerts et al. 2004. Meerts, Ilonka A. T. M., Saske Hoving, Johannes H. J. van den Berg, Bert M. Weijers, Hans J. Swarts, Eline M. van der Beek, Ake Bergman, Jan H. Koeman, and Abraham Brouwer. 2004. "Effects of In Utero Exposure to 4-hydroxy-2,3,3',4',5-pentachlorobiphenyl (4-OH-CB107) on Developmental Landmarks, Steroid Hormone Levels, and Female Estrous Cyclicity in Rats." *Toxicological Sciences* 82(1): 259-67.

Melkonian et al. 2010. Melkonian, Stephanie, Maria Argos, Brandon L. Pierce, Yu Chen, Tariqul Islam, Alauddin Ahmed, Emdadul H. Syed, Faruque Parvez, Joseph Graziano, Paul J. Rathouz, and Habibul Ahsan. 2010. "A Prospective Study of the Synergistic Effects of Arsenic Exposure and Smoking, Sun Expo-sure, Fertilizer Use, and Pesticide Use on Risk of Premalignant Skin Lesions in Bangladeshi Men." *American Journal of Epidemiology* 173(2): 183–91.

Merritt 2007. Merritt, Richard. 2007. "Negative Effects of Plastic Additive Blocked by Nutrient Supplements." *Gene Imprint,* July 29.

Michaels 2008. Michaels, David. 2008. *Doubt is Their Product: How Industry's Assault on Science Threatens Your Health.* Oxford, UK: Oxford University Press.

Mishamandani 2014. Mishamandani, Sara. 2014. "A New Approach to Determine Cancer Risk of Chemicals." *Environmental Factor by the National Institute of Environmental Health Sciences,* September.

Mondal et al. 2012. Mondal, Debapriya, Maria-Jose Lopez-Espinosa, Ben Armstrong, Cheryl R. Stein, and Tony Fletcher. 2012. "Relationships of Perfluorooctanoate and Perfluorooctane Sulfonate Serum Concentrations between Mother-Child Pairs in a Population with Perfluorooctanoate Exposure from Drinking Water." *Environmental Health Perspectives* 120(5): 752–7.

Monsanto 2013. Monsanto. 2013. *Monsanto Company 2013 Annual Report.* St. Louis, MO: Monsanto.

Monteiro and Boxall 2010. Monteiro, Sara C. and Alistair B. A. Boxall. 2010. "Occurrence and Fate of Human Pharmaceuticals in the Environment." *Reviews of Environmental Contamination and Toxicology* 202: 53-154.

Mooney 2004. Mooney, Chris. 2004. "Paralysis by Analysis: Jim Tozzi's Regulation to End All Regulation." *Washington Monthly,* May.

Motel 2014. Motel, Seth. 2014. "Polls Show That Most Americans Believe in Climate Change, But Give It Low Priority." *FactTank by PewResearchCenter,* September 23.

Mui 2008. Mui, Ylan Q. 2008. "Wal-Mart to Pull Bottles Made with Chemical BPA." *Washington Post,* April 18.

Muir, Kurt-Karakus, and Stow 2013. Muir, D., P. Kurt-Karakus, and J. Stow, eds. 2013. *Canadian Arctic Contaminants Assessment Report on Persistent Organic Pollutants – 2013.* Ottawa, ON: Northern Contaminants Program, Aboriginal Affairs and Northern Development.

Naidenko et al. 2008. Naidenko, Olga, Renee Sharp, Jane Houlihan, and Bill Walker. 2008. "Credibility Gap: Toxic Chemicals in Food Pack-aging." *Research by Environmental Working Group,* June 9.

NASA 2014. National Aeronautics and Space Administration. 2014. "Climate Change: How Do We Know?" Accessed October 10.

National Climate Assessment 2014. National Climate Assess-ment. 2014. "Overview." Accessed November 15.

National Geographic 2008. National Geographic. 2008. *Green Guide: The Complete Reference for Consuming Wisely.* Washington, DC: National Geographic Society.

National Heart, Lung, and Blood Institute 2012. National Heart, Lung, and Blood Institute. 2012. "Why Is Sleep Important?" Last modified February 22.

Nazaryan 2013. Nazaryan, Alex-ander. 2013. "World War Cancer." *New Yorker,* June 30.

NCI 2013. National Cancer Insti-tute. 2013. "Cell Phones and Cancer Risk." Last modified June 24.

NCI 2014. National Cancer Insti-tute. 2014. "Cancer in Children and Adolescents." Last modified May 12.

NIAID 2005. National Institute of Allergy and Infectious Diseases. 2005. *Progress in Autoimmune Diseases Research. NIH Publica-tion No. 05-5140.* Bethesda, MD: National Institutes of Health: National Institute of Allergy and Infectious Diseases.

NIEHS 2011. National Institute of Environmental Health Sciences. 2011. *Child Development and Environmental Toxins.* Research Triangle Park, NC: National Institutes of Health: National Institute of Environmental Health Sciences.

NIEHS 2012. National Institute of Environmental Health Sciences. 2012. "Dioxin Induces Disease and Reproductive Problems in Later Generations." Last modified December 14.

NIMH 2011. National Institute of Mental Health. 2011. *The Teen Brain: Still Under Construction. NIH Publication No. 11-4929.* Bethesda, MD: National Institutes of Health: National Institute of Mental Health.

Nobel Prize.org 1995. Nobel Prize.org. 1995. "Press Release: The 1995 Nobel Prize in Chemistry." Last modified October 11.

NRDC 2005. Natural Resources Defense Council. 2005. "The Cycle of Hazardous Chemicals." Last modified March 25.

NRDC 2010. Natural Resources Defense Council. 2010. "Press Release. Lawsuit Seeks to Ban BPA from Food Packaging." Last modified June 29.

NRDC 2011. Natural Resources Defense Council. 2011. "Press Release. NRDC, FDA Reach Settlement in BPA Lawsuit. Agency Set to Make Decision on BPA Ban from Food Packaging by March 31." Last modified December 7.

NRDC 2012. Natural Resources Defense Council. 2012. "Press Release. FDA Rejects NRDC Call to Eliminate BPA from Food Packaging." Last modified March 30.

NRDC 2014. Natural Resources Defense Council. 2014. "Toxic Chemicals in Our Couches." Accessed October 23.

NTP 2008. National Toxicology Program. 2008. *NTP-CERHR Monograph on the Potential Human Reproductive and Developmental Effects of Bisphenol A. NIH Publication No. 08-5994.* Research Triangle Park, NC: National Toxicology Program. US Department of Health and Human Services.

NY DOH 2013. New York State Department of Health. 2013. "Fact Sheet: Tetrachloroethene (PERC) in Indoor and Outdoor Air." Last modified September.

O'Connor 2012. O'Connor, Anahad. 2012. "Really? The Claim: Eating Soy Increases the Risk of Breast Cancer." *Well by New York Times* (blog), June 25.

OECD 2009. Organization for Economic Cooperation and Development. 2009. *Emission Scenario Document on Plastic Additives. Environment Directorate, Joint Meeting of the Chemicals Committee and the Working Party on Chemicals, Pesticides and Biotechnology. ENV/JM/MONO(2004)8/REV1.* Paris: Organization for Economic Cooperation and Development.

OECD 2013. Organization for Economic Cooperation and Development. 2013. *Health at a Glance 2013: OECD Indicators.* Paris: OECD Publishing.

OECD 2014. Organization for Economic Cooperation and Development. 2014. "What Is the OECD." Accessed December 3.

Ontario College of Family Physicians 2004. Ontario College of Family Physicians. 2004. "Comprehensive Review of Pesticide Research Confirms Dangers: Family Doctors Highlight Link Between Pesticide Exposure and Serious Illnesses and Disease; Children Particularly Vulnerable." Last modified April 23.

Paul 2010a. Paul, Annie Murphy. 2010. "How the First Nine Months Shape the Rest of Your Life." *Time,* September 22.

Paul 2010b. Paul, Annie Murphy. 2010. "The Womb. Your Mother. Yourself." *Time,* October 4.

Paul 2011. Paul, Annie Murphy. 2011. *Origins: How the Nine Months before Birth Shape the Rest of Our Lives.* New York: Free Press.

PBS 2007. PBS. 2007. "Epigenetics." Video for *NOVA Science-NOW,* 13:02. Posted July 24.

Pearce 2008. Pearce, Elizabeth N. 2008. "Iodine in Pregnancy: Is Salt Iodization Enough?" *Journal of Clinical Endocrinology and Metabolism* 93(7): 2466-8.

Peeples 2013. Peeples, Lynne. 2013. "Lead Paint, Other Toxic Products Banned in US Still Exported to Unsuspecting Customers Abroad." *Huffington Post,* March 25.

Peralta 2012. Peralta, Eyder. 2012. "Study: Plastic Garbage in Pacific Ocean Has Increased 100-Fold in 40 Years." *The Two-Way by NPR* (blog), May 9.

Perrin, Bloom, and Gortmaker 2007. Perrin, James M., Sheila R. Bloom, and Steven L. Gortmaker. 2007. "The Increase of Childhood Chronic Conditions in the United States." *Journal of the American Medical Association* 297(24): 2755-9.

Pestano 2012. Pestano, Paul. 2012. "BPA Substitute Found on Store Receipts." *Enviroblog by Environmental Working Group,* July 13.

Pesticide Free BC 2013. Pesticide Free BC. 2013. "Laws in Canada." Last modified September 18.

Physicians for Social Responsibility 2014. Physicians for Social Responsibility. 2014. "Cancer and Toxic Chemicals." Accessed August 27.

Powell 2014. Powell, Eric A. 2014. "Byzantine Secret Ingredient." *Archaeology, A Publication of the Archaeological Institute of America,* June 9.

Rachel Carson – Prisen 2014. Rachel Carson - Prisen. 2014. "Award Winner 2009: Marie-Monique Robin." Accessed October 23.

Rahman et al. 2001. Rahman, F., K. H. Langford, M. D. Scrimshaw, and J. N. Lester. 2001. "Polybrominated Diphenyl Ether (PBDE) Flame Retardants." *The Science of the Total Environment* 275(1-3): 1-17.

Reinstein 2010. Reinstein, Linda. 2010. "Asbestos: Not Gone, Not Forgotten." *Enviroblog by Environmental Working Group,* March 25.

Reuben 2010. Reuben, Suzanne H. 2010. *2008 – 2009 Annual Report, President's Cancer Panel. Reducing Environmental Cancer Risk: What We Can Do Now.* Bethesda, MD: National Cancer Institute.

Reuters 2012. Reuters. 2012. "Update 2 – US FDA Denies Petition to Ban Common Chemical BPA." *Chicago Tribune,* March 30.

Rimer 2011. Rimer, Sara. 2011. "The Biology of Emotion-and What It May Teach Us About Helping People to Live Longer." *Happiness and Health by Harvard School of Public Health,* winter.

Riseborough 1990. Riseborough, R. W. 1990. "Beyond Long-Range Transport: A Model of a Global Gas Chromatographic System." In *Long Range Transport of Pesticides,* edited by David A. Kurtz, 417-26. Chelsea, MI: Lewis.

Roan 2010. Roan, Shari. 2010. "Household Chemicals Linked to Reduced Fertility." *Los Angeles Times,* January 27.

Roberts et al. 2009. Roberts, John W., Lance A. Wallace, David E. Camann, Philip Dickey, Steven G. Gilbert, Robert G. Lewis, and Tim K. Takaro. 2009. "Monitoring and Reducing Exposure of Infants to Pollutants in House Dust." In *Reviews of Environmental Contamination and Toxicology Volume 201,* edited by David M. Whitacre, 1–39. New York: Springer.

Robin 2010. Robin, Marie-Monique. 2010. *The World According to Monsanto.* New York: New Press.

Rogers et al. 2009. Rogers, Bonnie, Leyla Erk McCurdy, Katie Slavin, Kimberly Grubb, and James R. Roberts. 2009. "Children's Environmental Health Faculty Champions Initiative: A Successful Model for Integrating Environmental Health into Pediatric Health Care." *Environmental Health Perspectives* 117(5): 850-5.

Rosenberg 2014. Rosenberg, Daniel. 2014. "The Chemical Safety Improvement Act Will Not Solve the Problems Illustrated by the West Virginia Chemical Spill." *Switchboard by Natural Resources Defense Council* (blog), January 15.

Ross and Nolan 2003. Ross, Malcolm and Robert P. Nolan. 2003. "History of Asbestos Discovery and Use and Asbestos-Related Disease in Context with the Occurrence of Asbestos within Ophiolite Complexes." In *Ophiolite Concept and the Evolution of Geological Thought,* edited by Yildirim Dilek and Sally Newcomb, 447-70. Boulder, CO: The Geological Society of America.

Rudel 2000. Rudel, Ruthann. 2000. "Polycyclic Aromatic Hydrocarbons, Phthalates, and Phenols." In *Indoor Air Quality Handbook,* edited by John D. Spengler, Jonathan M. Samet, and John F. McCarthy. New York: McGraw Hill.

Runkle 2014. Runkle, Jennifer. 2014. "Parental Pesticide Exposure Linked to Childhood Cancer." *Environmental Health Policy Institute by Physicians For Social Responsibility*, accessed November 14.

Safer Chemicals 2014. Safer Chemicals, Healthy Families. 2014. "Persistent, Bioaccumulative and Toxic Chemicals (PBTs)." Accessed November 21.

Saunders, Liddelow, and Dziegielewska 2012. Saunders, Norman R., Shane A. Liddelow, and Katarzyna M. Dziegielewska. 2012. "Barrier Mechanisms in the Developing Brain." *Frontiers in Pharmacology* 3(46): 1-18.

Saviva Research 2013. Saviva Research. 2013. "Saviva Research Review. Hybrid Energy Systems for Telecom Towers." Last modified May.

Scheer and Moss 2011. Scheer, Roddy and Doug Moss. 2011. "Dirt Poor: Have Fruits and Vegetables Become Less Nutritious?" *Earth Talk by Scientific American Blog Network,* April 27.

Schenk et al. 1996. Schenk, Maryjean, Sharon M. Popp, Anne V. Neale, and Raymond Y. Demers. 1996. "Environmental Medicine Content in Medical School Curricula." *Academic Medicine* 71(5): 499-501.

Schettler et al. 2000. Schettler, Ted, Jill Stein, Fay Reich, Maria Valenti, and David Wallinga. 2000. *In Harm's Way: Toxic Threats to Child Development.* Cambridge: Greater Boston Physicians for Social Responsibility.

Schnoor 2014. Schnoor, Jerald L. 2014. "Re-Emergence of Emerging Contaminants." *Environmental Science and Technology* 48(19): 11019-20.

Schreder 2012. Schreder, Erika. 2012. *Hidden Hazards in the Nursery.* Seattle, WA: Washington Toxics Coalition/Safer States.

Scorecard 2014. Scorecard: The Pollution Information Site. 2014. "Health Effects, Carcinogens." Accessed August 27.

Searcey and Barry 2013. Searcey, Dionne and Rob Barry. 2013. "As Asbestos Claims Rise, So Do Worries About Fraud." *Wall Street Journal,* March 11.

Senate Committee on Environment and Public Works 2014a. United States Senate Committee on Environment and Public Works. 2014. "Press Release: Vitter Announces Growing Support for Bipartisan TSCA Reform Bill." Last modified April 15.

Senate Committee on Environment and Public Works 2014b. United States Senate Committee on Environment and Public Works. 2014. "Testimony of Lisa P. Jackson Administrator United States Environmental Protection Agency before the Committee on Environment and Public Works. United States Senate." Accessed October 15.

Shim, Mlynarek, and van Wijngaarden 2009. Shim, Youn K., Steven P. Mlynarek, and Edwin van Wijngaarden. 2009. "Parental Exposure to Pesticides and Childhood Brain Cancer: US Atlantic Coast Childhood Brain Cancer Study." *Environmental Health Perspectives* 117(6): 1002-6.

Shubin 2009. Shubin, Neil. 2009. *Your Inner Fish: A Journal into the 3.5-Billion-Year History of the Human Body.* New York: Vintage.

Shubin 2013. Shubin, Neil. 2013. *The Universe Within: Discovering the Common History of Rocks, Planets, and People.* New York: Pantheon Books.

Skin Cancer Foundation 2014. Skin Cancer Foundation. 2014. "Skin Cancer Facts." Last modified June 4.

Spivak 2015. Spivak, Marla. 2015. "What Will Happen if the Bees Disappear?" *CNN,* March 5.

Sprouse 2014. Sprouse, Elizabeth. 2014. "5 Notable Discoveries in Epigenetics Research." *Curiosity by Discovery Channel,* accessed November 1.

St Clair et al. 2005. St Clair, D., M. Xu, P. Wang, Y. Yu, Y. Fang, F. Zhang, X. Zheng, N. Gu, G. Feng, P. Sham, and L. He. 2005. "Rates of Adult Schizophrenia following Prenatal Exposure to the Chinese Famine of 1959-1961." *The Journal of the American Medical Association* 294(5): 557-62.

Statistic Brain 2013. Statistic Brain. 2013. "Cell Phone Tower Statistics." Last modified November 13.

Steingraber 2001. Steingraber, Sandra. 2001. *Having Faith.* Cambridge: Perseus.

Steingraber 2010. Steingraber, Sandra. 2010. *Living Downstream: An Ecologist's Investigation of Cancer and the Environment.* 2nd ed. Cambridge: Da Capo Press.

Steinhauer et al. 2014. Steinhauer, Nathalie A., Karen Rennich, Michael E. Wilson, Dewey M. Caron, Eugene J. Lengerich, Jeff S. Pettis, Robyn Rose, et al. 2014. "A National Survey of Managed Honey Bee 2012-2013 Annual Colony Losses in the USA: Results from the Bee Informed Partnership." *Journal of Apicultural Research* 53(1): 1-18.

Stephens 2014. Stephens, Stephanie. 2014. "Children with Chronic Health Conditions Less Likely to Graduate from High School." *Health Behavior News Service by Center for Advancing Health,* October 16.

Stockholm Convention 2014a. Stockholm Convention. Protecting Human Health and the Environment from Persistent Organic Pollutants. 2014. "The 12 Initial POPs under the Stockholm Convention." Accessed November 12.

Stockholm Convention 2014b. Stockholm Convention. Protecting Human Health and the Environment from Persistent Organic Pollutants. 2014. "Fifth Meeting of the Conference of the Parties to the Stockholm Convention." Accessed November 22.

Stockholm Convention 2014c. Stockholm Convention: Protecting Human Health and the Environment from Persistent Organic Pollutants. 2014. "The New POPs under the Stockholm Convention." Accessed October 3.

Stockholm Convention 2014d. Stockholm Convention. Protecting Human Health and the Environment from Persistent Organic Pollutants. 2014. "Status of Ratifications." Accessed November 26.

Stockholm Convention and UNEP 2012. Stockholm Convention and United Nations Environment Programme. 2012. *Success Stories: Stockholm Convention 2001-2011.* Geneva, Switzerland: Secretariat of the Stockholm Convention.

Stromberg 2014. Stromberg, Joseph. 2014. "Air Pollution in China Is Spreading across the Pacific to the US." *Smithsonian. com,* January 21.

Swan et al. 2005. Swan, S. H., K. M. Main, F. Liu, S. L. Stewart, R. L. Kruse, A. M. Calafat, C. S. Mao, J. B. Redmon, C. L. Temand, S. Sullivan, and J. L. Teague. 2005. "Decrease in Anogential Distance among Male Infants with Prenatal Phthalates Exposure." *Environmental Health Perspectives* 113(8): 1056-61.

Tai, Val Martin, and Heald 2014. Tai, Amos P. K., Maria Val Martin, and Colette L. Heald. 2014. "Threat to Future Global Food Security from Climate Change and Ozone Air Pollution." *Nature Climate Change* 4: 817-21.

TEDX 2007. The Endocrine Disruption Exchange. 2007. "Prenatal Origins of Cancer: Summary." Last modified October.

TEDX 2014a. The Endocrine Disruption Exchange. 2014. "About TEDX: Introduction." Accessed November 5.

TEDX 2014b. The Endocrine Disruption Exchange. 2014. "Prenatal Origins of Endocrine Disruption: Introduction." Accessed November 5.

TEDX 2014c. The Endocrine Disruption Exchange. 2014. "TEDX List of Potential Endocrine Disruptors." Accessed October 3.

Telecompaper 2014. Telecompaper. 2014. "Global Telecoms Industry Revenue to Hit 2.4 Tln in 2019." Last modified February 2.

Than 2014. Than, Ker. 2014. "How Much Is US to Blame for "Made-in-China" Pollution?" *National Geographic,* January 24.

Thornton 2000. Thornton, Joseph. 2000. *Pandora's Poison: Chlorine, Health, and a New Environmental Strategy.* Cambridge: MIT Press.

Thornton 2002. Thornton, Joseph. 2002. *Environmental Impacts of Polyvinyl Chloride Building Materials.* Washington, DC: Healthy Building Network.

Toms et al. 2009. Toms, Leisa-Maree L., Andreas Sjödin, Fiona Harden, Peter Hobson, Richard Jones, Emily Edenfield, and Jochen F. Mueller. 2009. "Serum Polybrominated Diphenyl Ether (PBDE) Levels Are Higher in Children (2-5 Years of Age) Than in Infants and Adults." *Environmental Health Perspectives* 117(9): 1461-5.

Tortorello 2012. Tortorello, Michael. 2012. "Is It Safe to Play Yet? Going to Extreme Lengths to Purge Household Toxins." *New York Times*, March 14.

Trasande 2008. Trasande, Leonardo. 2008. *The Urgent Need for Federal Policy Interventions to Prevent Diseases of Environmental Origin in American Children.* New York: Mount Sinai Children's Environmental Health Center.

Tweed 2013. Tweed, Katherine. 2013. "Why Cellular Towers in Developing Nations Are Making the Move to Solar Power." *Scientific American,* January 15.

Uhde et al. 2001. Uhde, E., M. Bednarek, F. Fuhrmann, and T. Salthammer. 2001. "Phthalic Esters in the Indoor Environment-Test Chamber Studies on PVC-Coated Wallcoverings." *Indoor Air* 11(3): 150-5.

UNEP 2005. United Nations Environment Programme. 2005. *Ridding the World of POPs: A Guide to the Stockholm Convention on Persistent Organic Pollutants.* Geneva, Switzerland: United Nations Environment Programme.

UNEP 2010. United Nations Environment Programme. 2010. *Ridding the World of POPs: A Guide to the Stockholm Convention on Persistent Organic Pollutants.* Geneva, Switzerland: United Nations Environment Programme.

Union of Concerned Scientists 2007. Union of Concerned Scientists. 2007. *Smoke, Mirrors and Hot Air: How ExxonMobil Uses Big Tobacco's Tactics to Manufacture Uncertainty on Climate Science.* Cambridge: Union of Concerned Scientists.

Urbina 2013. Urbina, Ian. 2013. "Think Those Chemicals Have Been Tested?" *New York Times,* April 13.

Van Cleave, Gortmaker, and Perrin 2010. Van Cleave, Jeanne, Steven L. Gortmaker, and James M. Perrin. 2010. "Dynamics of Obesity and Chronic Health Conditions among Children and Youth." *Journal of the American Medical Association* 303(7): 623–30.

van der Schalie et al. 1999. van der Schalie, William H., Hank S. Gardner Jr., John A. Bantle, Chris T. De Rosa, Robert A. Finch, John S. Reif, Roy H. Reuter, Lorraine C. Backer, Joanna Burger, Leroy C. Folmar, and William S. Stokes. 1999. "Animals as Sentinels of Human Health Hazards of Environmental Chemicals." *Environmental Health Perspectives* 107(4): 309-15.

Vandenberg 2008. Vandenberg, Laura N. 2008. *Fetal Origins of Adult Disease: Xenoestrogens and Breast Cancer Risk.* Ann Arbor, MI: ProQuest Information and Learning.

Viñas and Watson 2013. Viñas, Rene and Cheryl S. Watson. 2013. "Bisphenol S Disrupts Estradiol-Induced Nongenomic Signaling in a Rat Pituitary Cell Line: Effects on Cell Functions." *Environmental Health Perspectives* 121(3): 352–8.

Vinson et al. 2011. Vinson F., M. Merhi, I. Baldi, H. Raynal, and L. Gamet-Payrastre. 2011. "Exposure to Pesticides and Risk of Childhood Cancer: A Meta-Analysis of Recent Epidemiological Studies." *Occupational and Environmental Medicine* 68(9): 694-702.

Walsh 2010. Walsh, Bryan. 2010. "The Perils of Plastic." *Time,* April 1.

Weil 2012. Weil, Elizabeth. 2012. "Puberty before Age 10: A New 'Normal'?" *New York Times,* March 30.

Wheeler and Marcos 2015. Wheeler, Lydia and Cristina Marcos. 2015. "House Passes Bill Blocking States from Requiring GMO Labels on Food." *Floor Action from The Hill* (blog), July 23.

White 2004. White, Michelle J. 2004. "Asbestos and the Future of Mass Torts." *Journal of Economic Perspectives* 18(2): 183-204.

WHO 2003. World Health Organization. 2003. *Climate Change and Human Health – Risks and Responses. Summary.* Geneva, Switzerland: World Health Organization.

WHO 2005. World Health Organization. 2005. "Electromagnetic Fields and Public Health." Last modified December.

WHO 2010. World Health Organization: Yona Amitai, Hamed Bakir, Nida Besbelli, Stephan Boese-O'Reilly, Mariano Cebrian, Yaohua Dai, Paul Dargan, et al. 2010. *Childhood Lead Poisoning.* Geneva, Switzerland: World Health Organization.

WHO 2011a. World Health Organization. 2011. "Children and Neurodevelopmental Behavioral Intellectual Disorders (NDBID)." Last modified October.

WHO 2011b. World Health Organization. 2011. *Global Status Report on Noncommunicable Diseases 2010.* Geneva, Switzerland: World Health Organization.

WHO 2011c. World Health Organization. 2011. *Pharmaceuticals in Drinking-Water. Public Health and Environment Water, Sanitation, Hygiene and Health.* Geneva, Switzerland: World Health Organization.

WHO 2012. World Health Organization. 2012. *Pharmaceuticals in Drinking-Water.* Geneva, Switzerland: World Health Organization.

WHO 2013. World Health Organization. 2013. "What Are the Health Risks Associated with Mobile Phones and Their Base Stations?" Last modified September 20.

WHO 2014a. World Health Organization. 2014. "7 Million Premature Deaths Annually Linked to Air Pollution." Last modified March 25.

WHO 2014b. World Health Organization. 2014. "Ambient (Outdoor) Air Quality and Health." Last modified March.

WHO 2014c. World Health Organization. 2014. "Electromagnetic Fields." Accessed October 29.

WHO 2014d. World Health Organization. 2014. "The Top 10 Causes of Death." Last modified May.

WHO 2014e. World Health Organization. 2014. "What is the International EMF Project?" Last modified June 30.

WHO and UNEP 2013. World Health Organization and United Nations Environment Programme. 2013. *State of the Science of Endocrine Disrupting Chemicals – 2012.* Geneva, Switzerland: WHO Press.

WiFi in Schools Australia 2014. WiFi in Schools Australia. 2014. "Governments and Authorities around the World." Accessed September 2.

Wilson and Schwarzman 2009. Wilson, Michael P. and Megan R. Schwarzman. 2009. "Toward a New US Chemicals Policy: Rebuilding the Foundation to Advance New Science, Green Chemistry, and Environmental Health." *Environmental Health Perspectives* 117(8): 1202–9.

Wolff et al. 1993. Wolff, M. S., P. G. Toniolo, E. W. Lee, M. Rivera, and N. Dubin. 1993. "Blood Levels of Organochlorine Residues and Risk of Breast Cancer." *Journal of the National Cancer Institute* 85(8): 648-52.

Wong et al. 2013. Wong, Jeannette R., Jenine K. Harris, Carlos Rodriguez-Galindo, and Kimberly J. Johnson. 2013. "Incidence of Childhood and Adolescent Melanoma in the United States: 1973 – 2009." *Pediatrics* 131: 846-54.

World Bank 2014. World Bank. 2014. "Gross Domestic Product 2013." Last modified September 22.

World Economic Forum 2012. World Economic Forum. 2012. "What If the World's Soil Runs Out?" *Time,* December 14.

Yale Project on Climate Change Communication 2015. Yale Project on Climate Change Communication. 2015. "Estimated Percent of Adults Who Think Global Warming is Happening, 2014." Accessed June 28.

Zeller 2008. Zeller, Tom, Jr. 2008. "Bank of America to Stop Financing Mountaintop Mining." *Green by New York Times* (blog), December 4.

Zhang 2004. Zhang, Y. 2004. "Cancer-Preventive Isothiocyanates: Measurement of Human Exposure and Mechanism of Action." *Mutation Research* 555(1-2): 173-90.

Zsarnovszky et al. 2005. Zsarnovszky, Attila, Hoa H. Le, Hong-Sheng Wang, and Scott M. Belcher. 2005. "Ontogeny of Rapid Estrogen-Mediated Extracellular Signal-Regulated Kinase Signaling in the Rat Cerebellar Cortex: Potent Nongenomic Agonist and Endocrine Disrupting Activity of the Xenoestrogen Bisphenol A." *Endocrinology* 146(12): 5388–96.

Alexander et al. 2009. Alexander, Jan, Diane Benford, Alan Boobis, Sandra Ceccatelli, Jean-Pierre Cravedi, Alessandro Di Domenico, Daniel Doerge, et al. 2009. "Scientific Opinion on Arsenic in Food." *EFSA Journal* 7(10): 1351.

Alonso-Magdalena et al. 2010. Alonso-Magdalena, Paloma, Elaine Vieira, Sergi Soriano, Lorena Menes, Deborah Burks, Ivan Quesada, and Angel Nadal. 2010. "Bisphenol A Exposure during Pregnancy Disrupts Glucose Homeostasis in Mothers and Adult Male Offspring." *Environmental Health Perspectives* 118(9): 1243-50.

Andersen 2008. Andersen, F. Alan. 2008. "Final Amended Report on the Safety Assessment of Methylparaben, Ethylparaben, Propylparaben, Isopropylparaben, Butylparaben, Isobutylparaben, and Benzylparaben as Used in Cosmetic Products." *International Journal of Toxicology* 27(Suppl 4): 1-82.

Apelberg et al. 2007. Apelberg, Benjamin J., Frank R. Witter, Julie B. Herbstman, Antonia M. Calafat, Rolf U. Halden, Larry L. Needham, and Lynn R. Goldman. 2007. "Cord Serum Concentration of Perfluorooctane Sulfonate (PFOS) and Perfluorooctanoate (PFOA) in Relation to Weight and Size at Birth." *Environmental Health Perspectives* 115(11): 1670-6.

ATSDR 2000. Agency for Toxic Substances and Disease Registry. 2000. *Public Health Statement: Polychlorinated Biphenyls (PCBS)*. Atlanta, GA: Agency for Toxic Substances and Disease Registry.

ATSDR 2002. Agency for Toxic Substances and Disease Registry. 2002. *Di(2-ethylhexyl) Phthalate (DEHP) CAS #117-81-7*. Atlanta, GA: Agency for Toxic Substances and Disease Registry.

ATSDR 2004. Agency for Toxic Substances and Disease Registry. 2004. "Public Health Statement: Polybrominated Diphenyl Ethers." Last modified September.

ATSDR 2015a. Agency for Toxic Substances and Disease Registry. 2015. "Public Health Statement for 1,4 Dioxane." Last modified January 21.

ATSDR 2015b. Agency for Toxic Substances and Disease Registry. 2015. "Public Health Statement for Cadmium." Last modified January 21.

ATSDR 2015c. Agency for Toxic Substances and Disease Registry. 2015. "Public Health Statement for Methylene Chloride." Last modified January 21.

Bader 2011. Bader, Walter. 2011. *Sleep Safe in a Toxic World*. Topanga, CA: Freedom Press.

Betts 2008. Betts, Kellyn. 2008. "New Thinking on Flame Retardants." *Environmental Health Perspectives* 116(5): A211-3.

Bienkowski 2014. Bienkowski, Brian. 2014. "BPA Triggers Changes in Rats That May Lead to Breast Cancer." *Environmental Health News,* July 2.

Bienkowski and *Environmental Health News* 2014. Bienkowski, Brian and Environmental Health News. 2014. "BPA Exposure Linked to Prostate Cancer." *Scientific American,* January 7.

Bilbrey 2014. Bilbrey, Jenna. 2014. "BPA-Free Plastic Containers May Be Just as Hazardous." *Scientific American,* August 11.

Birnbaum 1994. Birnbaum, Linda S. 1994. "Endocrine Effects of Prenatal Exposure to PCBs, Dioxins, and Other Xenobiotics: Implications for Policy and Future Research." *Environmental Health Perspectives* 102(8): 676-9.

Birnbaum and Staskal 2004. Birnbaum, Linda S. and Daniele F. Staskal. 2004. "Brominated Flame Retardants: Cause for Concern?" *Environmental Health Perspectives* 112(1): 9-17.

Bornehag et al. 2004. Bornehag, Carl-Gustaf, Jan Sundell, Charles J. Weschler, Torben Sigsgaard, Bjorn Lundgren, Mikael Hasselgren, and Linda Hagerhed-Engman. 2004. "The Association between Asthma and Allergic Symptoms in Children and Phthalates in House Dust: A Nested Case-Control Study." *Environmental Health Perspectives* 112(14): 1393-7.

Bouchard et al. 2011. Bouchard, Maryse F., Jonathan Chevrier, Kim G. Harley, Katherine Kogut, Michelle Vedar, Norma Calderon, Celina Trujillo, et al. 2011. "Prenatal Exposure to Organophosphate Pesticides and IQ in 7-Year-Old Children." *Environmental Health Perspectives* 119(8): 1189-95.

Business Wire 2011. Business Wire. 2011. "Research and Markets: Polyvinyl Chloride (PVC) Global Supply Dynamics to 2020 – China Emerges as the Leader in Global Production." Last modified January 10.

CA EPA 2010. California Environmental Protection Agency. 2010. *Chemicals Known to the State to Cause Cancer or Reproductive Toxicity. April 2, 2010.* Sacramento, CA: State of California Environmental Protection Agency, Office of Environmental Health Hazard Assessment.

CA EPA 2015. California Environmental Protection Agency. 2015. "Composite Wood Products." Last modified April 23.

Calafat et al. 2007. Calafat, Antonia M., Lee-Yang Wong, Zsuzsanna Kuklenyik, John A. Reidy, and Larry L. Needham. 2007. "Polyfluoroalkyl Chemicals in the US Population: Data from the National Health and Nutrition Examination Survey (NHANES) 2003-2004 and Comparisons with NHANES 1999-2000." *Environmental Health Perspectives* 115(11): 1596-602.

California Air Resources Board 2005. California Air Resources Board. 2005. *Report to the California Legislature: Indoor Air Pollution in California.* Sacramento, CA: California Environmental Protection Agency, Air Resources Board.

California Department of Public Health 2015. California Department of Public Health. 2015. "Frequently Asked Questions About Lead Poisoning." Accessed April 21.

Campaign for Safe Cosmetics 2012. Campaign for Safe Cosmetics. 2012. *Retailer Therapy. Ranking Retailers on Their Commitment to Personal Care Product and Cosmetics Safety.* San Francisco, CA: Breast Cancer Fund and Commonweal.

Campaign for Safe Cosmetics 2015. Campaign for Safe Cosmetics. 2015. "Synthetic Musks." Accessed April 29.

Caress and Steinemann 2009. Caress, Stanley M. and Anne C. Steinemann. 2009. "Prevalence of Fragrance Sensitivity in the American Population." *Journal of Environmental Health* 71(7): 46-50.

Carwile et al. 2009. Carwile, Jenny L., Henry T. Luu, Laura S. Bassett, Daniel A. Driscoll, Caterina Yuan, Jennifer Y. Chang, Xiaoyun Ye, Antonia M. Calafat, and Karin B. Michels. 2009. "Polycarbonate Bottle Use and Urinary Bisphenol A Concentrations." *Environmental Health Perspectives* 117(9): 1368-72.

CDC 2010. Centers for Disease Control and Prevention. 2010. "Parabens." Last modified May.

CDC 2013a. Centers for Disease Control and Prevention. 2013. "National Biomonitoring Program. Biomonitoring Summary: Bisphenol A. CAS No. 80-05-7." Last modified December 4.

CDC 2013b. Centers for Disease Control and Prevention. 2013. "National Biomonitoring Program. Factsheet: Bisphenol A." Last modified July 23.

CDC 2013c. Centers for Disease Control and Prevention. 2013. "National Biomonitoring Program. Factsheet: Lead." Last modified July 12.

CDC 2013d. Centers for Disease Control and Prevention. 2013. "National Biomonitoring Program. Factsheet: Perfluorochemicals (PFCs)." Last modified July 23.

CDC 2013e. Centers for Disease Control and Prevention. 2013. "National Biomonitoring Program. Factsheet: Perfluorooctanoic Acid (PFOA)." Last modified July 23.

CDC 2013f. Centers for Disease Control and Prevention. 2013. "National Biomonitoring Program. Factsheet: Phthalates." Last modified July 16.

CDC 2015. Centers for Disease Control and Prevention. 2015. "PCBs: A Study of Breast Cancer among Workers from Three Manufacturing Plants." Accessed April 20.

Clean and Healthy New York 2011. Clean and Healthy New York. 2011. *The Mattress Matters: Protecting Babies from Toxic Chemicals While They Sleep.* Albany, NY: Clean and Healthy New York, American Sustainable Business Council.

Cone and *Environmental Health News* 2012. Cone, Marla and Environmental Health News. 2012. "Children May Be Exposed to Higher Chemical Concentrations Than Their Mothers." *Scientific American,* January 26.

Congleton 2013. Congleton, Johanna. 2013. "New Research Explores How a Widely Used Fire Retardant Could Trigger Cancer."

Enviroblog by Environmental Working Group, September 3.

Cox 2002. Cox, Caroline. 2002. *Pesticide Registration: No Guarantee of Safety.* Eugene, OR: Northwest Coalition for Alternatives to Pesticides.

CPSC 2013. United States Consumer Product Safety Commission. 2013. *An Update on Formaldehyde.* Bethesda, MD: United States Consumer Product Safety Commission.

CPSC 2015a. United States Consumer Product Safety Commission. 2015. "The Inside Story: A Guide to Indoor Air Quality." Accessed May 2.

CPSC 2015b. United States Consumer Product Safety Commission. 2015. "Phthalates." Accessed April 30.

de Groot and Frosch 1997. de Groot, Anton C. and Peter J. Frosch. 1997. "Adverse Reactions to Fragrances: A Clinical Review." *Contact Dermatitis* 36(2): 57-86.

Donohue et al. 2013. Donohue, Kathleen M., Rachel L. Miller, Matthew S. Perzanowski, Allan C. Just, Lori A. Hoepner, Srikesh Arunajadai, Stephen Canfield, et al. 2013. "Prenatal and Postnatal Bisphenol A Exposure and Asthma Development among Inner-City Children." *Journal of Allergy and Clinical Immunology* 131(3): 736-42.

Dufault et al. 2009. Dufault, Renee, Blaise LeBlanc, Roseanne Schnoll, Charles Cornett, Laura Schweitzer, David Wallinga, Jane Hightower, Lyn Patrick, and Walter J. Lukiw. 2009. "Mercury from Chlor-Alkali Plants: Measured Concentrations in Food Product Sugar." *Environmental Health* 8(2).

EHANS 2011. Environmental Health Association of Nova Scotia. 2011. "Guide to Less Toxic Products." Last modified in Spring.

EJNet 1996. Environmental Justice Net. 1996. "Eliminate the Use of Polystyrene." Last modified March 4.

Environmental Health Network 2008. Environmental Health Network. 2008. "Making Sense of Scents."

Environmental Justice Foundation 2007. Environmental Justice Foundation. 2007. *The Deadly Chemicals in Cotton.* London: Environmental Justice Foundation in Collaboration with Pesticide Action Network UK.

EPA 1985. United States Environmental Protection Agency. 1985. *Federal Register Vol. 50, No. 9. 40 CFR Parts 261, 264, 265, 270, and 775.* United States Environmental Protection Agency.

EPA 1994. United States Environmental Protection Agency. 1994. "Chemical Summary for Chlorine. EPA 749-F-94-010a." Last modified August.

EPA 2000. United States Environmental Protection Agency. 2000. *Healthy Indoor Painting Practices. EPA 744-F-00-011.* United States Environmental Protection Agency.

EPA 2007a. United States Environmental Protection Agency. 2007. "Formaldehyde: TEACH Chemical Summary." Last modified September 20.

EPA 2007b. United States Environmental Protection Agency. 2007. "Phthalates: TEACH Chemical Summary." Last modified October 10.

EPA 2009a. United States Environmental Protection Agency. 2009. "Benzene: TEACH Chemical Summary." Last modified February 27.

EPA 2009b. United States Environmental Protection Agency. 2009. "Polychlorinated Biphenyls (PCBs). TEACH Chemical Summary." Last modified October 8.

EPA 2011a. United States Environmental Protection Agency. 2011. "DDT." Last modified April 18.

EPA 2011b. United States Environmental Protection Agency. 2011. "Indoor Air: Pesticides in the Home – Additional Information." Last modified August 19.

EPA 2012a. United States Environmental Protection Agency. 2012. "Children Are at Greater Risks from Pesticide Exposure." Last modified May 9.

EPA 2012b. United States Environmental Protection Agency. 2012. "An Introduction to Indoor Air Quality (IAQ): Volatile Organic Compounds (VOCs)." Last modified July 9.

EPA 2012c. United States Environmental Protection Agency. 2012. "Phthalates Action Plan." Last modified March 14.

EPA 2013a. United States Environmental Protection Agency. 2013. "2006-2007 Pesticide Market Estimates: Usage." Last modified July 19.

EPA 2013b. United States Environmental Protection Agency. 2013. "Arsenic Compounds." Last modified October 18.

EPA 2013c. United States Environmental Protection Agency. 2013. "Health Effects of PCBs." Last modified June 13.

EPA 2013d. United States Environmental Protection Agency. 2013. "Lead Compounds." Last modified October 18.

EPA 2013e. United States Environmental Protection Agency. 2013. "Major Crops Grown in the United States." Last modified April 11.

EPA 2013f. United States Environmental Protection Agency. 2013. "Mercury Compounds." Last modified October 18.

EPA 2013g. United States Environmental Protection Agency. 2013. "Methylene Chloride (Dichloromethane)." Last modified October 18.

EPA 2013h. United States Environmental Protection Agency. 2013. "Questions and Answers on Health Effects of Disinfection Byproducts." Last modified October 31.

EPA 2013i. United States Environmental Protection Agency. 2013. "Toluene." Last modified October 18.

EPA 2013j. United States Environmental Protection Agency. 2013. *Toxicological Review of 1,4-Dioxane (with Inhalation Update) (CAS No 123-91-1).* Washington, DC: United States Environmental Protection Agency.

EPA 2014a. United States Environmental Protection Agency. 2014. "2,3,7,8-Tetrachlorodibenzo-p-dioxin (TCDD); CASRN 1746-01-6." Last modified October 31.

EPA 2014b. United States Environmental Protection Agency. 2014. "Chlorine Bleach." Last modified January 27.

EPA 2014c. United States Environmental Protection Agency. 2014. "Dye Facilities." Last modified October 31.

EPA 2015a. United States Environmental Protection Agency. 2015. "Bisphenol A (BPA) Action Plan Summary." Last modified January 8.

EPA 2015b. United States Environmental Protection Agency. 2015. "DDT – A Brief History and Status." Last modified January 6.

EPA 2015c. United States Environmental Protection Agency. 2015. "Persistent Organic Pollutants: A Global Issue, a Global Response." Last modified May 4.

EPA 2015d. United States Environmental Protection Agency. 2015. "Polybrominated Diphenyl Ethers (PBDEs) Action Plan Summary." Last modified January 8.

EPA 2015e. United States Environmental Protection Agency. 2015. "Technical Factsheet on: Dioxin (2,3,7,8-TCDD)." Accessed April 22.

EWG 2003a. Environmental Working Group. 2003. "PFCs: Global Contaminants: Consumers Instantly Recognize Them as Household Miracles of Modern Chemistry – Teflon, Scotchgard, Stainmaster, Gore-Tex." Last modified April 3.

EWG 2003b. Environmental Working Group. 2003. "PFCs: Global Contaminants: PFC Health Concerns." Last modified April 3.

EWG 2007. Environmental Working Group. 2007. "EWG Research Shows 22 Percent of All Cosmetics May Be Contaminated with Cancer-Causing Impurity." Last modified February 8.

EWG 2009. Environmental Working Group. 2009. "Pollution in Minority Newborns: BPA and Other Cord Blood Pollutants." Last modified November 23.

EWG 2010. Environmental Working Group. 2010. "Pesticides: Testing, Kids, Regulation and You." *Enviroblog by Environmental Working Group*, February 23.

EWG 2011. Environmental Working Group. 2011. "EWG to FDA, EPA: Expand Nano Investigations." Last modified August 17.

EWG 2013. Environmental Working Group. 2013. *Water Treatment Contaminants: Forgotten Toxics in American Water*. Washington, DC: Environmental Working Group.

EWG 2015a. Environmental Working Group. 2015. "Caramel Color." Accessed April 20.

EWG 2015b. Environmental Working Group. 2015. "EWG's Guide to Perfluorochemicals." Accessed April 20.

EWG 2015c. Environmental Working Group. 2015. "EWG's Guide to Triclosan." Accessed May 1.

EWG 2015d. Environmental Working Group. 2015. "Frequently Asked Questions." Accessed April 20.

EWG 2015e. Environmental Working Group. 2015. "Healthy Home Tips: Tip 3 – Pick Plastics Carefully." Accessed May 1.

EWG 2015f. Environmental Working Group. 2015. "Hexachlorinated Dioxin." Accessed April 20.

EWG 2015g. Environmental Working Group. 2015. "Myths on Cosmetics Safety." Accessed April 20.

EWG 2015h. Environmental Working Group. 2015. "Petroleum Distillates." Accessed April 20.

EWG 2015i. Environmental Working Group. 2015. "Propylene Glycol." Accessed April 20.

EWG 2015j. Environmental Working Group. 2015. "Surfactants." Accessed April 29.

EWG 2015k. Environmental Working Group. 2015. "Top Tips for Safer Products." Accessed April 20.

EWG 2015l. Environmental Working Group. 2015. "Nanoparticles in Sunscreens." Accessed February 8.

EWG and the Campaign for Safe Cosmetics 2010. Environmental Working Group and the Campaign for Safe Cosmetics. 2010. "Not So Sexy: Hidden Chemicals in Perfume and Cologne." Last modified May 12.

Farrow et al. 2003. Farrow, Alexandra, Hazel Taylor, Kate Northstone, and Jean Golding. 2003. "Symptoms of Mothers and Infants Related to Total Volatile Organic Compounds in Household Products." *Archives of Environmental Health* 58(10): 633-41.

FDA 2000. United States Food and Drug Administration. 2000. *Triclosan: What Consumers Should Know*. Silver Spring, MD: United States Food and Drug Administration.

FDA 2014a. United States Food and Drug Administration. 2014. "FDA Regulations No Longer Authorize the Use of BPA in Infant Formula Packaging Based on Abandonment; Decision Not Based on Safety." Last modified June 9.

FDA 2014b. United States Food and Drug Administration. 2014. "Hair Dyes: Fact Sheet." Last modified March 19.

Fisher et al. 2003. Fisher, Jane S., S. Macpherson, N. Marchetti, and Richard M. Sharpe. 2003. "Human 'Testicular Dysgenesis Syndrome': A Possible Model Using In-Utero Exposure of the Rat to Dibutyl Phthalate." *Human Reproduction* 18(7): 1383-94.

Freinkel 2011. Freinkel, Susan. 2011. *Plastic: A Toxic Love Story*. New York: Houghton Mifflin Harcourt.

Fuqua 1986. Fuqua, Don. 1986. *Neurotoxins: At Home and the Workplace. Report to the Committee on Science and Technology, US House of Representatives*. Washington, DC: Committee on Science and Technology.

Gerona et al. 2013. Gerona, Roy R., Tracey J. Woodruff, Carrie A. Dickenson, Janet Pan, Jackie M Schwartz, Saunak Sen, Matthew W. Friesen, Victor Y. Fujimoto, and Patricia A. Hunt. 2013. "Bisphenol-A (BPA), BPA Glucuronide, and BPA Sulfate in Mid-Gestation Umbilical Cord Serum in a Northern and Central California Population." *Environmental Science and Technology* 47(21): 12477-85.

Goldman, Shannon, and the Committee on Environmental Health 2001. Goldman, Lynn R., Michael W. Shannon, and the Committee on Environmental Health. 2001. "Technical Report: Mercury in the Environment: Implications for Pediatricians." *Pediatrics* 108(1): 197-205.

The Good Guide 2015. The Good Guide. 2015. "Sodium Benzoate Ingredient Information." Accessed April 29.

Grandjean et al. 2012. Grandjean, Philippe, Elisabeth Wreford Andersen, Esben Budtz-Jorgensen, Flemming Nielsen, Kare Molbak, Pal Weihe, and Carsten Heilmann. 2012. "Serum Vaccine Antibody Concentrations in Children Exposed to Perfluorinated Compounds." *The Journal of the American Medical Association* 307(4): 391-7.

Green Building Council 2007. Green Building Council. 2007. "Memorandum. TSAC Report on PVC." Last modified February 26.

Green Science Policy Institute 2015a. Green Science Policy Institute. 2015. "Health and Environment." Accessed May 19.

Green Science Policy Institute 2015b. Green Science Policy Institute. 2015. "The Safe Kids Buyer's Guide." Accessed April 21.

Greenop et al. 2013. Greenop, Kathryn R., Susan Peters, Helen D. Bailey, Lin Fritschi, John Attia, Rodney J. Scott, Deborah C. Glass, et al. 2013. "Exposure to Pesticides and the Risk of Childhood Brain Tumors." *Cancer Causes and Control* 24(7): 1269-78.

Gross 2013. Gross, Liza. 2013. "Flame Retardants in Consumer Products Are Linked to Health and Cognitive Problems." *Washington Post,* April 15.

Harley et al. 2013. Harley, Kim G., Robert B Gunier, Katherine Kogut, Caroline Johnson, Asa Bradman, Antonia M. Calafat, and Brenda Eskenazi. 2013. "Prenatal and Early Childhood Bisphenol A Concentrations and Behavior in School-Aged Children." *Environmental Research* 126: 43-50.

Hawthorne, Nieland, and Eads 2012. Hawthorne, Michael, Katie Nieland, and David Eads. 2012. "Flame Retardants and Their Risks." *Chicago Tribune,* May 10.

Healthy Building Network 2008. Healthy Building Network 2008. *Fact Sheet: Alternative Resin Binders for Particleboard, MDF and Wheatboard.* Washington, DC: Healthy Building Network.

HealthyStuff.org 2015. Healthy Stuff. 2015. "Cadmium: Health Effects." Accessed April 22.

Hendricks 2000. Hendricks, Melissa. 2000. "Home, Sick Home." Last modified September.

Henry 2013. Henry, Trish. 2013. "BPA, Phthalate Exposure May Cause Fertility Problems." *CNN,* October 15.

Hiroi et al. 2004. Hiro, H., O. Tsutsumi, T. Takeuchi, M. Momoeda, Y. Ikezuki, A. Okamura, H. Yokota, and Y. Taketani. 2004. "Differences in Serum Bisphenol A Concentrations in Premenopausal Normal Women and Women with Endometrial Hyperplasia." *Endocrine Journal* 51(6): 595-600.

Hollender and Zissu 2010. Hollender, Jeffrey and Alexandra Zissu. 2010. *Planet Home: Conscious Choices for Cleaning and Greening the World You Care About Most.* New York: Clarkson Potter.

Hollender et al. 2006. Hollender, Jeffrey, Geoff Davis, Meika Hollender, and Reed Doyle. 2006. *Naturally Clean: The Seventh Generation Guide to Safe and Healthy, Non-Toxic Cleaning.* Gabriola Island, BC: New Society.

Houlihan 2015. Houlihan, Jane. 2015. "Why This Matters – Cosmetics and Your Health." Accessed April 29.

HUD 2003. United States Department of Housing and Urban Development. 2003. *Simple Steps to Protect Your Family from Lead Hazards.* Washington, DC: United States Department of Housing and Urban Development.

IARC 1997. International Agency for Research on Cancer. 1997. *IARC Monographs on the Evaluation of Carcinogenic Risks to Humans. Volume 69. Polychlorinated Dibenzo-para-Dioxins and Polychlorinated Dibenzofurans.* Lyon, France: International Agency for Research on Cancer.

IARC 1999. International Agency for Research on Cancer. 1999. *IARC Monographs on the Evaluation of Carcinogenic Risks of Humans. Volume 71. Re-Evaluation of Some Organic Chemicals, Hydrazine and Hydrogen Peroxide.* Lyon, France: International Agency for Research on Cancer.

IARC 2002. International Agency for Research on Cancer. 2002. *IARC Monographs on the Evaluation of Carcinogenic Risks of Humans. Some Traditional Herbal Medicines, Some Mycotoxins, Naphthalene and Styrene. Volume 82.* Lyon, France: International Agency for Research on Cancer.

IARC 2004. International Agency for Research on Cancer. 2004. "IARC Classifies Formaldehyde as Carcinogenic to Humans." Last modified June 15.

IFRA 2015. International Fragrance Association. 2015. "Ingredients." Accessed April 22.

Imo et al. 2014. Imo, T., F. Latu, V. Varurasi, J. Yoshida, P. Amosa, and M. A. Sheikh. 2014. "Distribution of Heavy Metals in Sediments at the Commercial and Fishing Ports in Samoa." *International Journal of Environmental Science and Development* 5(6): 517-21.

Jones and Miller 2008. Jones, D. C. and G. W. Miller. 2008. "The Effects of Environmental Neurotoxicants on the Dopaminergic System: A Possible Role in Drug Addiction." *Biochemical Pharmacology* 76(5): 569-81.

Jurewicz and Hanke 2008. Jurewicz, J. and W. Hanke. 2008. "Prenatal and Childhood Exposure to Pesticides and Neurobehavioral Development: Review of Epidemiological Studies." *International Journal of Occupational Medicine and Environmental Health* 21(2): 121-32.

Kaur et al. 2014. Kaur, K., V. Chauhan, F. Gu, and A. Chauhan. 2014. "Bisphenol A Induces Oxidative Stress and Mitochondrial Dysfunction in Lymphoblasts from Children with Autism and Unaffected Siblings." *Free Radical Biological Medicine* 76: 25-33.

Lee 2003. Lee, Jennifer S. 2003. "EPA Orders Companies to Examine Effects of Chemicals." *New York Times,* April 15.

Lessenger 2001. Lessenger, James E. 2001. "Occupational Acute Anaphylactic Reaction to Assault by Perfume Spray in the Face." *Journal of the American Board of Family Medicine* 14(2): 137-40.

Liu, Schade, and Simpson 2008. Liu, Jeannie, Michael Schade, and Heather Simpson. 2008. *Pass Up* the Poison Plastic: The PVC – Free Guide for Your Family and Home. Falls Church, VA: The Center for Health, Environment and Justice.

Lorber 2008. Lorber, Matthew. 2008. "Exposure of Americans to Polybrominated Diphenyl Ethers." *Journal of Exposure Science and Environmental Epidemiology* 18: 2-19.

Martin 2010. Martin, David S. 2010. "Companies, Hospitals Move Away from Toxic Material." *CNN,* May 26.

Mattsson et al. 2015. Mattsson, Karin, Mikael T. Ekvall, Lars-Anders Hansson, Sara Linse, Anders Malmendal, and Tommy Cedervall. 2015. "Altered Behavior, Physiology, and Metabolism in Fish Exposed to Polystyrene Nanparticles." *Environmental Science and Technology* 49(1): 553-61.

McCann et al. 2007. McCann, Donna, Angelina Barrett, Alison Cooper, Debbie Crumpler, Lindy Dalen, Kate Grimshaw, Elizabeth Kitchin, et al. 2007. "Food Additives and Hyperactive Behavior in 3-Year-Old and 8/9-Year-Old Children in the Community: A Randomized, Double-Blinded, Placebo-Controlled Trial." *The Lancet* 370(9598): 1560-7.

McGinn 2000. McGinn, Anne Platt. 2000. *POPs Culture.* Washington, DC: Worldwatch Institute.

Meeker and Stapleton 2010. Meeker, John D. and Heather M. Stapleton. 2010. "House Dust Concentrations of Organophosphate Flame Retardants in Relation to Hormone Levels and Semen Quality Parameters." *Environmental Health Perspectives* 118(3): 318-23.

Meharg, Deacon, et al. 2008. Meharg, Andrew A., Claire Deacon, Robert C. J. Campbell, Anne-Marie Carey, Paul N. Williams, Joerg Feldmann, and Andrea Raab. 2008. "Inorganic Arsenic Levels in Rice Milk Exceed EU and US Drinking Water Standards." *Journal of Environmental Monitoring* 10(4): 428-31.

Meharg, Sun, et al. 2008. Meharg, Andrew A., Guoxin Sun, Paul N. Williams, Eureka Adomako, Claire Deacon, Yong-Guan Zhu, Joerg Feldmann, and Andrea Raab. 2008. "Inorganic Arsenic Levels in Baby Rice Are of Concern." *Environmental Pollution* 152(3): 746-9.

Melzer et al. 2012. Melzer, David, Phil Gates, Nicholas J. Osborn, William E. Henley, Ricardo Cipelli, Anita Young, Cathryn Money, et al. 2012. "Urinary Bisphenol A Concentration and Angiography-Defined Coronary Artery Stenosis." *PLoS ONE* 7(8): e43378.

Mendonca et al. 2014. Mendonca, K., R. Hauser, A. M. Calafat, T. E. Arbuckle, and S. M. Duty. 2014. "Bisphenol A Concentrations in Maternal Breast Milk and Infant Urine." *International Archives of Occupational and Environmental Health* 87(1): 13-20.

Minnesota Department of Health 2015. Minnesota Department of Health. 2015. "Volatile Organic Compounds in Your Home." Last modified February 17.

National Association of State Fire Marshals 2015. National Association of State Fire Marshals. 2015. "National Furniture Flammability Standard. Frequently Asked Questions." Accessed February 12.

National Environmental Trust 2004. National Environmental Trust. 2004. *Cabinet Confidential: Toxic Products in the Home.* Washington, DC: National Environmental Trust.

National Geographic **2008.** National Geographic. 2008. *Green Guide: The Complete Reference for Consuming Wisely.* Washington, DC: National Geographic Society.

National Research Council 2008. National Research Council. 2008. *Phthalates and Cumulative Risk Assessment: The Tasks Ahead.* Washington, DC: National Academies Press.

NCI 2014. National Cancer Institute. 2014. "Aromatherapy and Essential Oils (PDQ)." Last modified December 17.

Newbold, Jefferson, and Banks 2007. Newbold, Retha R., Wendy N. Jefferson, and Elizabeth Padilla Banks. 2007. "Long-Term Adverse Effects of Neonatal Exposure to Bisphenol A on the Murine Female Reproductive Tract." *Reproductive Toxicology* 24(2): 253-8.

NIEHS 2012. National Institute of Environmental Health Sciences. 2012. *Perfluorinated Chemicals (PFCs).* Research Triangle Park, NC: National Institute of Environmental Health Sciences.

NIEHS 2015. National Institute of Environmental Health Sciences. 2015. "Bisphenol A (BPA)." Last modified January 21.

NIEHS and EPA 2013. National Institute of Environmental Health Sciences and the United States Environmental Protection Agency. 2013. *NIEHS/EPA Children's Environmental Health and Disease Prevention Research Centers: Protecting Children's Health for a Lifetime.* Research Triangle Park, NC: National Institute of Environmental Health Sciences.

NRDC 1997. Natural Resources Defense Council. 1997. "Our Children at Risk: The Five Worst Environmental Threats to Their Health." Last modified November 25.

NRDC 2011a. Natural Resources Defense Council. 2011. "Guide to Greener Fibers." Last modified November 8.

NRDC 2011b. Natural Resources Defense Council. 2011. "Nanomaterials." Last modified December 27.

NRDC 2012. Natural Resources Defense Council. 2012. "From Field to Store: Your T-Shirt's Life Story." Last modified January 18.

NRDC 2014. Natural Resources Defense Council. 2014. "Methylene Chloride." Last modified October 14.

NRDC 2015a. Natural Resources Defense Council. 2015. "Endocrine Disruption: An Overview and Resource List." Accessed April 20.

NRDC 2015b. Natural Resources Defense Council. 2015. "Toxic Chemicals in Our Couches." Accessed April 20.

NTP 2008. National Toxicology Program. 2008. *NTP-CERHR Monograph on the Potential Human Reproductive and Developmental Effects of Bisphenol A. NIH Publication No. 08-5994.* Research Triangle Park, NC: National Toxicology Program. US Department of Health and Human Services.

NTP 2014. National Toxicology Program. 2014. *13th Report on Carcinogens.* US Department of Health and Human Services.

NY DOH 2011. New York State Department of Health. 2011. "Bisphenol A." Last modified February.

OSHA 2003. Occupational Safety and Health Administration. 2003. *Methylene Chloride. OSHA 3144-06R.* Washington, DC: US Department of Labor.

OSHA 2015. Occupational Safety and Health Administration. 2015. "OSHA Archive: Solvents." Accessed April 22.

Ostiguy et al. 2010. Ostiguy, Claude, Brigitte Roberge, Catherine Woods, and Brigitte Soucy. 2010. *Chemical Substances and Biological Agents: Studies and Research Projects Report R-656. Engineered Nanoparticles: Current Knowledge About OHS Risks and Prevention Measures, Second Edition.* Montreal: Institut de recherche Robert-Sauve.

Perera et al. 2012. Perera, Frederica, Julia Vishnevetsky, Julie B. Herbstman, Antonia M. Calafat, Wei Xiong, Virginia Rauh, and Shuang Wang. 2012. "Prenatal Bisphenol A Exposure and Child Behavior in an Inner-City Cohort." *Environmental Health Perspectives* 120(8): 1190-4.

Physicians for Social Responsibility 2015. Physicians for Social Responsibility. 2015. "Examples of Environmental Carcinogens." Accessed April 22.

Pitre 2014. Pitre, Simone. 2014. "Phthalates Are out of Children's Toys, but in Your Food." *Enviroblog by Environmental Working Group,* July 16.

Porrini et al. 2005. Porrini, Stefania, Virginia Belloni, Daniele Della Seta, Francesca Farabollini, Giuletta Giannelli, and Francesco Dessi-Fulgheri. 2005. "Early Exposure to a Low Dose of Bisphenol A Affects Socio-Sexual Behavior of Juvenile Female Rats." *Brain Research Bulletin* 65(3): 261-6.

Reuben 2010. Reuben, Suzanne H. 2010. *2008 – 2009 Annual Report, President's Cancer Panel. Reducing Environmental Cancer Risk: What We Can Do Now.* Bethesda, MD: National Cancer Institute.

Rier and Foster 2002. Rier, Sherry and Warren G. Foster. 2002. "Environmental Dioxins and Endometriosis." *Toxicological Sciences* 70(2): 161-70.

Sagiv et al. 2012. Sagiv, Sharon K., Sally W. Thurston, David C. Bellinger, Larisa M. Altshul, and Susan A. Korrick. 2012. "Neuropsychological Measures of Attention and Impulse Control among 8-Year-Old Children Exposed Prenatally to Organochlorines." *Environmental Health Perspectives* 120(6): 904-9.

Schell et al. 2014. Schell, Lawrence M., Mia V. Gallo, Glenn D. Deane, Kyrie R. Nelder, Anthony P. DeCaprio, Agnes Jacobs, and the Akwesasne Task Force on the Environment. 2014. "Relationships of Polychlorinated Biphenyls and Dichlorodiphenyldichloroethylene (p,p'DDE) with Testosterone Levels in Adolescent Males." *Environmental Health Perspectives* 122(3): 304-9.

Schettler 2006. Schettler, Ted. 2006. "Human Exposure to Phthalates via Consumer Products." *International Journal of Andrology* 29(1): 181-5.

Schreder 2012. Schreder, Erika. 2012. *Hidden Hazards in the Nursery.* Seattle, WA: Washington Toxics Coalition/Safer States.

Sigurdson 2014. Sigurdson, Tina. 2014. "Expert Panel Confirms That Fragrance Ingredient Can Cause Cancer." *Enviroblog by Environmental Working Group,* August 7.

Silas, Hansen, and Lent 2007. Silas, Julie, Jean Hansen, and Tom Lent. 2007. *The Future of Fabric: Health Care.* Healthy Building Network.

Sjodin et al. 2008. Sjodin, Andreas, Lee-Yang Wong, Richard S. Jones, Annie Park, Yalin Zhang, Carolyn Hodge, Emily DiPietro, et al. 2008. "Serum Concentrations of Polybrominated Diphenyl Ethers (PBDEs) and Polybrominated Biphenyl (PBB) in the United States Population: 2003-2004." *Environmental Science and Technology* 42(2): 1377-84.

Smith and Lourie 2009. Smith, Rick and Bruce Lourie. 2009. *Slow Death by Rubber Duck: The Secret Danger of Everyday Things.* Berkeley, CA: Counterpoint.

Srogi 2007. Srogi, K. 2007. "Monitoring of Environmental Exposure to Polycyclic Aromatic Hydrocarbons: A Review." *Environmental Chemistry Letters* 5(4): 169-95.

Stafford 2009. Stafford, Ned. 2009. "New Nano Rule for EU Cosmetics." *Chemistry World by Royal Society of Chemistry,* November 27.

Stahlhut et al. 2007. Stahlhut, Richard W., Edwin van Wijngaarden, Timothy D. Dye, Stephen Cook, and Shanna H. Swan. 2007. "Concentrations of Urinary Phthalate Metabolites Are Associated with Increased Waist Circumference and Insulin Resistance in Adult US Males." *Environmental Health Perspectives* 115(6): 876-82.

Stapleton et al. 2011. Stapleton, Heather M., Susan Klosterhaus, Alex Keller, P. Lee Ferguson, Saskia van Bergen, Ellen Cooper, Thomas F. Webster, and Arlene Blum. 2011. "Identification of Flame Retardants in Polyurethane Foam Collected from Baby Products." *Environmental Science and Technology* 45(12): 5323-31.

Stapleton et al. 2012. Stapleton, Heather M., Smriti Sharma, Gordon Getzinger, P. Lee Ferguson, Michelle Gabriel, Thomas F. Webster, and Arlene Blum. 2012.

"Novel and High Volume Use Flame Retardants in US Couches Reflective of the 2005 PentaBDE Phase Out." *Environmental Science and Technology* 46(24): 13432-9.

Steinemann et al. 2010. Steinemann, Anne C., Ian C. MacGregor, Sydney M. Gordon, Lisa G. Gallagher, Amy L. Davis, Daniel S. Ribeiro, and Lance A. Wallace. 2010. "Fragranced Consumer Products: Chemicals Emitted, Ingredients Unlisted." *Environmental Impact Assessment Review* 31(3): 328–33.

Steingraber 2010. Steingraber, Sandra. 2010. *Living Downstream: An Ecologist's Investigation of Cancer and the Environment.* 2nd ed. Cambridge: Da Capo Press.

Stockholm Convention 2015. Stockholm Convention. 2015. "Listing of POPs in the Stockholm Convention." Accessed April 21.

Sun et al. 2009. Sun, Guo-Xin, Paul N. Williams, Yong-Guan Zhu, Claire Deacon, Anne-Marie Carey, Andrea Raab, Joerg Feldmann, and Andrew A. Meharg. 2009. "Survey of Arsenic and Its Speciation in Rice Products Such as Breakfast Cereals, Rice Crackers and Japanese Rice Condiments." *Environment International* 35(3): 473-5.

Swan et al. 2005. Swan, Shanna H., Katharina M. Main, Fan Liu, Sara L. Stewart, Robin L. Kruse, Antonia M. Calafat, Catherine S. Mao, et al. 2005. "Decrease in Anogenital Distance among Male Infants with Prenatal Phthalate Exposure." *Environmental Health Perspectives* 113(8): 1056-61.

Takeda et al. 2009. Takeda, Ken, Ken-ichiro Suzuki, Aki Ishihara, Miyoko Kubo-Irie, Rie Fujimoto, Masako Tabata, Shigeru Oshio, Yoshimasa Nihei, Tomomi Ihara, and Masao Sugamata. 2009. "Nanoparticles Transferred from Pregnant Mice to Their Offspring Can Damage the Genital and Cranial Nerve Systems." *Journal of Health Science* 55(1): 95-102.

TEDX 2009. The Endocrine Disruption Exchange. 2009. "Endocrine Disruption: Bisphenol A." Last modified September.

Teitelbaum et al. 2012. Teitelbaum, Susan L., Nancy Mervish, Erin L. Moshier, Nita Vangeepuram, Maida P. Galvez, Antonia M. Calafat, Manori J. Silva, Barbara L. Brenner, Mary S. Wolff. 2012. "Associations between Phthalate Metabolite Urinary Concentrations and Body Size Measures in New York City Children." *Environmental Research* 112: 186-93.

Tox Town 2014a. Tox Town. 2014. "Formaldehyde." Last modified October 27.

Tox Town 2014b. Tox Town. 2014. "Solvents." Last modified November 17.

Trasande, Attina, and Blustein 2012. Trasande, Leonardo, Teresa M. Attina, and Jan Blustein. 2012. "Association between Urinary Bisphenol A Concentration and Obesity Prevalence in Children and Adolescents." *The Journal of the American Medical Association* 308(11): 1113-21.

Trouiller et al. 2009. Trouiller, B., R. Reliene, A. Westbrook, P. Solaimani, and R. H. Schiestl. 2009. "Titanium Dioxide Nanoparticles Induce DNA Damage and Genetic Instability In Vivo in Mice." *Cancer Research* 69(22): 8784-9.

Urban Green Council 2010. Urban Green Council. 2010. *NYC Green Codes Task Force: A Report to Mayor Michael R. Bloomberg and Speaker Christine C. Quinn.* New York: Urban Green Council, New York Chapter of the US Green Building Council.

Urban Green Council 2015. Urban Green Council. 2015. *Green Codes Task Force Report.* New York: Urban Green Council.

USDA 2014. United States Department of Agriculture. 2014. "Cotton and Wool. Overview." Last modified October 17.

Villanueva et al. 2004. Villanueva, C. M., K. P. Cantor, S. Cordier, J. J. Jaakkola, W. D. King, C. F. Lynch, S. Porru, and M. Kogevinas. 2004. "Disinfection Byproducts and Bladder Cancer: A Pooled Analysis." *Epidemiology* 15(3): 357-67.

Wallinga et al. 2009. Wallinga, David, Janelle Sorensen, Pooja Mottl, and Brian Yablon. 2009. *Not So Sweet: Missing Mercury and High Fructose Corn Syrup.* Minneapolis, MN: Institute for Agriculture and Trade Policy.

Wallis 2007. Wallis, Claudia. 2007. "Hyper Kids? Cut Out Preservatives." *Time,* September 6.

Washington Toxics Coalition 2009. Washington Toxics Coalition. 2009. "Statement of Washington Toxics Coalition Regarding EPA Announcement of Deca Flame Retardant Phase-Out and Federal Legislation Introduced Today." Last modified December 18.

Wassener 2011. Wassener, Bettina. 2011. "Raising Awareness of Plastic Waste." *New York Times,* August 14.

Weil 2012. Weil, Elizabeth. 2012. "Puberty before Age 10: A New 'Normal'?" *New York Times Magazine,* March 30.

WHO 2010a. World Health Organization: Yona Amitai, Hamed Bakir, Nida Besbelli, Stephan Boese-O'Reilly, Mariano Cebrian, Yaohua Dai, Paul Dargan, et al. 2010. *Childhood Lead Poisoning.* Geneva, Switzerland: World Health Organization.

WHO 2010b. World Health Organization. 2010. *WHO Guidelines for Indoor Air Quality: Selected Pollutants.* Copenhagen, Denmark: World Health Organization.

WHO 2012. World Health Organization. 2012. "Arsenic." Last modified December.

WHO 2014. World Health Organization. 2014. "Dioxins and Their Effects on Human Health." Last modified June.

WHO and UNEP 2013. World Health Organization and United Nations Environment Programme. 2013. *State of the Science of Endocrine Disrupting Chemicals – 2012.* Geneva, Switzerland: WHO Press.

Williams et al. 2005. Williams, P. N., A. H. Price, A. Raab, S. A. Hossain, J. Feldmann, and A. A. Meharg. 2005. "Variation in Arsenic Speciation and Concentration in Paddy Rice Related to Dietary Exposure." *Environmental Science and Technology* 39(15): 5531-40.

Worldwatch Institute 2000. Worldwatch Institute. 2000. "POPs Culture." Last modified April.

Yang et al. 2011. Yang, Chun Z., Stuart I. Yaniger, V. Craig Jordan, Daniel J. Klein, and George D. Bittner. 2011. "Most Plastic Products Release Estrogenic Chemicals: A Potential Health Problem That Can Be Solved." *Environmental Health Perspectives* 119(7): 989-96.

Yazar et al. 2011. Yazar, K, S. Johnsson, M. L. Lind, A. Boman, and C. Liden. 2011. "Preservatives and Fragrances in Selected Consumer-Available Cosmetics and Detergents." *Contact Dermatitis* 64(5): 265-72.

Works Cited: Parts III and IV

AAP 2015. American Academy of Pediatrics. 2015. "Poison Prevention and Treatment Tips National Poison Prevention Week, March 15-21, 2015." Last modified March 10.

Ackerman 2015. Ackerman, Jennifer. 2015. "Food: How Altered?" *National Geographic,* accessed May 7.

ADA 2014. American Dental Association. 2014. "Taking Care of Your Child's Smile." Last modified May.

ADA 2015a. American Dental Association. 2015. "Fluoride and Instant Formula." Accessed February 7.

ADA 2015b. American Dental Association. 2015. "Oral Health Topics. Fluoride Supplements. Facts About Fluoride." Accessed February 7.

American Heart Association 2015. American Heart Association. 2015. "Know Your Fats." Last modified April 29.

American Lung Association 2015. American Lung Association. 2015. "Tobacco." Accessed May 11.

Anderson and Anderson 2000. Anderson, R. C. and J. H. Anderson. 2000. "Respiratory Toxicity of Mattress Emissions in Mice." *Archives of Environmental Health* 55(1): 38-43.

Andrews et al. 2002. Andrews, Linda S., Anna M. Key, Roy L. Martin, Robert Grodner, and Douglas L. Park. 2002. "Chlorine Dioxide Wash of Shrimp and Crawfish an Alternative to Aqueous Chlorine." *Food Microbiology* 19: 261-7.

Asthma and Allergy Foundation of America 2015. Asthma and Allergy Foundation of America. 2015. "Sick Building Syndrome." Accessed May 11.

ATSDR 1997. Agency for Toxic Substances and Disease Registry. 1997. *Public Health Statement Chloroform. CAS# 67-66-3.* Atlanta, GA: US Department of Health and Human Services, Public Health Service, Agency for Toxic Substances and Disease Registry.

ATSDR 2000. Agency for Toxic Substances and Disease Registry. 2000. *Toxicological Profile for Methylene Chloride.* Atlanta, GA: US Department of Health and Human Services, Public Health Service, Agency for Toxic Substances and Disease Registry.

ATSDR 2012. Agency for Toxic Substances and Disease Registry. 2012. *Public Health Statement Styrene.* Atlanta, GA: US Department of Health and Human Services, Public Health Service, Agency for Toxic Substances and Disease Registry.

Bader 2009. Bader, Walter. 2009. *Sleep Safe in a Toxic World: Your Guide to a Safe Night's Sleep.* Topanga, CA: Freedom Press.

Bader 2011. Bader, Walter. 2011. *Sleep Safe in a Toxic World.* Topanga, CA: Freedom Press.

Barry 2009. Barry, Carolyn. 2009. "Plastic Breaks Down in Ocean, after All – and Fast." *National Geographic News,* August 20.

BBC 2001. BBC. 2001. "Carpets Harbour 'Toxic Dust.'" *BBC News,* May 3.

Bellieni et al. 2012. Bellieni, C. V., I. Pinto, A. Bogi, N. Zoppetti, D. Andreuccetti, and G. Buonocore. 2012. "Exposure to Electromagnetic Fields from Laptop Use of 'Laptop' Computers." *Archives of Environmental and Occupational Health* 67(1): 31-6.

Benenson 1985. Benenson, Abram S. 1985. *Control of Communicable Disease in Man.* Washington, DC: American Public Health Association.

Betts 2008. Betts, Kellyn S. 2008. "Unwelcome Guest: PBDEs in Indoor Dust." *Environmental Health Perspectives* 116(5): A202-8.

Bhatia and Greer 2008. Bhatia, Jatinder and Frank Greer. 2008. "Use of Soy Protein-Based Formulas in Infant Feeding." *Pediatrics* 121: 1062–8.

Black 2010. Black, Rosemary. 2010. "85 Percent of Childrens' Drinks Contain Lead Exceeding Federal Limits for Young Kids." *NY Daily News,* June 14.

Blanchard et al. 2014. Blanchard, Olivier, Philippe Glorennec, Fabien Mercier, Nathalie Bonvallot, Cecile Chevrier, Olivier Ramalho, Corinne Mandin, and Barbara Le Bot. 2014. "Semivolatile Organic Compounds in Indoor Air and Settled Dust in 30 French Dwellings." *Environmental Science and Technology* 48(7): 3959-69.

Bliss 2012. Bliss, Rosalie. 2012. "The Stealth Sodium Revolution." *Agricultural Research* 60(3): 22.

Blount et al. 2000. Blount, Benjamin C., Manori J. Silva, Samuel P. Caudill, Larry L. Needham, Jim L. Pirkle, Eric J. Sampson, George W. Lucier, Richard J. Jackson, and John W. Brock. 2000. "Levels of Seven Urinary Phthalate Metabolites in a Human Reference Population." *Environmental Health Perspectives* 108(10): 979-82.

Blum and Ames 1977. Blum, Arlene and Bruce N. Ames. 1977. "Flame-Retardant Additives as Possible Cancer Hazards." *Science* 195(4273): 17-23.

Bocarsly et al. 2010. Bocarsly, Miriam E., Elyse S. Powell, Nicole M. Avena, and Bartley G. Hoebel. 2010. "High-Fructose Corn Syrup Causes Characteristics of Obesity in Rats: Increased Body Weight, Body Fat and Triglyceride Levels."

Pharmacology, Biochemistry and Behavior 97(1): 101-6.

Boesler 2013. Boesler, Matthew. 2013. "Bottled Water Costs 2000 Times as Much as Tap Water." *Business Insider,* July 12.

Bornehag et al. 2005. Bornehag, Carl-Gustaf, Bjorn Lundgren, Charles J. Weschler, Torben Sigsgaard, Linda Hagerhed-Engman, and Jan Sundell. 2005. "Phthalates in Indoor Dust and Their Association with Building Characteristics." *Environmental Health Perspectives* 113(10): 1399-404.

Brunekreef et al. 1989. Brunekreef, Bert, Douglas W. Dockery, Frank E. Speizer, James H. Ware, John D. Spengler, and Benjamin G. Ferris. 1989. "Home Dampness and Respiratory Morbidity in Children." *American Review of Respiratory Disease* 140(5): 1363-7.

Building Green 2015. Building Green. 2015. "Checklist for Minimizing IAQ Problems with Carpets." Accessed May 7.

Burros 1999. Burros, Marian. 1999. "Eating Well; Plastic Wrap and Health: Studies Raise Questions." *New York Times,* January 13.

Butte and Heinzow 2002. Butte, Werner and Birger Heinzow. 2002. "Pollutants in House Dust as Indicators of Indoor Contamination." *Reviews of Environmental Contamination and Toxicology* 175: 1-46.

CA EPA 2015. California Environmental Protection Agency. 2015. *Chemicals Known to the State to Cause Cancer or Reproductive Toxicity. March 27, 2015.* Sacramento, CA: California Environmental Protection Agency, Office of Environmental Health Hazard Assessment.

Calafat et al. 2007. Calafat, Antonia M., Lee-Yang Wong, Zsuzsanna Kulklenyik, John A. Reidy, and Larry L. Needham. 2007. "Polyfluoroalkyl Chemicals in the US Population: Data from the National Health and Nutrition Examination Survey (NHANES) 2003-2004 and Comparisons with NHANES 1999-2000." *Environmental Health Perspectives* 115(11): 1596-602.

Callahan and Roe 2012. Callahan, Patricia and Sam Roe. 2012. "Chemical Makers Fan the Flames of Fear." *Los Angeles Times,* May 12.

Campbell and Campbell 2006. Campbell, T. Colin and Thomas M. Campbell II. 2006. *The China Study: The Most Comprehensive Study of Nutrition Ever Conducted. Startling Implications for Diet, Weight Loss, and Long-Term Health.* Dallas, TX: BenBella.

Cao et al. 2008. Cao, Xu-Liang, Guy Dufresne, Stephane Belisle, Genevieve Clement, Mirka Falicki, Franca Beraldin, and Anastase Rulibikiye. 2008. "Levels of Bisphenol A in Canned Liquid Infant Formula Products in Canada and Dietary Intake Estimates." *Journal of Agricultural and Food Chemistry* 56(17): 7919–24.

CDC 1997. Centers for Disease Control and Prevention. 1997. "Update: Blood Lead Levels – United States, 1991-1994." Last modified February 21.

CDC 2011. Centers for Disease Control and Prevention. 2011. "Chemicals in Tobacco Smoke." Last modified March 21.

CDC 2012a. Centers for Disease Control and Prevention. 2012. "Flavorings-Related Lung Disease: Exposures to Flavoring Chemicals." Last modified August 29.

CDC 2012b. Centers for Disease Control and Prevention. 2012. "Where's the Sodium?" Last modified February.

CDC 2013. Centers for Disease Control and Prevention. 2013. "Facts About Chlorine." Last modified April 10.

CDC 2014a. Centers for Disease Control and Prevention. 2014. "Handwashing: Clean Hands Save Lives. Show Me the Science – How to Wash Your Hands." Last modified October 17.

CDC 2014b. Centers for Disease Control and Prevention. 2014. "The National Institute for Occupational Safety and Health (NIOSH): Protect Your Family: Reduce Contamination at Home." Last modified June 6.

CDC 2014c. Centers for Disease Control and Prevention. 2014. "Smoking and Tobacco Use: Tobacco-Related Mortality." Last modified November 21.

CDPH 2007. California Department of Public Health. 2007. "California Department of Public Health Advises Consumers Not to Use CDPH Lunch Boxes." Last modified September 20.

Chan 2009. Chan, W. H. 2009. "Impact of Genistein on Maturation of Mouse Oocytes, Fertilization, and Fetal Development." *Reproductive Toxicology* 28(1): 52-8.

Chang 2001. Chang, John C. S. 2001. *Capstone Report on the Development of a Standard Test Method for VOC Emission from Interior Latex and Alkyd Paints.* Research Triangle Park, NC: United States Environmental Protection Agency.

Claiborne, Childs, Siegel 2010. Claiborne, Ron, Dan Childs, and Hanna Siegel. 2010. "Report Says Contaminated Meat Is in Supermarkets." *ABC News,* April 14.

Clean and Healthy New York 2011. Clean and Healthy New York. 2011. *The Mattress Matters: Protecting Babies from Toxic Chemicals While They Sleep.* Albany, NY: Clean and Healthy New York, American Sustainable Business Council.

Cohen, Janssen, and Solomon 2007. Cohen, Alison, Sarah Janssen, and Gina Solomon. 2007. *Clearing the Air. Hidden Hazards of Air Fresheners.* New York: Natural Resources Defense Council.

Colt et al. 2004. Colt, Joanne S., Jay Lubin, David Camann, Scott Davis, James Cerhan, Richard K. Severson, Wendy Cozen, and Patricia Hartge. 2004. "Comparison of Pesticide Levels in Carpet Dust and Self-Reported Pest Treatment Practices in Four US Sites." *Journal of Exposure Analysis and Environmental Epidemiology* 14(1): 74-83.

Colt et al. 2005. Colt, Joanne S., Richard K. Severson, Jay Lubin, Nat Rothman, David Camann, Scott Davis, James R. Cerhan, Wendy Cozen, and Patricia Hartge. 2005. "Organochlorines in Carpet Dust and Non-Hodgkin Lymphoma." *Epidemiology* 16(4): 516-25.

Consumer Reports **2009.** Consumer Reports. 2009. "Interior Paints: Our New Tests Reveal Surprises About What Paint Makers Claim and What You Get." *Consumer Reports Magazine*, March.

Consumer Reports **2012.** Consumer Reports. 2012. "Arsenic in Your Food: Our Findings Show a Real Need for Federal Standards for This Toxin." *Consumer Reports Magazine,* November.

Consumer Reports **2014.** Consumer Reports. 2014. "How Much Arsenic Is in Your Rice? Consumer Reports' New Data and Guidelines are Important for Everyone But Especially for Gluten Avoiders." Last modified November.

Consumers Union 1998. Consumers Union. 1998. "Report to the FDA Regarding Plastic Packaging." Last modified June 5.

Costner, Thorpe, and McPherson 2005. Costner, Pat, Beverley Thorpe, and Alexandra McPherson. 2005. *Sick of Dust: Chemicals in Common Products – A Needless Health Risk in Our Homes.* Spring Brook, NY: Clean Production Action.

CotLife2000 2015. CotLife2000. 2015. "Statistics: Results of the New Zealand Mattress-Wrapping Campaign." Accessed May 17.

CPSC 1996. United States Consumer Product Safety Commission. 1996. "CPSC Finds Lead Poisoning Hazard for Young Children in Imported Vinyl Miniblinds." Last modified June 25.

CPSC 2013. United States Consumer Product Safety Commission. 2013. *An Update on Formaldehyde.* Bethesda, MD: US Consumer Product Safety Commission.

CPSC 2015a. United States Consumer Product Safety Commission. 2015. "Carbon Monoxide Questions and Answers." Accessed May 11.

CPSC 2015b. United States Consumer Product Safety Commission. 2015. "FAQs: Lead in Paint (and Other Surface Coatings)." Accessed February 15.

CPSC 2015c. United States Consumer Product Safety Commission. 2015. "The Inside Story: A Guide to Indoor Air Quality." Accessed May 11.

Dadd 2011. Dadd, Debra Lynn. 2011. *Toxic Free: How to Protect Your Health and Home from the Chemicals That Are Making You Sick.* New York: Penguin.

Davies et al. 1990. Davies, D. J. A., I. Thornton, J. M. Watt, E. B. Culbard, P. G. Harvey, H. T. Delves, J. C. Sherlock, G. A. Smart, J. F. A. Thomas, and M. J. Quinn. 1990. "Lead Intake and Blood Lead in Two-Year-Old UK Urban Children." *Science of the Total Environment* 90: 13-29.

Davis 2010. Davis, Devra. 2010. *Disconnect: The Truth About Cell Phone Radiation, What the Industry Has Done to Hide It, and How to Protect Your Family.* New York: Dutton.

de Vendomois et al. 2009. de Vendomois, Joel Spiroux, Francois Roullier, Dominique Cellier, and Gilles-Eric Seralini. 2009. "A Comparison of the Effects of Three GM Corn Varieties on Mammalian Health." *International Journal of Biological Sciences* 5(7): 706-26.

Delclos et al. 2009. Delclos, K. B., C. C. Weis, T. J. Bucci, G. Olson, P. Mellick, N. Sadovova, J. R. Latendresse, B. Thorn, and R. R. Newbold. 2009. "Overlapping But Distinct Effects of Genistein and Ethinyl Estradiol (EE(2)) in Female Sprague-Dawley Rats in Multigenerational Reproductive and Chronic Toxicity Studies." *Reproductive Toxicology* 27(2): 117-32.

Discovery News **2011.** Discovery News. 2011. "Food Packaging Harbors Harmful Chemicals." *Discovery News,* March 29.

Division of Sleep Medicine at Harvard Medical School 2007a. Division of Sleep Medicine at Harvard Medical School. 2007. "Healthy Sleep: Sleep and Disease Risk." Last modified December 18.

Division of Sleep Medicine at Harvard Medical School 2007b. Division of Sleep Medicine at Harvard Medical School. 2007. "Healthy Sleep: Sleep, Learning, and Memory." Last modified December 18.

Dodson et al. 2012. Dodson, Robin E., Laura J. Perovich, Adrian Covaci, Nele Van den Eede, Alin C. Ionas, Alin C. Dirtu, Julia Green Brody, and Ruthann A. Rudel. 2012. "After the PBDE Phase-Out: A Broad Suite of Flame Retardants in Repeat House Dust Samples from California." *Environmental Science and Technology* 46(24): 13056-66.

Downs 2008. Downs, Martin. 2008. "The Truth About 7 Common Food Additives." *CBS News,* August 5.

Dudley, Nassar, and Hartman 2009. Dudley, Susan, Salwa Nassar, and Emily Hartman. 2009. "Tampon Safety." *National Center for Health Research,* July.

Dufault et al. 2009. Dufault, Renee, Blaise LeBlanc, Roseanne Schnoll, Charles Cornett, Laura Schweitzer, David Wallinga, Jane Hightower, Lyn Patrick, and Walter J. Lukiw. 2009. "Mercury from Chlor-Alkali Plants: Measured Concentrations in Food Product Sugar." *Environmental Health* 8(2).

Duty et al. 2005. Duty, Susan M., Robin M. Ackerman, Antonia M. Calafat, and Russ Hauser. 2005. "Personal Care Product Use Predicts Urinary Concentrations of Some Phthalate Monoesters." *Environmental Health Perspectives* 113(11): 1530-5.

Easton, Luszniak, and Von der Geest 2002. Easton, M. D. L., D. Luszniak, and E. Von der Geest. 2002. "Preliminary Examination of Contaminant Loadings in Farmed Salmon, Wild Salmon and Commercial Salmon Feed." *Chemosphere* 46(7): 1053-74.

ECHA 2010. European Chemicals Agency. 2010. "Member State Committee Draft Support Document for Identification of Disodium Tetraborate, Anhydrous as a Substance of Very High Concern Because of Its CMR Properties." Last modified June 9.

ECHA 2015. European Chemicals Agency. 2015. "Candidate List of Substances of Very High Concern for Authorisation." Last modified December 17.

Ecology Center 2012a. The Ecology Center. 2012. "Ecology Center Report on Toxic Chemicals in Jewelry Covered by Media Outlets across the Country." Last modified March 24.

Ecology Center 2012b. The Ecology Center. 2012. *Model Year 2011/2012 Guide to New Vehicles.* Ann Arbor, MI: The Ecology Center.

EHANS 2015. Environmental Health Association of Nova Scotia. 2015. "Guide to Less Toxic Products: Household Cleaners." Accessed February 7.

Eng 2012. Eng, Monica. 2012. "Cooking Tips to Possibly Lessen Risk of Arsenic in Rice." *Chicago Tribune,* October 3.

EPA 1988. United States Environmental Protection Agency. 1988. *The Inside Story: A Guide to Indoor Air Quality. EPA/400/1-88/004.* Washington, DC: United States Environmental Protection Agency.

EPA 1994. United States Environmental Protection Agency. 1994. *Project Summary: Characterization of Emissions from Carpet Samples Using a 10-Gallon Aquarium as the Source Chamber. EPA/800/ SR-94/141.* Research Triangle Park, NC: United States Environmental Protection Agency.

EPA 1997. United States Environmental Protection Agency. 1997. *Summary and Assessment of Published Information on Determining Lead Exposures and Mitigating Lead Hazards Associated with Dust and Soil in Residential Carpets, Furniture, and Forced Air Ducts.* Washington, DC: United States Environmental Protection Agency.

EPA 2000a. United States Environmental Protection Agency. 2000. "Chloroform Hazard Summary." Last modified January.

EPA 2000b. United States Environmental Protection Agency. 2000. *Healthy Indoor Painting Practices. EPA 744-F-00-011.* United States Environmental Protection Agency.

EPA 2006. United States Environmental Protection Agency. 2006. "Action Memorandum: Inert Reassessment – Ethyl Acetate (CAS Reg. No. 141-78-6) and Amyl Acetate (CAS Reg. No 628-63-7.)" Last modified July 31.

EPA 2007a. United States Environmental Protection Agency. 2007. "Nitrates and Nitrites TEACH Chemical Summary." Last modified May 22.

EPA 2007b. United States Environmental Protection Agency. 2007. "Phthalates TEACH Chemical Summary." Last modified October 10.

EPA 2009. United States Environmental Protection Agency. 2009. "Buildings and Their Impact on the Environment: A Statistical Summary." Last modified April 22.

EPA 2010. United States Environmental Protection Agency. 2010. *Toxicological Review of Formaldehyde – Inhalation Assessment. CAS No. 50-00-0.* Washington, DC: United States Environmental Protection Agency.

EPA 2011. United States Environmental Protection Agency. 2011. "Outdoor Air – Industry, Business, and Home: Paint and Coating Manufacturing." Last modified August 19.

EPA 2012a. United States Environmental Protection Agency. 2012. "Air and Radiation: Basic Information." Last modified July 16.

EPA 2012b. United States Environmental Protection Agency. 2012. "Healthy Hair Care and the Environment: Know What's in Your Hair Products." Last modified February 14.

EPA 2012c. United States Environmental Protection Agency. 2012. "An Introduction to Indoor Air Quality (IAQ)." Last modified June 21.

EPA 2012d. United States Environmental Protection Agency. 2012. "Mold and Moisture: A Brief Guide to Mold, Moisture, and Your Home." Last modified March 5.

EPA 2012e. United States Environmental Protection Agency. 2012. "Remodeling Your Home? Have You Considered Indoor Air Quality?" Last modified July 3.

EPA 2013a. United States Environmental Protection Agency. 2013. "Basic Information about Fluoride in Drinking Water: Review of Fluoride Drinking Water Standard." Last modified July 23.

EPA 2013b. United States Environmental Protection Agency. 2013. "Mercury Compounds." Last modified October 18.

EPA 2013c. United States Environmental Protection Agency. 2013. "Naphthalene." Last modified October 18.

EPA 2013d. United States Environmental Protection Agency. 2013. "The Original List of Hazardous Air Pollutants as Follows:." Last modified August 8.

EPA 2013e. United States Environmental Protection Agency. 2013. "Water: Consumer Confidence Report Rule. Frequent Questions." Last modified September 10.

EPA 2014a. United States Environmental Protection Agency. 2014. "2,3,7,8-Tetrachlorodibenzo-p-dioxin (TCDD); CASRN 1746-01-6." Last modified October 31.

EPA 2014b. United States Environmental Protection Agency. 2014. "Basic Information About Lead in Drinking Water." Last modified February 5.

EPA 2014c. United States Environmental Protection Agency. 2014. "Greening Your Purchase of Carpet: A Guide for Federal Purchasers." Last modified on September 11.

EPA 2014d. United States Environmental Protection Agency. 2014. "Ground-Level Ozone." Last modified November 26.

EPA 2014e. United States Environmental Protection Agency. 2014. "Nitrogen Dioxide: Health." Last modified August 15.

EPA 2014f. United States Environmental Protection Agency. 2014. "Climate Change: What You Can Do." Last modified March 18.

EPA 2015a. United States Environmental Protection Agency. 2015. "Detailed Fact Sheet: Architectural Coating Rule for Volatile Organic Compounds." Accessed February 12.

EPA 2015b. United States Environmental Protection Agency. 2015. "Evaluation of the Potential Carcinogenicity of Phenacetin." Last modified March 25.

EPA 2015c. United States Environmental Protection Agency. 2015. "Fact Sheet on Perchloroethylene, Also Known as Tetrachloroethylene." Last modified January 8.

EPA 2015d. United States Environmental Protection Agency. 2015. "Radon (Rn): Health Risks." Last modified January 16.

EPA 2015e. United States Environmental Protection Agency. 2015. "Technical Fact Sheet on: Dioxin (2,3,7,8–TCDD)." Accessed May 13.

Epstein 2015. Epstein, Samuel. 2015. "Talcum Powder: The Hidden Dangers." *Dr. Frank Lipman* (blog), accessed May 14.

Eskenazi et al. 2013. Eskenazi, Brenda, Jonathan Chevrier, Stephen A. Rauch, Katherine Kogut, Kim G. Harley, Caroline Johnson, Celina Trujillo, Andreas Sjodin, and Asa Bradman. 2013. "In Utero and Childhood Polybrominated Diphenyl Ether (PBDE) Exposures and Neurodevelopment in the CHAMACOS Study." *Environmental Health Perspectives* 121(2): 257-62.

EWG 2003. Environmental Working Group. 2003. "Mother's Milk: Breast Milk is Still Best." Last modified September 23.

EWG 2004. Environmental Working Group. 2004. "Rocket Fuel in Cows' Milk – Perchlorate: Milk Consumption Not Safe?" Last modified June 22.

EWG 2007a. Environmental Working Group. 2007. "FDA Warns Cosmetics Industry to Follow Law on Untested Ingredients." Last modified September 27.

EWG 2007b. Environmental Working Group. 2007. "Safety Guide to Children's Personal Care Products." Last modified November.

EWG 2007c. Environmental Working Group. 2007. "Bisphenol A – Toxic Plastics Chemical in Canned Food." Last modified, March 5.

EWG 2008a. Environmental Working Group. 2008. "CDC: Americans Carry Body Burden of Toxic Sunscreen Chemical." Last modified March 25.

EWG 2008b. Environmental Working Group. 2008. "EWG Comments on the FDA's Draft Assessment of Bisphenol A (BPA)." Last modified October 30.

EWG 2008c. Environmental Working Group. 2008. "Guide to Baby-Safe Bottles and Formula." Last modified October 11.

EWG 2008d. Environmental Working Group. 2008. "Reducing Your Exposure to PBDEs in Your Home." Last modified October 15.

EWG 2009. Environmental Working Group. 2009. "EWG's 10 Tips for a Less Toxic Pregnancy." *Enviroblog by Environmental Working Group*, December 7.

EWG 2010. Environmental Working Group. 2010. "Test Your Knowledge of Cosmetics Safety: 8 Myths Debunked." Last modified July 23.

EWG 2011. Environmental Working Group. 2011. "Brands That Hide Formaldehyde: The Chemical Name Game." Last modified April.

EWG 2013a. Environmental Working Group. 2013. "Regulation of New Chemicals, Protection of Confidential Business Information, and Innovation." Last modified July 11.

EWG 2013b. Environmental Working Group. 2013. *Water Treatment Contaminants: Forgotten Toxics in American Water*. Washington, DC: Environmental Working Group.

EWG 2015a. Environmental Working Group. 2015. "20 Mule Team Borax Natural Laundry Booster and Multi-Purpose Household Cleaner." Accessed February 2.

EWG 2015b. Environmental Working Group. 2015. "Cleaning Supplies: Secret Ingredients, Hidden Hazards." Accessed February 4.

EWG 2015c. Environmental Working Group. 2015. "Cleaning Supplies and Your Health." Accessed May 13.

EWG 2015d. Environmental Working Group. 2015. "Coal Tar." Accessed May 12.

EWG 2015e. Environmental Working Group. 2015. "Decoding the Labels." Accessed February 4.

EWG 2015f. Environmental Working Group. 2015. "EWG's Guide to Healthy Cleaning. Frequently Asked Questions." Accessed February 4.

EWG 2015g. Environmental Working Group. 2015. "EWG's Guide to PFCs." Accessed May 12.

EWG 2015h. Environmental Working Group. 2015. "EWG's Methodology for Assessing Sunscreens." Accessed February 9.

EWG 2015i. Environmental Working Group. 2015. "Exposures Add Up – Survey Results." Accessed February 6.

EWG 2015j. Environmental Working Group. 2015. "Fact Sheets: How Many Chemicals Are in Me?" Accessed March 24.

EWG 2015k. Environmental Working Group. 2015. "Hexachlorinated Dioxin." Accessed May 13.

EWG 2015l. Environmental Working Group. 2015. "Misleading Marketing Claims on Products for Children." Accessed March 16.

EWG 2015m. Environmental Working Group. 2015. "Nanoparticles in Sunscreens." Accessed February 8.

EWG 2015n. Environmental Working Group. 2015. "Oxybenzone." Accessed February 9.

EWG 2015o. Environmental Working Group. 2015. "The Problem with Vitamin A." Accessed February 8.

EWG 2015p. Environmental Working Group. 2015. "Safety Guide to Children's Personal Care Products." Accessed March 16.

EWG 2015q. Environmental Working Group. 2015. "The Story of Skin Deep." Accessed February 6.

EWG 2015r. Environmental Working Group. 2015. "Top Tips for Safer Products." Accessed February 5.

EWG 2015s. Environmental Working Group. 2015. "The Toxic Truth About a New Generation of Nonstick and Waterproof Chemicals." Last modified May 1.

EWG 2015t. Environmental Working Group. 2015. "The Trouble with Sunscreen Chemicals." Accessed February 25.

EWG 2015u. Environmental Working Group. 2015. "What's Wrong with High SPF?" Accessed April 8.

EWG 2015v. Environmental Working Group. 2015. "Why This Matters – Cosmetics and Your Health." Accessed December 22.

Fairfield 2010. Fairfield, Hannah. 2010. "Factory Food." *New York Times,* April 3.

FAO 2012. Food and Agriculture Organization of the United Nations. 2012. *FAO Statistical Yearbook 2012.* Rome, Italy: Food and Agriculture Organization of the United Nations.

FDA 1996. United States Food and Drug Administration's Allan B. Bailey Memorandum to G. Diachenko. 1996. "Cumulative Exposure Estimates for Bisphenol A (BPA), Individually for Adults and Infants, from Its Use in Epoxy-Based Can Coatings and Polycarbonate (PC) Articles. Verbal Request of 10-23-95." United States Food and Drug Administration.

FDA 2011. United States Food and Drug Administration. 2011. *21 CFR Parts 201 and 310 [Docket No. FDA-1978-N-0018] (Formerly Docket No. 1978-0038) RIN 0910-AF43. Labeling and Effectiveness Testing; Sunscreen Drug Products for Over-the-Counter Human Use.* United States Department of Health and Human Services.

FDA 2012. United States Food and Drug Administration. 2012. "Questions and Answers on Monosodium Glutamate (MSG.)" Last modified November 19.

FDA 2013a. United States Food and Drug Administration. 2013. "Everything Added to Food in the United States (EAFUS)." Last modified April 23.

FDA 2013b. United States Food and Drug Administration. 2013. "FDA Statement on Testing and Analysis of Arsenic in Rice and Rice Products." Last modified September 6.

FDA 2013c. United States Food and Drug Administration. 2013. "Phasing Out Certain Antibiotic Use in Farm Animals." Last modified December 13.

FDA 2013d. United States Food and Drug Administration. 2013. "Questions and Answers: Apple Juice and Arsenic." Last modified July 15.

FDA 2014a. United States Food and Drug Administration. 2014. "Dioxin." Last modified June 5.

FDA 2014b. United States Food and Drug Administration. 2014. "Everything Added to Food in the United States (EAFUS)." Last modified November 26.

FDA 2014c. United States Food and Drug Administration. 2014. "Pediatric X-Ray Imaging." Last modified June 5.

FDA 2014d. United States Food and Drug Administration. 2014. "Radiology and Children: Extra Care Required." Last modified October 14.

FDA 2014e. United States Food and Drug Administration. 2014. "Tobacco Products." Last modified August 27.

FDA 2015. United States Food and Drug Administration. 2015. "Prohibited and Restricted Ingredients." Last modified January 26.

Franck 1963. Franck, Heinz-Gerhard. 1963. "The Challenge in Coal Tar Chemicals." *Industrial and Engineering Chemistry* 55(5): 38-44.

Frey 2012. Frey, Allan H. 2012. "Opinion: Cell Phone Health Risk?" *The Scientist,* September 25.

FSIS 2009. Food Safety and Inspection Service. 2009. *Dioxin 08 Survey: Dioxins and Dioxin-Like Compounds in the US Domestic Meat and Poultry Supply.* Risk Assessment Division, Office of Public Health Science Food Safety and Inspection Service, United States Department of Agriculture.

Fuhrman 2006. Fuhrman, Joel. 2006. *Disease-Proof Your Child: Feeding Kids Right.* New York: St. Martin's Press.

Fuhrman 2015. Fuhrman, Joel. 2015. "Pesticides and Produce: What You Need to Know." *Dr. Fuhrman: Smart Nutrition. Superior Health* (blog), accessed May 14.

Furst 2006. Furst, P. 2006. "Dioxins, Polychlorinated Biphenyls and Other Organohalogen Compounds in Human Milk. Levels, Correlations, Trends and Exposure through Breastfeeding." *Molecular Nutrition and Food Research* 50(10): 922-33.

Gago-Dominguez et al. 2001. Gago-Dominguez, Manuela, J. Esteban Castelao, Jian-Min Yuan, Mimi C. Yu, and Ronald K. Ross. 2001.

"Use of Permanent Hair Dyes and Bladder-Cancer Risk." *International Journal of Cancer* 91(4): 575-9.

Gavigan 2008. Gavigan, Christopher. 2008. *Healthy Child, Healthy World: Creating a Cleaner, Greener, Safer Home.* New York: Dutton.

Goldstein and Emami 2010. Goldstein, Katherine and Gazelle Emami. 2010. "Monsanto's GMO Corn Linked to Organ Failure, Study Reveals." *Huffington Post,* March 18.

Goodland and Anhang 2009. Goodland, Robert and Jeff Anhang. 2009. "Livestock and Climate Change: What if the Key Actors in Climate Change are Cows, Pigs, and Chickens?" *Worldwatch Magazine,* November/December.

Gram 1993. Gram, David. 1993. "Carpet Fumes Suspected in a Rash of Illnesses: Environment: Complaints of Health Problems Have Come from Homes, Schools, Offices and Factories, But No Hard Evidence Exists. A Federal Hearing Is Set for This Week." *Los Angeles Times,* June 6.

Grube et al. 2011. Grube, Arthur, David Donaldson, Timothy Kiely, and La Wu. 2011. *Pesticides Industry Sales and Usage: 2006 and 2007 Market Estimates.* Washington, DC: United States Environmental Protection Agency.

Gunn et al. 2010. Gunn, J. Peralez, E. V. Kuklina, N. L. Keenan, and D. R. Labarthe. 2010. "Sodium Intake among Adults – United States, 2005 – 2006." In *Centers for Disease Control and Prevention MMWR Morbidity and Mortality Weekly Report, Vol 59 No 24,* edited by Frederic E. Shaw, 746-749. Atlanta, GA: United States Department of Health and Human Services, Centers for Disease Control and Prevention.

Gupta 2012. Gupta, Sanjay. 2012. "6 Tips for Minimizing Cell Phone Radiation." *The Chart by CNN* (blog), June 8.

Hamerschlag 2011. Hamerschlag, Kari. 2011. *Meat Eater's Guide to Climate Change and Health.* Oakland, CA: Environmental Working Group.

Haug et al. 2011. Haug, Line S., Sandra Huber, Georg Becher, and Cathrine Thomsen. 2011. "Characterisation of Human Exposure to Perfluorinated Compounds-Comparing Exposure Estimates with Biomarkers of Exposure." *Environment International* 37(4): 687-93.

Hauser et al. 2006. Hauser, R., J. D. Meeker, S. Duty, M. J. Silva, and A. M. Calafat. 2006. "Altered Semen Quality in Relation to Urinary Concentrations of Phthalate Monoester and Oxidative Metabolites." *Epidemiology* 17(6): 682-91.

Hauser et al. 2007. Hauser, R., J. D. Meeker, N. P. Singh, M. J. Silva, L. Ryan, S. Duty, and A. M. Calafat. 2007. "DNA Damage in Human Sperm Is Related to Urinary Levels of Phthalate Monoester and Oxidative Metabolites." *Human Reproductive* 22(3): 688-95.

Hawthorne 2012. Hawthorne, Michael. 2012. "Flame Retardants Hard to Avoid at Home." *Chicago Tribune,* May 6.

Healthy Child Healthy World 2013. Healthy Child Healthy World. 2013. "Avoid Alkylphenol Ethoxylates (APES) in Cleaning Products and More!" Last modified March 29.

Healthy Stuff 2015. Healthy Stuff. 2015. "FAQs." Accessed March 16.

Hepp 2012. Hepp, Nancy M. 2012. "Determination of Total Lead in 400 Lipsticks on the US Market Using a Validated Microwave-Assisted Digestion, Inductively Coupled Plasma-Mass Spectrometric Method." *Journal of Cosmetic Science* 63(3): 159-76.

Hirshberg 2015. Hirshberg, Joel. 2015. "The Truth About Paint." *Learning Center by Green Building Supply* (blog), accessed February 11.

Hites et al. 2004. Hites, Ronald A., Jeffery A. Foran, David O. Carpenter, M. Coreen Hamilton, Barbara A. Knuth, and Steven J. Schwager. 2004. "Global Assessment of Organic Contaminants in Farmed Salmon." *Science* 303(5655): 226-9.

Hollender and Zissu 2010. Hollender, Jeffrey and Alexandra Zissu. 2010. *Planet Home: Conscious Choices for Cleaning and Greening the World You Care About Most.* New York: Clarkson Potter.

Hollender et al. 2006. Hollender, Jeffrey, Geoff Davis, Meika Hollender, and Reed Doyle. 2006. *Naturally Clean: The Seventh Generation Guide to Safe and Healthy, Non-Toxic Cleaning.* Gabriola Island, BC: New Society.

Houlihan 2015. Houlihan, Jane. 2015. "Why This Matters- Cosmetics and Your Health." Accessed March 24.

IARC 2001. International Agency for Research on Cancer. 2001. *IARC Summary Recommendations for Public Health Action.* Lyon, France: International Agency for Research on Cancer, World Health Organization.

IARC 2011. International Agency for Research on Cancer. 2011. *IARC Classifies Radiofrequency Electromagnetic Fields as Possibly Carcinogenic to Humans.* Lyon, France: International Agency for Research on Cancer, World Health Organization.

IATP 2009a. Institute for Agriculture and Trade Policy. 2009. "Much High Fructose Corn Syrup Contaminated with Mercury, New Study Finds." Last modified January 26.

IATP 2009b. Institute for Agriculture and Trade Policy. 2009. *Smart Guide to Food Dyes: Buying Foods That Can Help Learning.* Minneapolis, MN: Institute for Agriculture and Trade Policy.

Institute of Medicine 2000. Institute of Medicine. 2000. *Clearing the Air: Asthma and Indoor Air Exposures.* Washington, DC: National Academy Press.

Institute of Medicine 2003. Institute of Medicine. 2003. *Dioxins and Dioxin-Like Compounds in the Food Supply: Strategies to Decrease Exposure.* Washington, DC: National Academy of Sciences.

Israel 2011. Israel, Brett. 2011. "Brominated Battle: Soda Chemical Has Cloudy Health History." *Environmental Health News,* December 12.

Jones et al. 2009. Jones, Robert L., David M. Homa, Pamela A. Meyer, Debra J. Brody, Kathleen L. Caldwell, James L. Pirkle, and Mary Jean Brown. 2009. "Trends in Blood Lead Levels and Blood Lead Testing among US Children Aged 1 to 5 Years, 1988-2004." *Pediatrics* 123(3): e376-85.

Juice Products Association 2012. Juice Products Association. 2012. "Juice Products Association Q and A: Orange Juice Standards." *DoctorOz. com,* January 17.

Karlstrom and Dell'Amore 2010. Karlstrom, Solvie and Christine Dell'Amore. 2010. "Why Tap Water Is Better Than Bottled Water." *National Geographic,* March 13.

Kelly, Smith, and Satola 1999. Kelly, Thomas J., Deborah L. Smith, and Jan Satola. 1999. "Emission Rate of Formaldehyde from Materials and Consumer Products Found in California Homes." *Environmental Science and Technology* 33(1): 81-8.

Kluger 2010. Kluger, Jeffrey. 2010. "Organic Eggs: More Expensive, But No Healthier." *Time,* July 8.

Koch 2011. Koch, Jared. 2011. *Clean Plates Manhattan: A Guide to the Healthiest Tastiest and Most Sustainable Restaurants for Vegetarians and Carnivores.* Cliffside Park, NJ: Craving Wellness.

Konkel and *Environmental Health News* 2009. Konkel, Lindsey and Environmental Health News. 2009. "Could Eating Too Much Soy Be Bad for You?" *Scientific American,* November 3.

Kristof 2012. Kristof, Nicholas. 2012. "Are You Safe on That Sofa?" *New York Times,* May 19.

Kummeling et al. 2008. Kummeling, Ischa, Carel Thijs, Machteld Huber, Lucy P. L. van de Vijver, Bianca E. P. Snijders, John Penders, Foekje Stelma, Ronald van Ree, Pier A. van den Brandt, and Pieter

C. Dagnelie. 2008. "Consumption of Organic Foods and Risk of Atopic Disease during the First 2 Years of Life in the Netherlands." *British Journal of Nutrition* 99: 598-605.

Landrigran and Etzel 2014. Landrigan, Philip J. and Ruth A. Etzel, eds. 2014. *Textbook of Children's Environmental Health.* New York: Oxford University Press.

Lanphear et al. 1996. Lanphear, Bruce P., Michael Weitzman, Nancy L. Winter, Shirley Eberly, Benjamin Yakir, Martin Tanner, Mary Emond, and Thomas D. Matte. 1996. "Lead-Contaminated House Dust and Urban Children's Blood Lead Levels." *American Journal of Public Health* 86(10): 1416-21.

Latendresse et al. 2009. Latendresse, J. R., T. J. Bucci, G. Olson, P. Mellick, C. C. Weis, B. Thorn, R. R. Newbold, and K. B. Delclos. 2009. "Genistein and Ethinyl Estradiol Dietary Exposure in Multigenerational and Chronic Studies Induce Similar Proliferative Lesions in Mammary Gland of Male Sprague-Dawley Rats." *Reproductive Toxicology* 28(3): 342-53.

LEAD Group Inc 2000. The LEAD Group Inc. 2000. "US Scented Candles Study." *LEAD Action News* 7(4).

Leonard 2015. Leonard, Annie. 2015. "Story of Stuff, Reference and Annotated Script by Annie Leonard." Accessed February 11.

Lewis 1998. Lewis, Carol. 1998. "Clearing Up Cosmetic Confusion." *FDA Consumer Magazine,* May – June.

Lipka 2012. Lipka, Mitch. 2012. "Could Your Valentine's Kiss Give You Lead Poisoning?" *Reuters,* February 14.

Liu, Schade, and Simpson 2008. Liu, Jeannie, Michael Schade, and Heather Simpson. 2008. *Pass Up the Poison Plastic: The PVC – Free Guide for Your Family and Home.* Falls Church, VA: The Center for Health, Environment and Justice.

Lorber 2008. Lorber, Matthew. 2008. "Exposure of Americans to Polybrominated Diphenyl Ethers." *Journal of Exposure Science and Environmental Epidemiology* 18(1): 2-19.

Lorber et al. 2015. Lorber, Matthew, Arnold Schecter, Olaf Paepke, William Shropshire, Krista Christensen, and Linda Birnbaum. 2015. "Exposure Assessment of Adult Intake of Bisphenol A (BPA) with Emphasis on Canned Food Dietary Exposures." *Environment International* 77: 55-62.

Lu et al. 2006. Lu, Chensheng, Kathryn Toepel, Rene Irish, Richard A. Fenske, Dana B. Barr, and Roberto Bravo. 2006. "Organic Diets Significantly Lower Children's Dietary Exposure to Organophosphorus Pesticides." *Environmental Health Perspectives* 114(2): 260-3.

Lu et al. 2008. Lu, Chensheng, Dana B. Barr, Melanie A. Pearson, and Lance A. Waller. 2008. "Dietary Intake and Its Contribution to Longitudinal Organophosphorus Pesticide Exposure in Urban/Suburban Children." *Environmental Health Perspectives* 116(4): 537-42.

Lunder 2011. Lunder, Sonya. 2011. "What Scientists Say About Vitamin A in Sunscreen." *Research by Environmental Working Group,* June 27.

Lunder 2012. Lunder, Sonya. 2012. "Toxic Fire Retardants Are Everywhere in Homes, New Studies Find." *Enviroblog by Environmental Working Group,* November 28.

Magaziner, Bonvie, and Zolezzi 2003. Magaziner, Allan, Linda Bonvie, and Anthony Zolezzi. 2003. *Chemical-Free Kids: How to Safeguard Your Child's Diet and Environment.* New York: Kensington Books.

Mahler et al. 2010. Mahler, Barbara J., Peter C. Van Metre, Jennifer T. Wilson, and Marylynn Musgrove. 2010. "Coal-Tar-Based Parking Lot Sealcoat: An Unrecognized Source of PAH to Settled House Dust." *Environmental Science and Technology* 44(3): 894-900.

Main et al. 2007. Main, Katharina Maria, Hannu Kiviranta, Helena Eeva Virtanen, Erno Sundqvist, Jouni Tapio Tuomisto, Jouko Tuomisto, Terttu Vartiainen, Niels Erik Skakkebaek, and Jorma Toppari. 2007. "Flame Retardants in Placenta and Breast Milk and Cryptorchidism in Newborn Boys." *Environmental Health Perspectives* 115(10): 1519-26.

Mayo Clinic 2013. Mayo Clinic. 2013. "Humidifiers: Air Moisture Eases Skin, Breathing Symptoms." Last modified May 18.

Mayo Clinic 2015. Mayo Clinic. 2015. "What Is MSG? Is It Bad for You?" Accessed May 7.

Mazdai et al. 2003. Mazdai, Anita, Nathan G. Dodder, Mary Pell Abernathy, Ronald A. Hites, and Robert M. Bigsby. 2003. "Polybrominated Diphenyl Ethers in Maternal and Fetal Blood Samples." *Environmental Health Perspectives* 111(9): 1249-52.

McCann et al. 2007. McCann, Donna, Angelina Barrett, Alison Cooper, Debbie Crumpler, Lindy Dalen, Kate Grimshaw, Elizabeth Kitchin, et al. 2007. "Food Additives and Hyperactive Behavior in 3-Year-Old and 8/9-Year-Old Children in the Community: A Randomized, Double-Blinded, Placebo-Controlled Trial." *The Lancet* 370(9598): 1560-7.

McCaustland et al. 1982. McCaustland, Karen A., Walter W. Bond, Daniel W. Bradley, James W. Ebert, and James E. Maynard. 1982. "Survival of Hepatitis A Virus in Feces after Drying and Storage for 1 Month." *Journal of Clinical Microbiology* 16(5): 957-8.

McCollough et al. 2007. McCollough, Cynthia H., Beth A. Schueler, Thomas D. Atwell, Natalie N. Braun, Dawn M. Regner, Douglas L. Brown, and Andrew J. LeRoy. 2007. "Radiation Exposure and Pregnancy: When Should We Be Concerned?" *RadioGraphics* 27(4): 909-18.

McDonald 2007. McDonald, Libby. 2007. *The Toxic Sandbox: The Truth About Environmental Toxins and Our Children's Health.* New York: Perigee Trade.

McKenzie et al. 2010. McKenzie, Lara B., Nisha Ahir, Uwe Stolz, and Nicolas G. Nelson. 2010. "Household Cleaning Product-Related Injuries Treated in US Emergency Departments in 1990-2006." *Pediatrics* 126(3): 509-16.

Micha, Wallace, and Mozaffarian 2010. Micha, Renata, Sarah K. Wallace, and Dariush Mozaffarian. 2010. "Red and Processed Meat Consumption and Risk of Incident Coronary Heart Disease, Stroke, and Diabetes Mellitus: A Systematic Review and Meta-Analysis." *Circulation: Journal of the American Heart Association* 121: 2271-83.

Miller et al. 2004. Miller, Rachel L., Robin Garfinkel, Megan Horton, David Camann, Frederica P. Perera, Robin M. Whyatt, and Patrick L. Kinney. 2004. "Polycyclic Aromatic Hydrocarbons, Environmental Tobacco Smoke, and Respiratory Symptoms in an Inner-City Birth Cohort." *Chest* 126(4): 1071-8.

Naidenko et al. 2008. Naidenko, Olga, Nneka Leiba, Renee Sharp, and Jane Houlihan. 2008. "Bottled Water Quality Investigation: 10 Major Brands, 38 Pollutants." *Research by Environmental Working Group*, October 15.

National Geographic 2008. National Geographic. 2008. *Green Guide: The Complete Reference for Consuming Wisely.* Washington, DC: National Geographic Society.

Nicole 2014. Nicole, Wendee. 2014. "A Question for Women's Health: Chemicals in Feminine Hygiene Products and Personal Lubricants." *Environmental Health Perspectives* 122(3): A71-5.

Nishioka et al. 1996. Nishioka, Marcia G., Hazel M. Burkholder, Marielle C. Brinkman, and Sydney M. Gordon. 1996. "Measuring Transport of Lawn-Applied Herbicide Acids from Turf to Home: Correlation of Dislodgeable 2, 4-D Turf Residues with Carpet Dust and Carpet Surface Residues." *Environmental Science and Technology* 30(11): 3313-20.

NRDC 2005. Natural Resources Defense Council. 2005. "Healthy Milk, Healthy Baby, Chemical Pollution and Mother's Milk: Chemicals in Mother's Milk." Last modified March 25.

NRDC 2011. Natural Resources Defense Council. 2011. "Smarter Living: Shopping Wise. Food Storage Containers." Last modified November 22.

NRDC 2015. Natural Resources Defense Council. 2015. "Smarter Business: Greening Advisor. Low-VOC Products." Accessed April 9.

NTP 2012. National Toxicology Program. 2012. *NTP Technical Report on the Photococarcinogenesis Study of Retinoic Acid and Retinyl Palmitate [CAS No. 302-79-4 (All-trans-retinoic acid) and 79-81-2 (All-trans-retinyl palmitate)].* Research Triangle Park, NC: National Institutes of Health, United States Department of Health and Human Services.

NTP 2014. National Toxicology Program. 2014. *Thirteenth Report on Carcinogens.* Research Triangle Park, NC: United States Department of Health and Human Services, Public Health Service.

Olson 2003. Olson, Elizabeth. 2003. "US Is Urged by Panel to Tell Women About Dioxins." *New York Times,* July 2.

Organic Consumers Association 2015. Organic Consumers Association. 2015. "All About Organics – OCA's Organic Resource Center. Why We Should Eat More Organic Food." Accessed February 24.

Perera et al. 2006. Perera, Frederica P., Virginia Rauh, Robin M. Whyatt, Wei-Yann Tsai, Deliang Tang, Diurka Diaz, Lori Hoepner, et al. 2006. "Effect of Prenatal Exposure to Airborne Polycyclic Aromatic Hydrocarbons on Neurodevelopment in the First 3 Years of Life among Inner-City Children." *Environmental Health Perspectives* 114(8): 1287-92.

Perrone 2013. Perrone, Matthew. 2013. "FDA: Anti-Bacterial Soaps May Not Curb Bacteria." *Associated Press,* December 16.

Pesticide Action Network 2008. Pesticide Action Network. 2008. *Message in a Bottle.* London: Pesticide Action Network Europe.

Polder, Gabrielsen, et al. 2008. Polder, A., G. W. Gabrielsen, J. O. Odland, T. N. Savinova, A. Tkachev, K. B. Loken, and J. U. Skaare. 2008. "Spatial and Temporal Changes of Chlorinated Pesticides, PCBs, Dioxins (PCDDs/PCDFs) and Brominated Flame Retardants in Human Breast Milk from Northern Russia." *The Science of the Total Environment* 391(1): 41-54.

Polder, Thomsen, et al. 2008. Polder, A., C. Thomsen, G. Lindstrom, K. B. Loken, and J. U. Skaare. 2008. "Levels and Temporal Trends of Chlorinated Pesticides, Polychlorinated Biphenyls and Brominated Flame Retardants in Individual Human Breast Milk Samples from Northern and Southern Norway." *Chemosphere* 73(1): 14-23.

Pollan 2007. Pollan, Michael. 2007. *The Omnivore's Dilemma: A Natural History of Four Meals.* New York: Penguin Books.

Potera 2011. Potera, Carol. 2011. "Scented Products Emit a Bouquet of VOCs." *Environmental Health Perspectives* 119(1): A16.

Rao et al. 2007. Rao, Manish, Shu-Li Wang, Wen-Jhy Lee, and Ya-Fen Wang. 2007. "Levels of Polybrominated Diphenyl Ethers (PBDEs) in Breast Milk from Central Taiwan and Their Relation to Infant Birth Outcome and Maternal Menstruation Effects." *Environment International* 33(2): 239-45.

Rasmussen, Subramanian, and Jessiman 2001. Rasmussen, P. E., K. S. Subramanian, and B. J. Jessiman. 2001. "A Multi-Element Profile of Housedust in Relation to Exterior Dust and Soils in the City of Ottawa, Canada." *Science of the Total Environment* 267(1-3): 125-40.

Redberg and Smith-Bindman 2014. Redberg, Rita F. and Rebecca Smith-Bindman. 2014. "We Are Giving Ourselves Cancer." *New York Times,* January 30.

Reuben 2010. Reuben, Suzanne H. 2010. *2008 – 2009 Annual Report, President's Cancer Panel. Reducing Environmental Cancer Risk: What We Can Do Now.* Bethesda, MD: National Cancer Institute.

Richardson 1994. Richardson, B. A. 1994. "Sudden Infant Death Syndrome: A Possible Primary Cause." *Journal - Forensic Science Society* 34(3): 199-204.

Rier and Foster 2002. Rier, Sherry and Warren G. Foster. 2002. "Forum: Environmental Dioxins and Endometriosis." *Toxicological Sciences* 70: 161-70.

Roberts et al. 1999. Roberts, J. W., W. S. Clifford, G. Glass, and P. G. Hummer. 1999. "Reducing Dust, Lead, Dust Mites, Bacteria, and Fungi in Carpets by Vacuuming." *Archives of Environmental Contamination and Toxicology* 36(4): 477-84.

Roberts et al. 2009. Roberts, John W., Lance A. Wallace, David E. Camann, Philip Dickey, Steven G. Gilbert, Robert G. Lewis, and Tim K. Takaro. 2009. "Monitoring and Reducing Exposure of Infants to Pollutants in House Dust." In *Reviews of Environmental Contamination and Toxicology Volume 201,* edited by David M. Whitacre, 1–39. Springer US.

Rock 2011. Rock, Andrea. 2011. "Consumer Reports Tests Juices for Arsenic and Lead." *Consumer Reports News by Consumer Reports,* November 30.

Rudel et al. 2003. Rudel, Ruthann A., David E. Camann, John D. Spengler, Leo R. Korn, and Julia G. Brody. 2003. "Phthalates, Alkylphenols, Pesticides, Polybrominated Diphenyl Ethers, and Other Endocrine-Disrupting Compounds in Indoor Air and Dust." *Environmental Science and Technology* 37(20): 4543-53.

Rudel et al. 2011. Rudel, Ruthann A., Janet M. Gray, Connie L. Engel, Teresa W. Rawsthorne, Robin E. Dodson, Janet M. Ackerman, Jeanne Rizzo, Janet L. Nudelman, and Julia Green Brody. 2011. "Food Packaging and Bisphenol A and Bis(2-Ethyhexyl) Phthalate Exposure: Findings from a Dietary Intervention." *Environmental Health Perspectives* 119(7): 914-20.

Sage 2014. Sage, Cindy, ed. 2014. *BioInitiative 2012: Summary for the Public (2014 Supplement).* Santa Barbara, CA: BioInitiative Working Group.

Saltzman and Hatlelid 2000. Saltzman, Lori E. and Kristina M. Hatlelid. 2000. *CPSC Staff Report on Asbestos Fibers in Children's Crayons.* Washington, DC: United States Consumer Product Safety Commission.

Sathyanarayana et al. 2008. Sathyanarayana, Sheela, Catherine J. Karr, Paula Lozano, Elizabeth Brown, Antonia M. Calafat, Fan Liu, and Shanna Swan. 2008. "Baby Care Products: Possible Sources of Infant Phthalate Exposure." *Pediatrics* 121(2): e260-8.

Schade 2012. Schade, Michael. 2012. *Hidden Hazards: Toxic Chemicals inside Children's Vinyl Back-to-School Supplies.* Falls Church, VA: Center for Health, Environment and Justice (CHEJ).

Schantz et al. 2007. Schantz, Michele M., Jennifer M. Lynch, John R. Kucklick, Dianne L. Poster, H. M. Stapleton, S. S. Vander Pol, and Stephen A. Wise. 2007. "Spotlighting NIST Standard Reference Materials – New Standard Material (SRM) 2585 Organic Contaminants in House Dust to Support Exposure Assessment Measurements." *American Laboratory* 39(15): 22-8.

Schettler et al. 2000. Schettler, Ted, Jill Stein, Fay Reich, Maria Valenti, and David Wallinga. 2000. *In Harm's Way: Toxic Threats to Child Development.* Cambridge: Greater Boston Physicians for Social Responsibility.

Schreder 2012. Schreder, Erika. 2012. *Hidden Hazards in the Nursery.* Seattle, WA: Washington Toxics Coalition/Safer States.

Schlosser 2001. Schlosser, Eric. 2001. *Fast Food Nation: The Dark Side of the All-American Meal.* New York: Houghton Mifflin.

Scranton 2011. Scranton, Alexandra. 2011. *Dirty Secrets: What's Hiding in Your Cleaning Products?* Missoula, MT: Women's Voices for the Earth.

Seattle Times **2008.** Seattle Times. 2008. "John W. 'Dr. Dust' Roberts." *Seattle Times,* November 2–3.

Selgrade et al. 2006. Selgrade, MaryJane K., Robert F. Lemanske, Jr., M. Ian Gilmour, Lucas M. Neas, Marsha D. W. Ward, Paul K. Henneberger, David N. Weissman, et al. 2006. "Induction of Asthma and the Environment: What We Know and Need to Know." *Environmental Health Perspectives* 114(4): 615-9.

Seltzer 1994. Seltzer, J. M. 1994. "Building-Related Illness." *The Journal of Allergy and Clinical Immunology* 94(2 Pt 2): 351-61.

Seventh Generation 2010. Seventh Generation. 2010. "Optical Brighteners: Just Say No to the Glow!" *7Gen Blog by Seventh Generation,* October 13.

Shaw et al. 2010. Shaw, S. D., A. Blum, R. Weber, K. Kannan, D. Rich, D. Lucas, C. P. Koshland, D. Dobraca, S. Hanson, and L. S. Birnbaum. 2010. "Halogenated Flame Retardants: Do the Fire Safety Benefits Justify the Risks?" *Reviews on Environmental Health* 25(4): 261-306.

Sheppard 2014. Sheppard, Jane. 2014. "The Best Organic Crib Mattress Is Safe and Non-Toxic for Your Baby: Toxic Chemicals in Baby Crib Mattresses?" *Healthy Child* (blog), May.

Sheppard 2015. Sheppard, Jane. 2015. "Toxic Gases in Baby Crib Mattresses." *Healthy Child* (blog), accessed March 16.

Silent Spring Institute 2015. Silent Spring Institute. 2015. "Tip Sheet: 6 Simple Steps to Avoid BPA and Phthalates in Food." Accessed February 20.

Skin Cancer Foundation 2015. Skin Cancer Foundation. 2015. "Sunscreens Explained." Accessed February 9.

Smith and Lourie 2009. Smith, Rick and Bruce Lourie. 2009. *Slow Death by Rubber Duck: The Secret Danger of Everyday Things.* Berkeley, CA: Counterpoint.

Smith-Bindman et al. 2009. Smith-Bindman, R., J. Lipson, R. Marcus, K. P. Kim, M. Mahesh, R. Gould, A. Berrington de Gonzalez, and D. L. Miglioretti. 2009. "Radiation Dose Associated with Common Computed Tomography Examinations and the Associated Lifetime Attributable Risk of Cancer." *Archives of Internal Medicine* 169(22): 2078-86.

Soffritti et al. 2006. Soffritti, Morando, Fiorella Belpoggi, Davide Degli Esposti, Luca Lambertini, Eva Tibaldi, and Anna Rigano. 2006. "First Experimental Demonstration of the Multipotential Carcinogenic Effects of Aspartame Administered in the Feed to Sprague-Dawley Rats." *Environmental Health Perspectives* 114(3): 379-85.

Soyfoods Association of North America 2015. Soyfoods Association of North America. 2015. "Consumer Demand for Protein Leads Soyfoods Sales to $4.5 Billion." Accessed April 10.

Stapleton et al. 2009. Stapleton, Heather M., Susan Klosterhaus, Sarah Eagle, Jennifer Fuh, John D. Meeker, Arlene Blum, and Thomas F. Webster. 2009. "Detection of Organophosphate Flame Retardants in Furniture Foam and US House Dust." *Environmental Science and Technology* 43(19): 7490-5.

Steinemann 2008. Steinemann, Anne C. 2008. "Fragranced Consumer Products and Undisclosed Ingredients." *Environmental Impact Assessment Review* 29(1): 32-8.

Steinemann et al. 2010. Steinemann, Anne C., Ian C. MacGregor, Sydney M. Gordon, Lisa G. Gallagher, Amy L. Davis, Daniel S. Ribeiro, and Lance A. Wallace. 2010. "Fragranced Consumer Products: Chemicals Emitted, Ingredients Unlisted." *Environmental Impact Assessment Review* 31(3): 328–33.

Steinfeld et al. 2006. Steinfeld, Henning, Pierre Gerber, Tom Wassenaar, Vincent Castel, Mauricio Rosales, Cees de Haan. 2006. *Livestock's Long Shadow: Environmental Issues and Options.* Rome, Italy: The Livestock, Environment and Development (LEAD) Initiative and the Food and Agriculture Organization of the United Nations (FAO).

Steingraber 2001. Steingraber, Sandra. 2001. *Having Faith.* Cambridge: Perseus.

Steingraber 2010. Steingraber, Sandra. 2010. *Living Downstream: An Ecologist's Investigation of Cancer and the Environment.* 2nd ed. Cambridge: Da Capo Press.

Stop SIDS Now 2015. Stop SIDS Now. 2015. "What You Need to Know About SIDS." Accessed March 17.

Sutton 2011. Sutton, Rebecca. 2011. "Your Best Air Freshener Isn't an Air Freshener." *Enviroblog by Environmental Working Group,* September 30.

Tan et al. 2002. Tan, L., N. H. Nielsen, D. C. Young, and Z. Trizna. 2002. "Recommendations of the Council on Scientific Affairs for the American Medical Association on Consumer Antiseptic Products." *Archives of Dermatology* 138: 1082-6.

Tappin et al. 2002. Tappin, D., H. Brooke, R. Ecob, and A. Gibson. 2002. "Used Infant Mattresses and Sudden Infant Death Syndrome in Scotland: Case-Control Study." *BMJ* 325(7371): 1007.

Tavernise 2012. Tavernise, Sabrina. 2012. "Farm Use of Antibiotics Defies Scrutiny." *New York Times,* September 3.

Thorne et al. 2005. Thorne, Peter S., Katarina Kulhankova, Ming Yin, Richard Cohn, Samuel J. Arbes, Jr., and Darryl C. Zeldin. 2005. "Endotoxin Exposure Is a Risk Factor for Asthma: The National Survey for Endotoxin in United States Housing." *American Journal of Respiratory and Critical Care Medicine* 172(11): 1371-7.

Tsumura et al. 2001. Tsumura, Y., S. Ishimitsu, A. Kaihara, K. Yoshii, Y. Nakamura, and Y. Tonogai. 2001. "Di(2-Ethylhexyl) Phthalate Contamination of Retail Packed Lunches Caused by PVC Gloves Used in the Preparation of Foods." *Food Additives and Contaminants* 18(6): 569-79.

Turner, Gibson, and Reed 2010. Turner, Pamela R., Sharon M. S. Gibson, and Ambre Latrice Reed. 2010. *Leave It at the Door.* Athens, GA: University of Georgia, Cooperative Extension, Colleges of Agricultural and Environmental Sciences and Family and Consumer Sciences.

USDA 2010. United States Department of Agriculture. 2010. *FSIS National Residue Program for Cattle. Audit Report 24601-08-KC.* Washington DC: United States Department of Agriculture.

USDA 2014. United States Department of Agriculture. 2014. "Recent Trends in GE Adoption." Last modified July 14.

Varlet, Smith, and Augsburger 2014. Varlet, V., F. Smith, and M. Augsburger. 2014. "New Trends in the Kitchen: Propellants Assessment of Edible Food Aerosol Sprays Used on Food." *Food Chemistry* 142: 311-7.

Villanueva et al. 2004. Villanueva, C. M., K. P. Cantor, S. Cordier, J. J. Jaakkola, W. D. King, C. F. Lynch, S. Porru, and M. Kogevinas. 2004. "Disinfection Byproducts and Bladder Cancer: A Pooled Analysis." *Epidemiology* 15(3): 357-67.

Wallinga et al. 2009. Wallinga, David, Janelle Sorensen, Pooja Mottl, and Brian Yablon. 2009. *Not So Sweet: Missing Mercury and High Fructose Corn Syrup.* Minneapolis, MN: Institute for Agriculture and Trade Policy.

Walsh 2011. Walsh, Bryan. 2011. "Why Air Fresheners Can Trigger Respiratory Problems." *Time,* November 8.

Washington Toxics Coalition 2000. Washington Toxics Coalition. 2000. "Carpeting and Children's Health: How Flooring Decisions Can Affect Home's Indoor Air Quality." Last modified October.

WHO 2008. World Health Organization. 2008. "Pesticides: Children's Health and the Environment: WHO Training Package for the Health Sector." Last modified July.

WHO 2010. World Health Organization: Yona Amitai, Hamed Bakir, Nida Besbelli, Stephan Boese-O'Reilly, Mariano Cebrian, Yaohua Dai, Paul Dargan, et al. 2010. *Childhood Lead Poisoning.* Geneva, Switzerland: World Health Organization.

WHO 2014. World Health Organization. 2014. "Dioxins and Their Effects on Human Health." Last modified June.

WHO and UNEP 2013. World Health Organization and United Nations Environment Programme. 2013. *State of the Science of Endocrine Disrupting Chemicals – 2012.* Geneva, Switzerland: WHO Press.

Williams 2005. Williams, Florence. 2005. "Toxic Breast Milk?" *New York Times,* January 9.

Wilson and Piepkorn 2008. Wilson, Alex and Mark Piepkorn, eds. 2008. *Green Building Products: The GreenSpec Guide to Residential Building Materials.* 3rd ed. Brattleboro, VT: BuildingGreen and New Society.

Wolverton 1997. Wolverton, B. C. 1997. *How to Grow Fresh Air: 50 House Plants That Purify Your Home or Office.* New York: Penguin Books.

Worland 2015. Worland, Justin. 2015. "Investigation Finds Asbestos in Crayons and Kids' Toys." *Time,* July 8.

Xie et al. 2013. Xie, Lulu, Hongyi Kang, Qiwu Xu, Michael J. Chen, Yonghong Liao, Meenakshisundaram Thiyagarajan, John O'Donnell, et al. 2013. "Sleep Drives Metabolite Clearance from the Adult Brain." *Science* 342(6156): 373-7.

Index

Acknowledgements

For all the personal virtues it has required to create a book like this, I must thank the many wonderful people in my personal universe. First, and foremost, my husband and children: You are the green grass that ground me, the lush trees that soothe me, and the sunshine and stars that light me up. My parents and my brother: You are my moon and my sun. My friends, greater family, and childcare providers: You are the flowers and butterflies in my life. Maggie: I never could have completed this book without your special role in our family. JK: You are my compass.

In the logistical process of creating this book:

Ashley Cooke: This book project would have taken too many more years without your diligent and multi-faceted help. Thank you for your detail-oriented and responsible help with research, fact-checking, and the works cited sections. I know that you worked with care and thoughtfulness.

There were several editorial reviews of various versions and portions of this manuscript over the years, some informal and some professional. Informally, the following reviewers provided important feedback at various stages of the process: Gregory Gushee, David Ruan MD, Julia and Jonathan Ruan MD, Eden Connelly, Michelle Choo, Darin Eydenberg, Adrienne Goldthorpe, Emily Alexander, Anna Saporito MD, Britta Soltan, Maggie Wnek, Rainbow Rubin PhD, and Mary Gushee. Professionally: Sheila Buff, thank you for helping to direct my young manuscript; Julia R. Barrett, thank you for your smart, informed, and supportive editorial feedback of part I; Elise Marton, thank you for your smart, informed and critical copyedits; Robert Coe, thank you for your honest, insightful feedback; Barbara Merchant, thank you for polishing my work as a proofreader; and Linda Herr Hallinger for the index.

There were many who helped me in finalizing the book cover. Unfortunately, there are too many to mention. A few key people I must note include Rafi Musher and Lara Seligman. Thank you for your exceptionally thoughtful feedback! Anurag Nema, I can't thank you enough for connecting me to Olya Domoradova. Olya, thank you for elevating and supporting my book's content with smart, beautiful book design. I love the cover and interior design! Thank you, Julia Movchan, for beautiful illustrations that complement the book.

Jonathan Albano, thank you for your generous help. Felicia Zekauskas of Zinc Design: Your brilliant ideas were an important part of my creative process; thank you for helping with the book's title.

Lisa Blau, a lunch many years ago helped jump-start my healthier path. Thank you for your help in launching my research. Charlotte Matthews and Ken Hillman, thank you both for carving time to share your expertise.

All the mentors and colleagues that I've worked with: I've learned so much from all of you.

Many organizations and individuals have made invaluable contributions towards advancing human and environmental health. While they all should be recognized, commended, and supported, I feel special gratitude for the contributions of Rachel Carson, Sandra Steingraber PhD, and Philip J. Landrigan MD MSc. Additional influences can be found through my website, NontoxicLiving.tips, for you to learn more and support them.

Collectively, you have all helped to create this book.

THE BOOK

Health-conscious mother of three, Sophia Ruan Gushée thought she knew how to be healthy. Only after she became a mother did she become aware of an overlooked influence on health: toxic exposures. These pervade not just our outdoor environments but also our homes, bodies, and diet. Their impact on health can be most influential during periods of rapid biological development, which makes protecting children a top priority.

Inspired to become a truly conscious parent and to provide her young family with a healthy foundation, Sophia spent more than five years identifying practical approaches for reducing her family's unnecessary exposures. In *A to Z of D-Toxing: The Ultimate Guide to Reducing Our Toxic Exposures*, Sophia shares what she learned.

Created to be the only reference book that a head of household needs, it includes hundreds of tips, as well as ten ideas to implement today—Sophia's D-Tox Strategy. These tips help increase the odds for more resilient health—not just for individuals, but for our planet as well. This is an empowering resource that will lay the groundwork for leading a healthy life.

THE AUTHOR

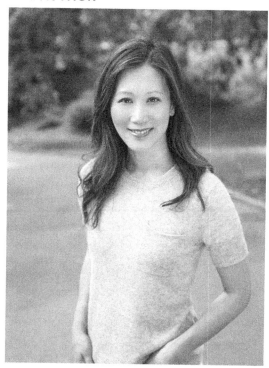

Sophia earned a Bachelor of Arts from Brown University and a Master in Business Administration from Columbia University. Formerly in private equity, she is an author, certified yoga teacher, devoted mother and wife, and lives in NYC. This is her first book.

For more practical information on D-Toxing and to follow Sophia's ongoing journey, sign up for her email newsletter at NontoxicLiving.tips.

Sophia will be donating 10 percent of her profits to advocacy groups. You can learn more on her website.

Made in the USA
Las Vegas, NV
22 December 2020

14448095R00254